Pediatric Emergency Nursing Manual

Deborah Parkman Henderson, RN, MA, CEN, has a background in the areas of mental health and emergency nursing. She did her undergraduate study at Vassar College and received her nursing degree, with honors, at Pasadena City College, Pasadena, CA. After completing a Bachelor of Science in Human Relations and Organizational Behavior at the University of San Francisco in 1983, she earned a Master's degree in Human Development at Pacific Oaks College Pasadena; and is currently enrolled in the doctoral program in Medical Education at the University of Southern California, School of Education.

Ms. Henderson has worked as a staff counselor at a mental health center, staff nurse and charge nurse in the emergency department, and as Crisis Intervention Nurse and Trauma Coordinator at Childrens Hospital of Los Angeles. Since 1986 she has been responsible for coordinating EMSC (Emergency Medical Services for Children) grant activities, which have included research, education, and pediatric emergency care system implementation. Currently Co-director and administrator of the National EMSC Resource Alliance (NERA), a grant funded by the U.S. Department of Health and Human Resources, Health Resources Services Administration, she also has a faculty appointment as Lecturer in the Department of Pediatrics, UCLA School of Medicine. Ms. Henderson is the author of numerous articles and chapters on pediatric emergency care.

Dena Brownstein, MD, received her undergraduate degree from Yale University and attended medical school at the University of Washington. She completed a residency in Pediatrics at the Children's Hospital and Medical Center in Seattle, and received fellowship training in Pediatric Emergency Medicine at the Children's Hospital of Philadelphia.

Dr. Brownstein has a special interest in pediatric prehospital care. She served as Director of the Washington EMS for Children Project, and as a member of the Washington State EMS and Trauma Steering Committee, chairing its Pediatric Technical Advisory Committee. She is currently an attending physician in Emergency Services at the Children's Hospital and Medical Center in Seattle, and is an Assistant Professor of Pediatrics at the University of Washington School of Medicine.

Pediatric Emergency Nursing Manual

Deborah P. Henderson, RN, MA, CEN

Dena Brownstein, MD

Editors

 Springer Publishing Company
New York

Springer Publishing Company, Inc.
536 Broadway
New York, NY 10012

Cover and interior design by Holly Block

Production Editor: Pam Ritzer

94 95 96 97 98 / 5 4 3 2 1

Library of Congress Cataloging-in-Publication Data

Pediatric emergeny nursing manual / Deborah P. Henderson
   Dena Brownstein, editors ; sponsored by the Emergency Nurses Association.
      p. cm.
   Includes bibliographical references and index.
   ISBN 0–8261–8330–1
   1. Pediatric emergencies.   2. Pediatric nursing.   3. Emergency
nursing.   I. Henderson, Deborah P.   II. Brownstein, Dena.
III. Emergency Nurses Association.
      DNLM: 1. Emergencies—in infancy, & childhood—nurses'
instruction.   2. Pediatric Nursing—methods—programmed instruction.
3. Emergency Nursing—methods—programmed instruction.   4. Nursing
Assessment—programmed instruction.   WY 18 P3702 1994
RJ370.P454   1994
618.92'0025—dc20
DNLM/DLC
for library of Congress   93–38206
                                                 CIP

Printed in the United States of America

This project was supported in part by project MCH #064001–01–3 from the Emergency Medical Services
for Children program (Section 1910, U.S. Public Health Service Act), Health Resources and Services Administration, Department of Health and Human Services, Maternal and Child Health Bureau in collabo-
ration with the U.S. Department of Transportation, National Highway Traffic Safety Administration.
Support was also provided by the Emergency Nurses Association.

To my children, Graeme, Nina, and Frances, with love. I have learned so much from you.

D.P.H.

To my little sweeties, Sophie and Madeleine, who define joy; my husband, David Williams, whose unflagging love and support make it all possible; and my mother, Barbara Brownstein, who showed me that women can do it all.

D.B.

Contents

Contributors

ASSESSMENT AND TRIAGE

Treesa Soud, RN, BSN
Children's Emergency Nurse Consultant
Baptist Medical Center
Jacksonville, FL 32207

Melissa L. Taylor, RN, BSN, CEN
Nurse Manager of Emergency Services
 and Life Flight
Baptist Medical Center
Jacksonville, FL 32207

RESPIRATORY

Donna Ojanen Thomas, RN, MSN, CEN
Director of Emergency Nursing
Primary Children's Hospital
Salt Lake City, UT 84113

Laurel S. Campbell, RN, MSN, CEN
Education Coordinator
Bozeman Deaconess Hospital
Bozeman, MT 59715

**Deborah Parkman Henderson, RN, MA,
 CEN**
Lecturer, UCLA School of Medicine
Co-Director, National EMSC Resources Alliance
Harbor-UCLA Medical Center
Torrance, CA 90502

Casie Williams, RN, MEd
Director, Nursing Education
Alaska Native Medical Center
Anchorage, AK 99501

CARDIOVASCULAR

Dawne W. Orgeron, RN, EMT-P
EMS Administrator
New Orleans Health Department
New Orleans, LA 70119

Joycelyn Jeansonne, RNC, CCRN, MN, NNT
Pediatric Nursing Instructor
Louisiana State University in Alexandria
Alexandria, LA 71302–9632

**Deborah Parkman Henderson, RN, MA,
 CEN**
Lecturer, UCLA School of Medicine
Co-Director, National EMSC Resource Alliance
Harbor-UCLA Medical Center
Torrance, CA 90502

NEUROLOGICAL

June C. Winnie, RN, BS
Trauma Coordinator
Wausau Hospital Centerr
Wausau, WI 54401

Colleen Cantlon, RN, MEd
Maternal and Child Health Program Liaison
MCH Section—Bureau of Public Health
Madison, WI 53703

Mary Salassi-Scotter, RN, MNSc,
Director of Nursing Education
Arkansas Children's Hospital
Little Rock, AR 72202

MEDICAL EMERGENCIES

Sara J. Zimmerman, RN, MEd, CEN
Clinical Educator, Emergency Medical Trauma
  Center
Children's National Medical Center
Washington, DC 20010

Dena Brownstein, MD
Assistant Professor, University of Washington
  School of Medicine
Children's Hospital
Seattle, WA 98105

NONTRAUMATIC SURGICAL EMERGENCIES

Dena Brownstein, MD
Assistant Professor, University of Washington
  School of Medicine
Children's Hospital
Seattle, WA 98105

William D. Hardin, Jr., MD
Associate Professor of Surgery
University of Alabama at Birmingham
Department of Pediatric Surgery
Children's Hospital of Alabama
Birmingham, AL 35233

**Deborah Parkman Henderson, RN, MA,
  CEN**
Lecturer, UCLA School of Medicine
Co-Director, National EMSC Resource Alliance
Harbor-UCLA Medical Center
Torrance, CA 90502

TRAUMA

**Patricia A. Moloney-Harmon, RN, MS,
  CCRN**
Clinical Nurse Specialist
Children's Services
Sinai Hospital of Baltimore
Baltimore, MD 21215

**GROWTH AND DEVELOPMENT:
PSYCHOSOCIAL ASPECTS**

Kathy MacPherson, RN, MA
Nurse Educator/Coordinator for the Pediatric
  Arthritis Center of Hawaii
Kapiolani Medical Center for Women &
  Children
Honolulu, HI 96826

Lisa Marie Bernardo, RN, PhD
Clinical Nurse Specialist, Emergency
  Department
Children's Hospital of Pittsburgh
Pittsburgh, PA 15261

Robert A. Wiebe, MD
Director of the Division of Emergency Medicine
Professor of Pediatrics, University of Texas
Southwestern Medical Center at Dallas
Dallas, TX 75235–9063

**Frederick M. Burkle, Jr., MD, MPH, FAAP,
  FACEP**
Professor of Pediatrics, Surgery (EMS) and
  Public Health
Chairman, Division of Emergency Medicine,
  Department of Surgery
Vice-Chairman, Department of Pediatrics
John A. Burns School of Medicine
Honolulu, HI 96822

CHILD MALTREATMENT

Mary Salassi-Scotter, RN, MNSc
Director of Nursing Education
Arkansas Children's Hospital
Little Rock, AR 72202

Jacqueline M. Jardine, RN
Nursing Manager, Emergency Department and
  Day Medicine
Arkansas Children's Hospital
Little Rock, AR 72204

Louanne Lawson, MNSc, RN
Instructor in Adult Health Department
  Psychology/Mental Health
University of Arkansas for Medical Sciences
College of Nursing
Little Rock, AR 72205

Preface

Emergency care of critically ill and injured children is one of the greatest challenges nursing has to offer. Because few pediatric patients with life-threatening conditions are seen in most emergency departments, emergency nurses generally have less experience and are uncertain about their knowledge and skills in meeting the needs of these patients. This manual is designed to provide a solid knowledge base in pediatric emergency assessment and intervention, and to help emergency nurses feel more at ease in caring for children in a variety of emergency settings.

The development of this self-learning text evolved as a result of California EMSC project experiences in rural areas. Research showed that when financial or personnel resources were limited, nurses could not attend traditional educational programs such as seminars and workshops. With cost-containment a continuing focus today, fewer hospitals are providing inservice education for nurses; the need for acquisition of reinforcement of knowledge and skills, however, remains constant. This manual provides an enjoyable and inexpensive alternative to traditional inservice programs and national courses in pediatric emergency care. It offers an opportunity for nurses to obtain information about pediatric emergency care conveniently, and at their own pace.

This manual was designed for use either as a self-study program or in a classroom setting with a facilitator. Nine specific areas of the emergency care of children are included:

Assessment of the Pediatric Patient

Respiratory Assessment and Intervention

Cardiovascular Assessment and Intervention

Neurologic Assessment and Intervention

Medical Emergencies

Surgical Emergencies

Trauma

Growth and Development

Child Maltreatment

The case study format is used to illustrate the various aspects of pediatric emergency care, engaging the learner and encouraging participation. The chapters are intended for sequential study—each chapter builds on knowledge gained in the previous one. The approach to initial assessment of the critically ill or injured child is consistent throughout, and information is provided in a simple, usable format, with tables or bulleted lists to aid in learning.

Throughout the development of this manual, nursing educators in many states have expressed their eagerness to use a self-learning program in pediatric emergency nursing. Many individual chapters of this manual were piloted in California, Missouri, Oklahoma, Pennsylvania, and Utah, receiving very positive comments; we hope that the entire program will be equally helpful. It is a great pleasure to offer this educational program to emergency nurses, who give so generously of their time and energies daily, often at personal risk, to provide nursing care for ill and injured patients in health care facilities across this country and internationally.

Acknowledgments

This manual could not have been completed without the involvement of many dedicated professionals. Every nurse and physician involved in writing the chapters made a unique and valuable contribution; their efforts are truly appreciated. Initial funding for the development of self-learning modules was provided by the Robert Wood Johnson Foundation, for the Pediatric Rural Emergency Systems and Education Project (PRESEP). During the course of this project and the EMSC project, James Seidel gave generously of his time, wisdom, and boundless enthusiasm in support of nursing education. The gentle help and constructive criticism of Neal D. Kaufman assured completion of the original project, and established a secure foundation for continued development. The first modules were piloted in Northern California with the able assistance of Sharon Avery and the Northern Sierra Health Care Consortium; mountains and snowstorms were not considered obstacles by these capable and resourceful professionals.

The EMSC-ENA Collaborative Curriculum project was funded in part by the U.S. Department of Health and Human Services, Maternal and Child Health Bureau. During the early stages of development, the Education Committee of the Washington Chapter of ENA tirelessly reviewed preliminary materials, enlisted support from the ENA, and offered many excellent suggestions for the educational format. Ann Manton, then Education Coordinator from ENA, assisted in the early conceptual development and was consistently encouraging and supportive. Once the project was well underway, Mary Scotter served as both writer and editor with extraordinary grace and diplomacy. Casie Williams contributed her experience as a nurse and rural educator, along with her writing and editing skills, good humor, and enthusiasm. Casie also located Peggy Hayashi, an emergency nurse whose excitement and interest in illustrating the manual came at the best possible time. Ruth Rea, Sue Budassi Sheehy, and Gail Pisarcick Lenahan provided moral support and wise counsel throughout. Jan Stephenson capably served as typist and proofreader, always willing to review materials one more time. Finally, this project could not have been completed without the assistance of Margy Emmons, who skillfully checked, revised and formatted each module, and all too often had to begin the whole process over once again.

Chapter One

Assessment and Triage of the Pediatric Patient

Prerequisite Skills

Before beginning this chapter, the learner should have

- The ability to triage adult patients in the emergency department correctly
- Knowledge of the *ABC*s of adult assessment in the emergency department
- The ability to recognize psychosocial issues related to patient care in the emergency department
- The ability to recognize important components of an emergency department discharge teaching plan

PREVIEW

Assessment of the pediatric patient is an art, but an art that can be cultivated and improved with experience. When assessing a child, the attributes of the child and of the parent must be taken into consideration, as well as the quality of the relationship between the two. The emergency nurse's first responsibility in assessment is to differentiate between well children and those needing urgent or emergent care. Most nurses with substantial experience in the emergency setting can intuitively distinguish the two. The purpose of this chapter is to help you identify the factors that this intuition comprises so that you can document your assessment effectively and be able to identify improvements or deterioration in a child's condition as it develops. Some general rules about approaching pediatric patients during the assessment process may be helpful.

Infants

Begin with the interview, then move to the physical; the most traumatic portions of the examination should be reserved for last. This includes the eye, ear, nose and throat examination (EENT). In early infancy the focus of the approach is on the parent or caretaker. Warmth and comfort are the key to keeping an infant contented. In later infancy, separation anxiety becomes an important issue. Allow the infant to stay on the parent's lap, and use toys and colorful objects for distraction.

Toddlers

Focus attention on both the caretaker and the child. The toddler's attitude can change rapidly—negativism is common. Complete the physical examination as quickly as possible following the interview. Useful techniques are to observe the child while in the mother's arms. The skilled examiner can learn much by observing a child's play. Palpation, percussion, and procedures considered invasive such as the EENT should be performed last.

Preschoolers

These visits can be very pleasant. Preschoolers are usually cooperative and can participate in their examination. It is always wise to reserve the EENT examination until the end.

School-Age Children

Involve the child in the interview with the parent. Explain all procedures in age-appropriate language and allow the child to participate in the examination as much as possible. Privacy is very important in this age group; during the physical examination attention to privacy is essential.

Case Study 1 Objectives

On completion of this case study, the learner will be able to

- State the components that are most helpful in forming a general impression of children who "look good" or "look bad"
- Prioritize the steps in pediatric assessment
- List two essential observations in assessing the neurologic status of a pediatric patient
- Given a set of pediatric vital signs, determine whether they are within normal limits for the child's age
- Determine whether a child's weight is within normal limits for his or her age
- Determine whether a child's development is within normal limits for his or her age
- Recognize important elements of a discharge teaching plan for the pediatric emergency patient

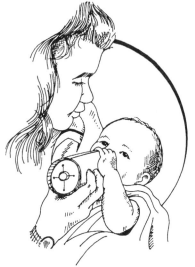

Figure 1.1

CASE STUDY 1

LaTisha Isn't Eating Well

LaTisha Freeman, a 6-month-old white female is carried into the emergency department at 11:30 P.M. by her mother (see Figure 1.1). You notice Ms. Freeman is wearing a uniform as she walks up to the triage desk holding LaTisha. Dressed in a flannel sleeper and wrapped in a blanket, with wispy blond hair sticking out, LaTisha appears to be sleeping.

Ms. Freeman says anxiously, "My baby hasn't been eating well for the last 3 days. I'd have brought her in sooner, but I couldn't get off work."

You take a quick glance at LaTisha, and you do not get the impression that she is seriously ill. You know from experience that this initial impression is often correct, but that you need to continue your assessment systematically.

Answer

Answer (1) is correct. Your initial first impression forms the basis for further evaluation. Because LaTisha is sleeping, her respiratory rate, work of breathing, and skin color contributed to your general impression that LaTisha was not acutely ill. If LaTisha were awake, an observation of her response to the environment would have provided additional valuable clues to her health status. Assessment of respiratory rate, work of breathing, skin color, and response to the environment can all be made without touching the child.

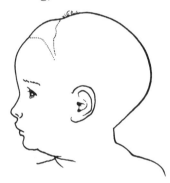

Figure 1.2

Touching the patient is required to assess capillary refill, skin temperature, and fontanel. Testing capillary refill and palpating peripheral pulses are useful means of determining perfusion in children. Normal capillary refill time is 2 seconds; any longer time may indicate cardiovascular compromise in a normothermic child. Skin temperature is difficult to assess, especially when the child is wrapped in several layers of clothing or blankets. The child may feel warm, even when he or she is afebrile. Palpating a young child's fontanel (see Figure 1.2) may help in assessing hydration or neurologic status. The anterior fontanel usually closes at about 14 to 18 months of age. Table 1.1 shows a useful sequence for triage assessment.

TABLE 1.1. Pediatric Initial Rapid Assessment

1. Initial impression or "across the room" assessment Does the child "look good" or "look bad"? • Respiratory rate. • Work of breathing. • Skin color (pallor, mottling, cyanosis). • Response to the environment.
2. Primary assessment: Evaluation of *ABCDEs* • Are the *ABCs* (airway, breathing, circulation) within normal limits? • Assessment of *D* = disability (neurologic status) *E* = exposure, and environment. Look for injuries and check body temperature. • A full set of vital signs may be taken if *ABCs* do not require immediate intervention.
3. Secondary assessment (brief history) Are there any underlying illnesses or psychosocial issues that may alter your initial triage impression? Are there cultural issues that require special attention during your assessment?

You ask Ms. Freeman to arouse LaTisha; her mother shakes her gently. LaTisha immediately begins to cry loudly but is easily consoled. Ms. Freeman continues to tell you how worried she is about LaTisha. She tells you again that she works in a local fast-food restaurant, and that they are running shorthanded, so she couldn't get off work any earlier. You say that LaTisha does not seem to be seriously ill right now, and that you don't think that her coming earlier would have made a difference. You assure her that you will tell her about what you find as you continue your assessment.

Your initial impression is that LaTisha's airway is clear (there are no unusual airway sounds), but there does seem to be some nasal congestion. Her breathing pattern is normal, respirations are nonlabored, and there is no nasal flaring. Her lips and skin are pink. Her skin color is normal, without mottling or bluish tinge. Her capillary refill is less than 2 seconds. When you touch LaTisha she is comfortably warm to touch and is not diaphoretic.

Because you have determined that the *ABC*s are adequate, you continue with *D* = disability and *E* = exposure. You assess her mental status.

Question

List two observations you might make in assessing a pediatric patient's neurologic status. (Fill in the blanks.)

1. _____

2. _____

Answer

Any of the observations listed in Table 1.2 would be appropriate for assessment of mental status. The infant or child's mental status is an essential component of the initial assessment. When a child is sleeping, you can ask the caretaker to awaken him or her gently to establish arousability.

TABLE 1.2.   Pediatric Neurologic Triage Assessment

Rapid pediatric neurologic assessment includes observation/evaluation of the following:

- Age-appropriate response to the environment and level of activity
- Arousability and response to comforting measures
- Recognition of and response to parents
- Condition of the anterior fontanel (under 14–18 months of age)
- Quality of cry: high–pitched, moaning or whimpering cries are abnormal
- Pupillary size and reaction
- Muscle tone: gait and posture

Note: "Paradoxic irritability" occurs when a child cries when comforted, and is quiet when left alone. This may be seen in children with meningitis. Children with **paradoxic irritability** and children who seem **unaware or unconcerned** with the hospital environment may be very ill and require immediate intervention.

TRIAGE DECISION

After this initial rapid assessment of the *ABC*s how would you triage LaTisha?

Emergent.   A life-threatening situation in need of immediate intervention.

Urgent.   Patient needs care within 1 hour to prevent further deterioration.

Nonurgent.   Patient is able to wait more than 1 hour without further deterioration.

TRIAGE DECISION ANSWER

At this point, LaTisha's condition appears to be nonurgent. Her history of sleepiness and fussiness needs some further exploration, but your initial findings (see Table 1.3) indicated to you that LaTisha is not acutely ill. She should therefore be triaged as nonurgent, although this may change as you obtain more information.

TABLE 1.3. *ABCDEs*

ABCDEs	Assessment parameters	Abnormal findings
Airway	Patency Posture	Audible airway sounds such as stridor, wheezing Positioning for best air entry (tripod position or "sniffing" position)
Breathing	Respiratory pattern Respiratory rate Respiratory effort	Grunting respirations Abnormal resting respiratory rate for age Retractions, nasal flaring, anxious facial expression
Circulation	Skin color and turgor Peripheral pulses Capillary refill	Pale, mottled, or cyanotic skin, presence of skin tenting Weak or absent peripheral pulses Capillary refill time > 2
Disability (neurologic status)	Arousability Consolability Response to environment Fontanel (infants)	Slow to arouse or unusual irritability Unable to console yet quiet when left alone Unaware or unconcerned with surroundings Bulging, tense fontanel when upright and not crying, sunken in the presence of other signs of dehydration
Exposure Environment	Skin temperature Skin color Skin abnormalities	Cool/clammy/cold skin Pallor, mottling, cyanosis Injuries, wounds, bruises

LaTisha's *ABCDEs* are normal, so you take her vital signs.

Apical pulse	140 beats/min
Respiratory rate	40 breaths/min
Temperature	101°F (38.3°C)
Blood pressure	86/55

LaTisha's peripheral pulses are strong and capillary refill is less than 2 seconds. While she is undressed, you note that LaTisha has no rashes, bruises or other lesions. You take her temperature, which is 101 °F. Your emergency department is just changing over to using centigrade temperatures, so you look this temperature up on the chart. (See Temperature Conversion Table at end of this chapter.)

In your emergency department, children's weights are obtained in the triage area. You escort Ms. Freeman into an examination room to obtain LaTisha's weight. You ask LaTisha's mother to undress her. LaTisha immediately begins to cry and protest. Her weight is 14 lb (6.4 kg). Ms. Freeman comforts LaTisha as you continue your assessment.

Question

Are LaTisha's pulse and respiratory rate normal for her age? (Choose yes or no for each rate.)

Normal pulse rate: ____Yes ____No

Normal respiratory rate: ____Yes ____No

Answer

The answer for both rates is No. Both LaTisha's pulse and respiratory rate are abnormal (see Table 1.4). Your major concern at this moment, however, is that there is no immediately apparent reason for these abnormalities. Before being undressed, she was resting quietly and seemed in no distress.

TABLE 1.4.   Pediatric Vital Signs[1]

Age	Heart Rate	Blood pressure (systolic)	Respiration (s)	Weight (kg)
Newborn	100–160	50–70	30–60	3
1–6 weeks	100–160	70–95	30–60	4
6 months	90–120	80–100	25–40	7
1 year	90–120	80–100	20–30	10
3 years	80–120	80–110	20–30	15
6 years	70–100	80–110	18–25	20
10 years	60–90	90–120	15–20	30

Question

Determine whether the following are true or false:

1. An 8-month-old infant has a fever of 103.6°F rectally. He is pink, but flushed, awake, tachycardic with brisk capillary refill, strong peripheral pulses, and his fontanel is flat. These physical findings are normal for a child of this age.

   True   False

2. A 6-month-old infant has a rectal temperature of 98°F. She is sleeping in her mother's arms. She is slow to arouse to tactile stimulation and her color is pale. Capillary refill is 5 s. Pulse is 80. Physical findings are normal for a sleeping child of this age.

   True   False

3. A 2-week-old infant has a rectal temperature of 101°F. Her color is pink, she arouses to tactile stimulation, and capillary refill is brisk. This infant can be referred to a health clinic.

   True   False

Answer

1. True. Physical findings are normal for a febrile infant of 8 months.
2. False. This infant, although afebrile, is slow to arouse, and has delayed capillary refill, pallor, and bradycardia.
3. False. This infant is only 2 weeks of age; therefore a septic workup may be indicated.

As you talk with LaTisha's mother, you are still concerned about her abnormally fast respiratory rate. You know that several factors can cause abnormal vital signs in children.

Question

Factors that can affect the respiratory rate in the nonemergently ill child include (Choose one answer.)

1. Fever, hypoxia, irritability

2. Fever, agitation, anxiety

3. Irritability, lethargy, fever

Answer

Fever, agitation, and anxiety, answer (2), can increase the respiratory rate of the nonemergently ill infant or child. Although fever is always a sign of illness, many children with fevers are not seriously ill. It is also important to remember that these signs may also indicate hypoxia and should not be dismissed without further consideration of the child's condition.[2]

ABNORMAL VITAL SIGNS

Assessment of vital signs is not the first priority when triaging children. Vital signs are important assessment parameters in the pediatric patient, but they must be interpreted in context with observational findings. Normal vital signs do not necessarily indicate the child is well. For example, blood pressure may remain normal in the hypovolemic child because the child has the ability to compensate with vasoconstriction, increased heart rate, and increased myocardial contractility. Even as blood volume is depleted, blood pressure tends to remain unchanged. When hypotension occurs, it is a late and ominous sign of cardiovascular decompensation.[3]

Fast Rates

- Tachycardia and tachypnea are often caused by fear, anxiety, agitation, fever, and crying, but they may also indicate hypoxia.

Slow Rates

- Bradycardia and bradypnea are abnormal findings in all infants and children. If the respiratory or heart rate seems close to a normal adult rate, it may be abnormally slow for the child.

Fevers

- Children with fevers may be cranky, tachypneic, irritable, and sleepy. They may also exhibit higher temperatures than adults because of an immature central nervous system. Children with high fevers may have benign illnesses and children with little or no fever may be significantly ill. McCarthy et al. found that **well-appearing**, febrile children with abnormal physical findings were seriously ill only 25% of the time.[4]

- Infants, less than 2 to 3 months of age are vulnerable to significant illness because they are reliant on maternal antibodies for protection. Any febrile infant less than 1 month of age should have a complete septic workup.[5] All febrile infants 1 to 3 months require extensive evaluation to determine the need for therapy.

Mental Status

- Lethargy and unusual irritability are also signs of hypoxia. Observing the child for age-appropriate behavior will assist with the identification of hypoxia-induced anxiety or lethargy.

You do not find anything acutely worrisome about LaTisha's assessment, and you wonder why Ms. Freeman chose to come to the emergency department tonight, and if there is a "hidden" agenda in this case. A brief history will help you to determine whether there are more serious underlying problems.

Question

Of the following, what information will be most useful to you in further assessment?

1. History of present illness or injury
2. The family's marital and socioeconomic status
3. The presence of an underlying illness
4. Observation of the parent–child interaction
5. Significant past medical history

Answer

The correct answers are, (1), (3), (4), and (5). A brief history obtained in the triage setting may reveal important information that would influence your triage decision. Questions should be designed to elicit the following information: (a) the presence of an underlying chronic illness (e.g., sickle cell disease, diabetes, or congenital heart disease); (b) significant past medical history (e.g., lengthy hospital stay); and (c) history of present illness.

If an underlying chronic process is present, it may be difficult to determine the need for emergent care (as with the cyanotic, congenital heart disease child). In these situations, asking the parent to compare the child's current appearance to normal (baseline) status may be helpful. Occasionally, the only clue to a significant past medical history is a lengthy hospital stay or frequent visits to a clinic, physician, or emergency department.

A useful tool in obtaining a rapid history in the critically ill or injured child is the mnemonic AMPLE, illustrated in Table 1.5.

TABLE 1.5.   AMPLE History[6]

A	*A*llergies
M	*M*edications (currently taking?)
P	*P*revious history of illness
L	*L*ast meal (time and contents)
E	*E*vents preceding injury

When obtaining this history, consideration should also be given to psychosocial and cultural aspects of the patient and family. A patient's family may inform you, for instance, that the child is the victim of a "spell," or that he or she failed to perform a certain ritual. These beliefs must be respected, and documented in your notes, regardless of your own beliefs. Such concerns may have a major effect on the care of the child and the family, so they must be taken seriously. It can be helpful for emergency departments to develop reference materials about cultures prevalent in the community, so recommended treatments and medications are coordinated as well as possible with cultural beliefs.

LaTisha is now awake, and she is drinking from her bottle as she sits, wrapped lightly in a towel in her mother's lap. You notice that Ms. Freeman is gently rocking LaTisha, looking into her little face and speaking quietly to her. These observations are important because they give you information about the relationship between parent and child. When the relationship is not a close and comfortable one, you usually consider ways in which dysfunctional relationships are manifested, such as child neglect or abuse. In such cases, you maintain a high degree of suspicion, obtaining a thorough history and observing parent–child interactions very carefully.

Question

List two signs that might indicate to you that Ms. Freeman's relationship with LaTisha is dysfunctional. (Fill in the blanks.)

1. _____

2. _____

Answer

Any of the signs listed in Table 1.6 would indicate a dysfunctional parent–child relationship.

TABLE 1.6.   Clues to an Unhealthy Maternal–Child Relationship[7]

- Holding the baby at a distance
- Maintaining little or no eye contact
- Not talking to the baby, or talking very little
- Calling the baby "it," and noting defects or undesirable traits
- Expressing dissatisfaction with caretaking
- Readily surrendering the baby to someone else
- Ignoring the baby's communication of needs
- Handling the baby roughly

You observe that Mrs. Freeman's interaction with LaTisha seems very normal. LaTisha now seems much more comfortable because she is less warmly wrapped. You tell Ms. Freeman about LaTisha's fever, and she wants to know if this is why LaTisha is acting differently. You discuss several points with her:

- Children with fevers may be cranky, tachypneic, irritable and sleepy.
- Children may have higher temperatures than adults because of an immature central nervous system.
- Children with high fevers sometimes have illnesses that are not serious, and children with little or no fever can be very sick.

You still have seen no reason for serious concern about LaTisha. Most well-appearing, febrile children, even with abnormal physical findings have been found to be seriously ill only 25% of the time.[4] Because Ms. Freeman seems so worried, however, you consider some additional possibilities.

Question

When triaging a child, what are some problems that would require immediate attention even though the child may "look good?" (Fill in the blanks.)

1. _____

2. _____

Answer

Any of the following situations might be serious, even with a child who seems to be in no distress on initial assessment:

- Ingestion of a toxic material
- Fever in an infant less than 3 months of age
- History of altered mental status
- Seizure (a child with a febrile seizure does not have a lengthy postictal state)
- Possible anaphylaxis
- History of trauma[8]

Note: Any febrile infant less than 1 month of age should have a complete septic workup.[5] All febrile infants 1 to 3 months of age require extensive evaluation to determine the need for therapy.

You observe Ms. Freeman sitting in the waiting area holding LaTisha who has fallen asleep. Because it is late and the evening is slow you are able to escort Ms. Freeman and LaTisha to an examination room in less than an hour. Ms. Freeman sits down on a chair, and you sit down facing her. She tells you once again that for the past 3 days LaTisha has been "fussy, sleepy, and has had a runny nose." She says, "I don't know what is wrong with her—she's too small to be sick!" You ask her about allergies, and she tells you that LaTisha does not seem to be allergic to anything.

Ms. Freeman does say that following her birth, LaTisha remained in the hospital for 1 week. She says that since then LaTisha visited the health clinic a week after being discharged from the hospital and then again when she was a month old. Ms. Freeman says everyone in the family is healthy and there is no family history of disease. She also informs you that she is only 16 years old, and proud of the fact that she is still managing to stay in school and hold a job. She says she is not married and never sees LaTisha's father.

Question

What three significant facts in the history would you consider the most important to question further? (Fill in the blanks.)

1. _____

2. _____

3. _____

Answer

Although Ms. Freeman presented you with a good deal of important information, the three issues that may have the most significance for LaTisha are

1. LaTisha remained in the hospital for 1 week following birth. You want to know whether her birth was premature. Because most normal newborns remain in the hospital for only 2 to 3 days, you might ask: Was LaTisha born early? Why did she remain in the hospital?

2. Ms. Freeman is a 16-year-old single parent. She goes to school during the day and works in the evening. This is a great deal of responsibility for such a young mother. It might be important to find out what social supports there are for Ms. Freeman.

3. LaTisha has only been to the health clinic twice. You realize that immunization history provides a historical clue as to the family's past compliance with medical care.

Obtaining more information, you learn that LaTisha's mother received no prenatal care. She says, "I didn't even know I was pregnant, I just thought I was sick." When asked if LaTisha was born early Ms. Freeman replies, "The doctor said LaTisha was small, only 4 lbs, 10 oz. She was born about a month before she should have been and then she had to stay in the hospital for a week because of breathing problems." Ms. Freeman says LaTisha did not have a "tube" helping her breathe but she did receive oxygen.

Question

Because LaTisha appears small and according to Ms. Freeman is not eating well you are concerned about her growth. Her weight is 14 lbs. Is this normal for an infant her age?

(Choose Yes or No.)

Answer

Yes, this is a normal weight for LaTisha. Infants generally double their birth weight by 6 months of age, and triple their birth weight by 1 year. Based on this rule, LaTisha is at the appropriate weight. In fact, she has tripled her birth weight.

If you have questions about her weight, a pediatric growth chart would be useful. Growth charts provide normal parameters for children based on the percentage of children that fall within a specific range. Premature infants must "catch up" with full-term infants so adjustments should be made when plotting their age and weight on the growth chart. LaTisha is just below the 25th percentile for a 6-month-old infant, and this probably accounts for her appearing small to you. When adjustments for age are made she falls just below the 50th percentile.

TABLE 1.7.   Physical Development of the Infant And Child[2, 7, 9, 10]

	Physical findings	Clinical implications
Head	• Rapid growth determined mainly by rate of brain expansion • Relatively large head compared with body • Open anterior fontanel until 14–18 months of age • Preferential nose breathing in infants < 2 months of age	• Two thirds of adult size by the end of the first year of life • Predisposition to head injuries from trauma • Rapid assessment for hydration status and intracranial pressure • Nasal obstruction leads to marked respiratory distress
Neck	• Short and narrow trachea (narrowest portion is the cricoid cartilage) • Soft cartilaginous larynx • Relatively hypermobile upper cervical spine and weak neck musculature	• Partial airway obstructions lead to marked compromise in airflow • Flexion and hyperextension will compress the airway • Increased risk of *upper* cervical-spine injuries from accelerative and torsional stresses
Chest, Pulmonary	• Poorly developed intercostal muscles • Highly elastic sternum and ribs • Primary muscle of respiration is the diaphragm	• Respiratory muscle fatigue occurs rapidly • Low risk of rib fractures, but significant underlying injury may be present; retractions are evident with increased work of breathing • Abdominal breathing is normal in the infant or young child; pressure from above (hyperexpanded lungs) or below (abdominal distention) will compromise effective respiration
Cardiovascular	• Fixed stroke volume	• Cardiac output (CO) is very heart rate dependent. Tachycardia increases CO only marginally in the infant; bradycardia will cause a significant decrease in CO (CO = HR × SV)
Abdomen	• Comparatively large liver and spleen, poor chest and abdominal muscle protection	• Increased risk of abdominal injuries owing to blunt trauma
Extremities	• Open epiphyses (growth plates) of the long bones	• When fractures occur they are frequently at the epiphysis and may be difficult to see on x-ray film; bone growth arrest can occur
Skin	• Large surface area to volume ratio	• High risk of environmental heat loss, hypothermia; susceptible to insensible fluid loss and dehydration
Neurologic	• Rapid changes in cognitive, language and motor skills	• Neurologic assessment must be age specific; knowledge of developmental milestones is essential

When asked who takes care of LaTisha, Ms. Freeman says she lives with her mother who takes care of LaTisha most of the time. Also living in the home are Ms. Freeman's 12-year-old sister, and 18-year-old brother. She talks about her family with some pleasure and says that her mother is very supportive, even though she was disturbed at first about Ms. Freeman's pregnancy. She says her sister likes to play with the baby.

You ask Ms. Freeman whether she takes LaTisha to the doctor regularly, and how many "shots" LaTisha has received. Ms. Freeman says LaTisha "has never been sick so she hasn't needed to see a doctor." She also tells you that LaTisha has not received any "childhood shots" and asks you when LaTisha is supposed to have them.

Question

Should LaTisha, at 6 months of age, have already received any of her childhood immunizations? (Check Yes or No.)

_____ Yes   _____ No

If yes, which ones should she have received at this point? (List types and ages.)

Age   Type of Immunization

_____   _____

_____   _____

_____   _____

_____   _____

Answer

Yes, LaTisha should have received diptheria, tetanus, and pertussis; and polio vaccine, usually three times by the age of 6 months.

TABLE 1.8. Immunizations[11]

2 months	DTP and OPV
4 months	DTP and OPV
6 months	DTP (OPV optional)
DTP = Diphtheria and tetanus toxoid with pertussis vaccine OPV = Oral polio vaccine containing attenuated poliovirus types 1, 2, and 3	

Note: Normal checkups for children in the first 6 months of life should occur within the first month of life, then at 2 months, 4 months, and 6 months of age.[12] (See "Recommended Routine Checkups and Immunizations" at the back of this chapter.)

You reassure Ms. Freeman that it is not too late to begin immunizations, and that you will give her more information before she leaves. Before the emergency physician comes in to examine LaTisha, you decide to complete your assessment. LaTisha's mother gently places her on the examination table. LaTisha's fontanel is flat (not sunken or bulging). While you are listening to her chest she grabs your stethoscope and tries to place it in her mouth.

As you palpate her abdomen you speak quietly to her, and she squeals with delight. When you reach over to pick up a tongue blade to distract her, LaTisha rolls over. You quickly grab her to prevent her from rolling off the bed.

LaTisha's breath sounds are clear to auscultation, except for some transmitted upper-airway sounds, and her abdomen is soft and nontender.

Question

Social development is of special concern to you in LaTisha's case both because she was premature and because of her environment. Of the following observations, which best leads you to believe that LaTisha is developing normally for her age? (Choose one answer.)

1. Flat fontanel, rolling over, ability to take bottle well

2. Rolling over, grasping the stethoscope, squealing with delight

3. Normal vital signs, normal size on the growth chart, drooling

---

Answer

Answer (2) is correct; these are all related to normal development. Normal development for a 6-month-old infant includes rolling over, grasping objects, babbling, laughing and squealing socially, and visually following objects.

A flat fontanel, normal vital signs, and taking the bottle give some indication of general health, but are not specific indications of age-appropriate development. A list of developmental milestones is included in Table 1.9 (facing page). These developmental milestones can be used to give an idea of whether a child is developing normally. Sick children and children who are afraid may regress slightly, so emergency department assessments should be considered very rough estimates of development.

During your interactions with LaTisha and her mother you have observed Ms. Freeman responding appropriately and lovingly to LaTisha's needs. You relay your findings to the emergency department physician, who, following a thorough examination, decides LaTisha has a mild upper respiratory infection (cold). His discharge orders include (a) cool mist humidifier in LaTisha's bedroom to relieve congestion; (b) acetaminophen (Tylenol), 80 mg every 4 hours as needed for fever; and (c) follow-up with a primary health care provider.

Question

Your nursing discharge teaching plan would include which of the following? (Mark each Yes or No.)

1. _____ Ask social services to check on Ms. Freeman to follow-up on LaTisha's primary health care needs.

2. _____ Teach Ms. Freeman how to suction LaTisha's nose to help her breath better because she has a cold.

3. _____ Teach Ms. Freeman how and when to administer the acetaminophen.

4. _____ Instruct Ms. Freeman to increase LaTisha's feedings because she is small for her age.

5. _____ Provide a mechanism, based on community resources, for LaTisha to receive primary health care.

6. _____ Stress the importance of childhood immunizations and recommend where they can be obtained.

7. _____ Explain the usefulness of a cool mist humidifier.

TABLE 1.9. Normal Childhood Development

Age	Activity	
Birth–1 month	• Visually tracks objects • Startle reflex (Moro)	• Turns head side to side • Responds to sounds
1–2 months	• Lifts chin • Coos	• Smiles socially • Reaches for objects
4–5 months	• Babbles/laughs/squeals • Rolls over • Visually follows objects 180°	• Moro reflex gone • Grasps toys • Pulls to sitting with little head lag
6–8 months	• Reaches for objects • Turns to voice • No head lag	• Hand–to–mouth activity • Transfers objects • Sits with support
9–11 months	• Sits alone • Plays pat–a–cake • Says "Mama" or "Dada"	• Crawls or scoots • Tries to find hidden objects
12–17 months	• Pulls to stand/cruises/walks • Drinks from a cup • Pincer response	• Tosses or rolls a ball • Speaks two to three words
18–23 months	• Walks well • Three or more words	• Feeds self
2 years	• Runs • Observes pictures	• Climbs stairs
3 years	• Knows first name • Counts three objects	• Stands momentarily on one foot
6 years	• Knows colors • Counts to ten	• Balances on one foot

Answer

1. No.   Your observations indicate that Ms. Freeman responds appropriately and lovingly to LaTisha's needs and has adequate support systems to assist with her care. You also know that LaTisha is developing normally and achieving developmental milestones appropriate for her age. Note, however, that if in your institution, social services is responsible for providing the family with a primary health care resource, then consulting a social worker would be a recommended intervention.

2. Yes.   You recognize that LaTisha's mother lacks the basic skills necessary to care for a sick infant. You therefore teach her how to suction LaTisha's nose. This is done by demonstrating the use of a bulb syringe, which is squeezed, placed fairly deeply in each nares, and released. Mucous should then be squeezed onto a tissue. This procedure should be repeated until LaTisha's nose is clear of mucous. If Ms. Freeman does not have a bulb syringe you provide one for her or tell her where one can be purchased.

3. Yes.   You provide Ms. Freeman with a syringe and show her, using water, how much acetaminophen should be placed in the syringe, then ask for a return demonstration. You inform Ms. Freeman that acetaminophen is used for fever and should not be given more frequently than every 4 hours. If she does not have a thermometer you provide her with one or tell her where to purchase one. You then demonstrate how to obtain both a rectal and axillary temperature.

4. No.   You know that LaTisha's growth is normal for a premature infant her age; in fact she is beginning to catch up to the size of normal 6-month-old infants. Ms. Freeman was concerned because LaTisha has not been eating well. You inform her that this is common for infants who do not feel well and smaller, more frequent feedings may be necessary.

5. Yes.   You know that adequate community resources are required to direct families to an ongoing source of care. Ongoing care is important because it provides an opportunity for specific health practitioners to know a child and family well, something difficult to accomplish in an emergency department setting. Many families see the emergency department as their primary source of care. You explain to Ms. Freeman why LaTisha should see a physician regularly.

6. Yes.   Many county health departments provide childhood immunizations. It is helpful to have a list of routine immunizations and where they can be obtained in your community available to give to parents.

7. Yes.   Explain to Ms. Freeman that a cool mist will keep LaTisha's breathing passages moist so that mucous can be suctioned easily, improving her breathing. The humidifier should be placed in LaTisha's bedroom and used when she sleeps. You inform Ms. Freeman that humidifiers must be cleaned often. You then inform Ms. Freeman where she can purchase a humidifier.

Ms. Freeman is told that her child has an upper-respiratory infection, and is given instructions to use a humidifier (which she says her mother has) and to suction LaTisha's nose to keep the air passages open. You also give Ms. Freeman a thermometer with an instruction sheet.

You also give her the name of two clinics near her home that accept patients who have state-supported insurance. Ms. Freeman puts LaTisha's sleeper back on, and thanks you for your help and advice.

Case Study 2 Objectives

On completion of this case study, the learner will be able to

- Choose the correct triage level for an afebrile patient with nasal discharge
- Identify appropriate interventions for a toddler resisting treatment
- Recognize the correct method of coping with anxious parents of a toddler
- Assess a pediatric patient for signs of dehydration
- Select appropriate responses to a parent who feels responsible for his or her child's illness
- Name the best method(s) of giving medication to an uncooperative toddler

CASE STUDY 2

Tommy Has Never Cried Like This

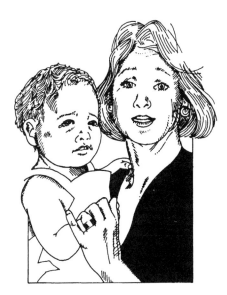

Figure 1.3

Tommy, a 20-month-old white toddler, is rushed into the emergency department triage area at 7:05 A.M. by his mother, Mrs. Jones. Mr. Jones runs in from the parking lot, looking tired and worried (see Figure 1.3). They both say Tommy must be really sick because he awakened frequently during the previous night with "inconsolable" crying. Mrs. Jones states, "I think Tommy is seriously ill. He's never cried like this before!" She tells you that she takes Tommy to a pediatrician, but his office doesn't open until 9:00 A.M., and she was very frightened by Tommy's crying.

Tommy screams and clings to his mother's neck as she approaches the triage desk. His airway appears to be clear as evidenced by his loud crying. His nose is running, but his breathing is not labored. He has no nasal flaring or retractions, his skin is pink, and his mucous membranes are pink and moist. Once he quiets down, you see him turning his head to watch every move you make.

Tommy's unusual irritability leads the triage nurse to triage him as emergent. You have special training in pediatric emergency care, and you disagree with this decision.

Question

From your "across the room" observations, list four reasons for your not agreeing with the triage nurse's impression. (*Hint:* think *ABCD*s)

1. _____

2. _____

3. _____

4. _____

Answer

Airway. Tommy's airway is clear except for nasal discharge.

Breathing. Tommy's breathing is nonlabored (no retractions or nasal flaring).

Circulation. Tommy's skin color is pink, and his mucous membranes are pink and moist. His skin feels very warm, and you suspect he has a fever.

Disability. Assessment of his neurologic status shows you Tommy is alert and very aware of his surroundings. He is frightened, which is normal behavior for a 20-month-old toddler. He is observant and moving his head from side to side, indicating there is no nuchal (neck) rigidity (one of the signs you might see if he had meningitis).

You talk with the emergency department nurse about your method of assessing pediatric patients (see Table 1.10, following page).

TABLE 1.10. Pediatric Triage Assessment

> Initial impression or "across-the-room" assessment
> - Does the child "look good" or "look bad"?
>
> Primary assessment
> - Are the *ABC*s within normal limits?
> - Assessment of *D* = disability (neurologic status); *E* = exposure and environment. Look for injuries and check body temperature.
> - Complete vital signs may be taken at this point if the *ABC*s are normal.
>
> Secondary assessment (brief history)
> - Are there any underlying illnesses or psychosocial issues that may alter your initial triage impression?

TRIAGE DECISION

Based on your assessment—initial impression, *ABC*s, and brief history, you would triage Tommy as

Emergent.   A life-threatening situation in need of immediate intervention.

Urgent.   Patient needs care within one hour to prevent further deterioration.

Nonurgent.   Patient is able to wait over one hour without further deterioration.

TRIAGE DECISION ANSWER

The correct answer is that on initial assessment Tommy's condition appears to be nonurgent. Although he may have a fever, in the absence of other symptoms this is not sufficient reason to triage Tommy as urgent. You would definitely be more concerned if he were less alert, if he were not actively moving around, or if he had a chronic illness. You are now ready to take Tommy's vital signs.

Question

Your emergency department requires that all patients have their vital signs taken in the triage area before being examined by the physician. Of the following list of approaches, choose those that are appropriate to gain Tommy's cooperation. (Mark appropriate answers with an **X**.)

_____   Ask Tommy's parents to step outside so Tommy will be more cooperative.

_____   Allow one of Tommy's parents to hold him while you obtain his vital signs.

_____   Reason with Tommy by offering him a treat if he cooperates.

_____   Provide Tommy with a distraction such as playing with the stethoscope or a toy.

_____   Remind Tommy that "big boys don't cry."

Answer

_____ It would not be helpful to ask Tommy's parents to step outside. You know that Tommy's behavior is normal for a toddler because toddlers commonly react to separation from their parents by protesting and crying. Separating Tommy from his parents will not gain his cooperation.

X Allow one of Tommy's parents to hold him while obtaining vital signs. Allowing Tommy to remain in his parent's arms fosters security and is more likely to lead to cooperation. It is not advisable to ask parents to help in restraining a child, but most young children will cooperate with an examination when held in a parent's arms.

_____ Reasoning with Tommy and offering him a treat for cooperation will probably not work. Because of their level of psychosocial development, toddlers do not respond to reasoning. They have not developed the ability to understand objective logic; instead, events are interpreted in terms of outward appearance only.

X Provide Tommy with a distraction such as playing with the stethoscope or a toy. Providing the toddler with a distraction is an acceptable approach to gain cooperation; allowing the child to play with equipment such as the stethoscope both familiarizes the child with the equipment in a nonthreatening manner and provides the child with a distraction.

_____ Reminding Tommy that "big boys don't cry" may foster guilt if he is not able to comply—in fact, this approach is not recommended for any age group. Toddlers have difficulty controlling their emotions. Older toddlers and preschoolers should be reassured that it is all right to cry with painful procedures.

Tommy's father has had to leave for work, so you ask Tommy's mother to assist you by holding Tommy in her arms and distracting him with a toy.

Tommy closely observes you as you obtain his vital signs.

Pulse	126 beats/min
Respiratory rate	30 breaths/min
Temperature	102°F (38.9°C)
Blood pressure	When you attempt to obtain Tommy's blood pressure, he fights and screams.

You notice that his capillary refill is brisk, peripheral pulses are strong, he has no rashes, but his skin feels hot. You begin taking Tommy's history to determine what seems to be happening. You ask his mother how long he has had this fever, and she tells you she thinks he has felt hot for the last 2 days. When you ask if he has had acetaminophen within the last 4 hours and if he is allergic to any medication, her answer is no to both questions. Because your emergency department has standing orders for acetaminophen, you obtain the medication and ask Tommy's mother to give it to him as you observe.

Question

Of the following, which information might influence your triage decision? (Choose answer 1, 2, or 3.)

   A. A history of chronic illness.

   B. A history of allergy to penicillin

   C. A lengthy, unexplained hospital stay

   D. A petechial rash

   E. A family history of asthma.

    (1) A, B, C   (2) A, C, E   (3) A, C, D

Answer

The correct answer is (3). A history of chronic illness such as a seizure disorder or congenital heart disease might lead you to perform an expanded triage assessment. A lengthy hospital stay may point to an underlying chronic illness. A petechial rash is a purpuric, nonblanching rash that may be associated with a serious underlying infection.

Neither a history of allergy to penicillin or a family history of asthma would influence your triage decision.

While Tommy is waiting in the bustling emergency department you notice that he is sitting curled up in his mother's lap sucking his thumb. He is clutching a worn, blue blanket and warily watching emergency department activities. Mrs. Jones asks several times "Can't you see my baby now? I know he's got a fever, so he must be sick."

Question

There is no need to explain to the Joneses that Tommy did not have a serious illness. That became evident during your initial triage assessment. (Choose True or False.)

_____ True   _____ False

Answer

The answer is False; you should have explained to the Joneses that Tommy was not seriously ill and offered them objective findings that might help to allay their fears. You should also have given them an estimate of how long they would have to wait to be seen.

The physicians in your emergency department do not insist that all children be totally undressed for the examination. You instruct Mrs. Jones to remove Tommy's shirt and put on the hospital "teddy bear" shirt. Tommy watches you closely but is not crying. You leave the room while his mother changes his shirt, but when you return Tommy looks at you and screams. Large tears run down his face (see Table 1.11).

Question

Which of the following methods is appropriate/inappropriate to gain Tommy's cooperation? (Mark **A** for appropriate, and **I** for inappropriate.)

_____ 1. Sit down with the family as you obtain a more complete history from Tommy's parents.

_____ 2. Maintain direct eye contact with Tommy as you speak with his parents.

_____ 3. Listen attentively to Tommy's parents' concerns.

_____ 4. Ask Tommy to tell you why he doesn't feel well.

_____ 5. Offer Tommy the small stuffed bear attached to your stethoscope when he sneaks a look at you.

Answer

1. **A**   A friendly, warm, unhurried, and informal attitude is often timesaving. "Children usually respond positively to those who they sense like them."[1]

2. **I**   Frightened toddlers often feel threatened when strangers maintain direct eye contact with them. Also, attentiveness to the parents (not necessarily to the child) is directly related to parental satisfaction with an emergency department visit.[2]

3. **A**   It is helpful to allow parents to express their concerns to an empathetic examiner. At times the parents may initially express one concern when their real concern is something else.

4. **I**   Tommy's cognitive abilities have not developed to a point where he can tell you why he does not feel well. Tommy would probably not respond to, "Do you feel bad?" because of distrust and fear.

5. **A**   Indirectly communicating with the toddler while speaking to the parents is often a useful technique for gaining cooperation.

TABLE 1.11. Hints for Gaining Cooperation with Toddlers

Allow the child to remain in the parent's lap for the examination. the child can lay across the parents lap and can also be hugged by the parent, facing away from the examiner.
If the child becomes fretful when spoken to, speak only to the parent initially.
It may be helpful to make the examination a game: Say, for example, "blow out the light" on the otoscope, look for "potatoes" or "turkey feathers" in the ears, "let me guess what you had for dinner" while looking in the throat or listening to the heart.
Adapt the examination to the situation; toe to head or head to toe may not be the best sequence for the examination. Save the most frightening procedures for last (e.g., ear examination).
Be observant! Much of the physical examination and the developmental examination can be performed through observation alone. Keep the examination as short as possible.
When possible give the child choices but *only* choices with which you can live. Say, for example, "Do you want me to look in this ear or that ear first?" instead of "Can I look in your ears?"

Tommy's tears subside as you sit in a chair across from his mother and begin to obtain a nursing history. As you ask his mother questions you notice that he is closely watching you out of the corner of his eye. Mrs. Jones says that Tommy has had a fever, diarrhea, and has been cranky for the last 2 days. She says he has had four loose (not watery) stools in the past 24 hours, soaking about half of his diaper each time. On the advice of her pediatrician 2 days ago, Mrs. Jones began giving Tommy clear liquids. During the night Tommy drank 8 oz of Gatorade.

Question Based on this history and your across-the-room assessment, you conclude that Tommy is probably dehydrated. (Choose True or False.) _____ True   _____ False

Answer

The correct answer is False. Tommy is crying large tears, he has moist mucous membranes, good capillary refill and his peripheral pulses are strong. He is alert, and has been drinking fluids well.

When asked about significant family history, Mrs. Jones confides that Tommy's family health history is unknown because he was adopted. Mrs. Jones says, "I'm so frightened. I know I'm doing everything wrong, because I don't know anything about children. I was a stockbroker for 10 years before we adopted Tommy. We waited so long for a child. If anything happens to him, I don't know what I'll do!"

Question

Of the following, which best describes the approach you should take with Tommy's mother at this time? (Choose one answer.)

1. Tell her that you are very concerned about her saying that, and that it may be helpful for her to talk this over with a counselor.

2. Call the hospital social worker to speak with her.

3. Listen to her concerns, and reassure her appropriately.

4. Ask Tommy's father to leave work and come back to the hospital to help in calming her.

Answer

The correct answer is (3); allowing Mrs. Jones to voice her concerns and providing positive reinforcement of her ability to care for Tommy may help allay her fears. It is also important to ask her more about her feelings of responsibility so that she can be reassured appropriately.

You know that Mrs. Jones panicked when Tommy became sick, and because of her need to "do the right thing" she will require a great deal of reassurance and support. You inform her that Tommy does not appear to be seriously ill, and that he is growing and developing normally. You patiently listen to Mrs. Jones's concerns and provide positive comments about her ability to care for Tommy.

Several minutes later your emergency physician enters the examination room, and Tommy anxiously watches her. She is skilled in examining uncooperative toddlers and quickly evaluates Tommy while he sits in his mother's arms. She finds that Tommy has bilateral otitis media and prescribes amoxicillin. You leave the room with her to begin discharge procedures while she calls Tommy's primary care physician to inform him of Tommy's emergency department visit.

When you return, Tommy is sitting on the examination room floor playing with a toy. He looks up at you and grins while holding up the toy. When you explain to Mrs. Jones that Tommy will need to take Amoxicillin for 10 days and then be checked by his pediatrician she says, "Oh no, it is so hard to get him to take medicine!"

Question

Of the following which best describe methods that can be used to administer medications to Tommy? (Choose one answer.)

A. Hold his nose so he will open his mouth allowing you to insert the medication.

B. Using a medication syringe slowly inject the medication in the posterior portion of the cheek.

C. Tell Tommy that the medication is candy and is good for him.

D. Disguise the medication in food to make it more palatable.

    1. A, B, D   2. B, C   3. B, D   4. All of the above

Answer

The best answer is (3). Administering medications to uncooperative children is often quite a challenge. Using a medication syringe and slowly injecting the medication in the *posterior portion of the cheek* (being careful not to aim toward the pharynx) is probably the most effective method (see Figure 1.4).

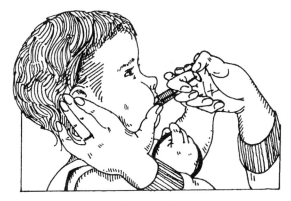

Figure 1.4

Parents often try to disguise the medication in food; however toddlers quickly catch on. When this method works, it works well and when it does not, the parent may wind up with a food and medicine mixture that the child refuses to eat. For infants, placing the medication in an empty nipple is a very effective way of administering liquid medications. Generally if a child's nose is held, he will cry (or scream). When the medication is administered the child often spits it out. There is also a risk of aspiration.

Note: Children should never be told that medication is candy because later children may associate potentially harmful colored pills or fluid with candy or Koolade.

Once you have shown Mrs. Jones how to give Tommy his medication, Mrs. Jones calms down quite a bit. She asks you many questions about why he has otitis media and seems very eager to give him his medication correctly. You give her some written information about fever in children, ways to treat upper-respiratory infections, and about otitis media. She seems very pleased.

Mr. Jones has returned to pick them up, and you suggest to them that they can come back in if Tommy seems worse, but that they should read the material carefully and discuss any questions they have with their pediatrician.

Case Study 3 Objectives

On completion of this case study, the learner will be able to

- Identify essential observations for initial rapid assessment of an adolescent
- Select the correct triage level for an adolescent with abdominal discomfort
- Recognize the significance of confidentiality and privacy issues for adolescent children
- Identify the major indications for a pelvic examination on a prepubescent female
- Name the best indicator that a female is approaching menarche
- Recognize interventions to enlist cooperation from an adolescent

CASE STUDY 3

Does Jenny Have Appendicitis?

As the triage nurse in a 200-bed hospital emergency department you notice an adolescent white female, with curly, auburn hair, walking rapidly toward the triage desk with her mother. They both appear extremely anxious. The mother, Mrs. Andrews, announces loudly, "My daughter needs to see a doctor immediately . . . She has appendicitis!" You quickly establish that the child's name is Jenny Andrews and she is 12 years old.

While obtaining a brief history of illness, you observe that Jenny is a well-dressed, well-developed adolescent. Jenny is standing erect, but is shyly hiding beside her mother. Her skin color is pink, respirations are even and unlabored, and she answers questions appropriately.

Question

As the triage nurse, what are three essential observations in your across-the-room assessment? (Fill in the blanks.)

1. _____

2. _____

3. _____

Answer

Initial rapid assessment involves obtaining a general impression. The most important initial observations are that (1) Jenny is able to breathe without difficulty, (2) her skin color seems normal, and (3) she is able to walk unaided. Your general impression is that she does not appear to be acutely ill at the moment.

Your next step is assessment of the *ABCDE*s

> Her airway is clear.
>
> She does not appear to have difficulty breathing.
>
> Her circulation is intact.
>
> Her mental status is apparently unimpaired.
>
> You defer examining her body until she is in an examination room.

Your assessment is that Jenny does not have a life-threatening emergency at this moment. The fact that she is able to walk without difficulty gives you an indication that she may not have severe abdominal pain at present.

Your third step is to take a brief history. You want to determine the urgency of Jenny's pain. On questioning, Jenny says she has not had any nausea, vomiting, diarrhea or pain on urination. She says that the stomach pain "comes and goes, hurts most around her belly button, and is worse in the daytime."

Mrs. Andrews says, "She's missed 3 days of school in the past 2 weeks, it must be serious."

TRIAGE DECISION

On the basis of your rapid, initial assessment, how would you triage Jenny?

Emergent.   A life-threatening situation in need of immediate intervention.

Urgent.   Patient needs care within 1 hour to prevent further deterioration.

Nonurgent.   Patient is able to wait over more than 1 hour without further deterioration.

TRIAGE DECISION ANSWER

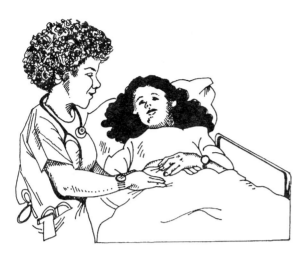

Figure 1.5

Jenny's condition appears on initial assessment to be nonurgent. Triage of a patient with abdominal pain should reflect severity, acuteness, and likely causes. Patients who must be seen immediately include those with prolonged, severe pain (causing them to double over), high temperatures (>39°C), constant crying, associated trauma, dehydration, tachypnea, or grunting.[1] Jenny displays none of these signs or symptoms.

You accompany Jenny to the pediatric room in your emergency department while her mother provides information to the registration desk. You explain to Jenny that she will need to put on a hospital gown so that a physical examination may be performed. She is reluctant to take off her clothes, but you reassure her that no one but you and the doctor will be in the room, and that she can keep her brassiere and panties on. Before she begins to undress, you use this opportunity alone with Jenny to begin the nursing history and physical examination. You leave briefly as she removes her clothes. When you return, she is sitting on the gurney. You look at her body, helping her to maintain her modesty as much as possible, and see no indication of injury or skin rashes (see Figure 1.5).

Question

Because she is so young, it is a good idea to ask Jenny about her menstrual history, sexual activity, or the possibility of sexually transmitted diseases with her mother present in the room. (Answer True or False.)

_____ True   _____ False

Answer

The answer is False. Confidentiality should be provided to all patients, regardless of age. Issues about bodily function, sexual activity, or drug use are often best asked away from the parent or guardian. Adolescents who fear punishment or disapproval from their parent may not answer questions truthfully in their presence. Attempt to interview the child alone and then the parent alone when seeking information about sensitive issues such as drug use, reproductive history, or sexual activity. This will not only establish a basis for trust, but also permits the child freedom to express concerns.

This is a good time to offer opportunities for questions and explanations, and help the adolescent understand bodily functions or teach preventive health information. After 12 years of age, adolescents are capable of verbalizing their medical concerns.[2]

After obtaining some history from Jenny, you tell her you know that talking about these things can be uncomfortable, but most women have some problems with their periods at various times in their lives. She looks nervous and asks you, "Will I have to be examined down . . . here?" as she gestures toward her lower body.

Question

In what instances might a pelvic examination be necessary for Jenny? (Circle all appropriate answers.)

1. Copious vaginal discharge
2. Missed menstrual period
3. Vomiting and diarrhea
4. Pain with history of sexual activity

Answer

Both answers (1) and (4) are correct. A copious or malodorous vaginal discharge is indicative of a vaginal or pelvic infection. A missed menstrual period coupled with abdominal pain might be a result of an ectopic pregnancy, but a missed menstrual period alone does not necessarily mean that a young girl needs a pelvic examination. An adolescent's menstrual periods are not always regular. Vomiting and diarrhea without other symptoms do not usually indicate a gynecologic problem in an adolescent.

Pelvic examinations **should** be done in all prepubescent females who have

- Acute abdominal pain
- Prolonged abdominal pain with unclear etiology
- Signs of pelvic disease[1]

You tell her that right now you are not sure, but you and the physician will be asking some questions to see what is causing her pain. As you question her further, Jenny says she has not begun to have periods and seems to have only a vague understanding about this physiologic process. She says she had some itching "down there" once but not recently. She denies having any discharge or blood on her panties, and seems shocked when you ask her if she's sexually active. She vehemently denies sexual activity. In fact, Jenny tells you she thinks all boys are "yucky and stupid" like her older brother. Jenny's vital signs are

Temperature	98.4°F (36.9°C)
Respirations	18 breaths/min
Blood pressure	100/72

As she talks to you, you note that she is moving well, sitting up and lying down easily, and without apparent pain.

Question

What physical signs or history would you expect to see in Jenny that will indicate she is approaching menarche? (Choose one answer.)

1. Breast development
2. Growth of pubic hair
3. Increase in height
4. All of the above

Answer

All of the above is the correct answer. Breast and pubic hair development occur before menarche; however, the best indicator that a girl is about to begin menstruating is an increase in height. The average peak growth period is at 12.4 years, and the average age for menarche is 12.5 years.[3]

Your feeling is that Jenny's responses are genuine. Because of her strong reaction, you explain to her that these are questions you always ask when a female has abdominal pain. You tell her that abdominal pain can come from many sources, and it is important for you to consider many different possibilities. While you wait for the physician, she says she needs to urinate, and you give her a urine cup.

Question

What urine tests do you think might be ordered for Jenny? (Fill in the blanks.)

1. _____

2. _____

3. _____

Answer

Probably a standard urinalysis will be needed, and possibly a urine culture and sensitivity. In addition, a urine pregnancy test might be appropriate to rule out pregnancy in the event that Jenny is confused about what causes pregnancy. Adolescents often are unaware that pregnancy may occur without complete penetration.

Note: It is important to remember that even an early adolescent could be pregnant or have a sexually transmitted disease.

Jenny has not begun menstruation, and she denies any vaginal discharge. Adolescents will probably perceive the examination of their reproductive organs as being different from the examination of other body parts. Instructions female children are sometimes given, such as "don't touch yourself" or "keep yourself covered up," may create self-consciousness and embarrassment when a pelvic examination is necessary. A first pelvic examination may be facilitated by the guidelines shown in Table 1.12.

TABLE 1.12. Guidelines for a First Pelvic Examination[2]

Action	Rationale
Perform the general physical before the gynecological examination	Allows the adolescent to become accustomed to the physician; develops trust
Explain what will occur including equipment that will be used	Shortens the time necessary to perform the examination; allays fears of the unknown
Teach relaxation techniques (e.g., deep breathing through the mouth)	Relaxes pelvic muscles
Allow adolescent to decide if parent will be present	Acknowledges the right to privacy and gives a sense of control
Ensure privacy of the examination room; expose only the necessary body parts	Adolescents may be embarrassed and modest about their body
Keep the examination room warm, and use a sheet to cover the patient	Shivering caused by a cold patient will cause pelvic muscles to tighten

The emergency physician tells you that he will do a brief visual pelvic examination. You explain to Jenny that you will be there with her, and she tells you she is very nervous about the examination, because she has not experienced this before.

Question

From the following, choose those actions that will help relieve Jenny's anxiety about the physical examination. (Circle all that apply.)

1. Ask Jenny if she wants her mother in the room during the examination.

2. Explain in advance what will occur during the physical examination.

3. Tell Jenny that you will help keep her body covered as much as possible during the examination.

4. Tell her that the examination will not be painful.

5. Tell Jenny that you or the doctor will answer all of her questions during and after the examination.

6. Describe the most common types of vaginal infections and their causes.

Answer

Answers (1), (2), (3), and (5) are correct. Adolescents should be given any opportunity possible to make decisions about their care. Give choices such as "do you want your parents present?" whenever possible because this allows an element of control. Adolescents are afraid of the unknown, so it is important to explain procedures or examinations to them to relieve the fear. Reassurance that they will be permitted privacy will reduce embarrassment. Never tell patients that they are silly to be afraid of the unknown.

It would not be helpful to say the examination will not be painful, but you could tell her that if she experiences pain, she should tell the physician, and he will stop. It is also not useful to tell her about the most common types of vaginal infections, because this may not be the cause of her distress.

When asked whether she would like her mother to be present during her examination, Jenny says that she would rather her mom waited outside the room. Mrs. Andrews is upset about this and says, "Jenny, I'm your mother! You're feeling sick, and I'm worried about you. I need to know what is wrong! I think I should stay with you." When Jenny looks at you helplessly, you ask Mrs. Andrews to step outside the room to talk with you. Hesitantly, she agrees.

You explain to Mrs. Andrews that many adolescents feel as Jenny does—they are learning to be independent.[4] Although it is sometimes worrisome to parents, it usually means that parents have done their job well; their child is growing up. You also tell her that Jenny may be embarrassed because her body is undergoing many changes at this stage of development. Mrs. Andrews calms down when you promise that the doctor will talk to her following the physical examination.

You are present as the emergency physician, Dr. Lewis, performs a full physical examination. He assesses Jenny's abdomen as symmetric; flat; and without lesions, rash, or visible peristaltic waves. Bowel sounds are normal in all four quadrants, and on palpation the organs are nontender and without masses. There is no complaint of flank pain. Jenny says that she has no complaints other than abdominal pain. During the examination, you consider how Jenny and her mother should be informed of the findings of the examination.

Question

In this situation, what would be the best way for the physician to discuss the results of the examination with Jenny and her mother? (Choose one answer.)

    1. Inform Mrs. Andrews first; then both the physician and Mrs. Andrews inform Jenny.
    2. Inform Jenny first; then tell Mrs. Andrews separately later.
    3. Inform both Jenny and Mrs. Andrews together.
    4. Inform Jenny first; then discuss with her how she wants her mother informed.
    5. Inform Jenny first; then ask what information she wants her mother to be given.
    6. Have the nurse inform Jenny, while the physician informs Mrs. Andrews.

Answer

The correct answer is (4). This decision should always be made on the basis of clinical judgment. In this case, you are not anticipating frightening results, so you could inform Jenny first and then ask her whether she wants her mother to be informed separately or with her. Because adolescents are becoming independent, it is important to treat them as adults as much as possible. If the results are very disturbing, however, it may be advisable to tell both parent and child together.

Note: In some states, a parent does not have to be informed when an emancipated minor is sexually active *and* has a sexually transmitted disease, or is pregnant.

On completion of the history and physical, Dr. Lewis orders lab work and X-rays films. The emergency department is rather quiet, and you have time to sit and talk with Jenny while waiting for her lab results. You suspect that the results will be negative and think that there may be an emotional basis for Jenny's discomfort.

Question

From the statements below, choose those that would enhance communication with Jenny and help determine factors contributing to her abdominal discomfort. (Circle any that apply.)

    1. "You mustn't worry about this Jenny. You'll probably feel much better tomorrow."

    2. "Tell me when you have the pain in your stomach. Does anything make it better or worse?"

    3. "Do you only have this pain on school days?"

    4. "Tell me about your school. It must be difficult to keep up with homework and help out at home, too."

Choose one of the following answers:

    a. 1, 2   b. 3, 4   c. 2, 4   d. All of the above

Answer

Answer (c) is correct. Try not to use stereotyped responses (such as 1) or ask leading questions (such as 3). Encourage client evaluation of a situation or event, and offer general leads that take more than a Yes or No answer.

Jenny's mother has gone for a cup of coffee. While sitting with Jenny you say, "Tell me about your school. I have a daughter who will be in the 7th grade next year. I wonder if she will like it." Jenny says, "I did at first, but then I got in Mrs. Lipski's math class. She's mean. Nothing I do is right. She yells at me all the time because I don't understand how to do decimals."

You ask, "Have you talked to your mom about this? She seems really worried about you. It must be nice to have a mother who cares about you so much." Jenny has tears in her eyes as she says, "She doesn't care about me. All she does is work all the time. She's never home. When I ask her to help me with my homework she always has something else to do."

Dr. Lewis enters the room with Mrs. Andrews. He tells Jenny that the physical examination, and lab and X-ray results were normal. He addresses Mrs. Andrews, saying that Jenny does not seem to have a physical basis for her pain. At that moment, he is stat paged to the trauma room. He quickly hands you the chart and asks you to discharge Jenny.

Question

Which of the following would be the best approach to this awkward situation? (Choose one answer.)

1. Tell Mrs. Andrews that Jenny has school phobia, and that her pain is psychosomatic.

2. Ask Jenny if you can share the information that she gave you with her mother.

3. Give Jenny and her mother the printed discharge instructions on viral gastroenteritis.

Answer

Answer (2) is correct. Development of somatic symptoms in response to stress is not uncommon in children. In order to best assist the family in dealing with the underlying issues, it is important to communicate a sense of respect. This can be facilitated by not violating Jenny's confidence, and by involving her in the discussion.

When you ask Jenny if she will share the information she gave you with her mother, she starts to cry. She tells her mother how unhappy she is at school, and how she misses her mother being at home. Mrs. Andrews seems shocked and says, "Jenny, I didn't know you felt that way," and puts her arm around her.

You explain to Jenny and Mrs. Andrews that stress is frequently manifested as pain, and that the pain can be very real. Mrs. Andrews seems taken aback initially but then relieved and says, "I'm so glad that there's nothing terribly wrong!"

Your assessment of Jenny results in the following nursing diagnoses: (a) anxiety; (b) ineffective individual coping; and (c) parental role conflict.

Question

Which of the following interventions will best help Jenny and Mrs. Andrews begin to deal with their problems? (Answer Yes or No.)

1. _____ Suggest referral sources available to Jenny and her family that may help enhance family communication (i.e., social worker, psychologist, or school counselor).

2. _____ Suggest that Mrs. Andrews take a leave of absence from her job.

3. _____ Suggest that Mrs. Andrews set aside a "protected time" at home together with Jenny.

4. _____ Reinforce the importance of school attendance.

Answer

1. Yes.　Suggest referral sources available to Jenny and her family that may help enhance family communication. It is often possible to identify a family communication problem in the emergency department; however, time factors make it difficult to help a family work through these problems. Emergency department nurses must realize they have an obligation to care for both the physical and emotional needs of a family. Referring clients to appropriate counseling sources is an important part of nursing practice.

2. No.　Mrs. Andrews may have chosen to work for financial reasons or for personal satisfaction. It is wrong to suggest that she leave her job. Instead, suggest ways to help the family cope with issues that arise as a result of having parents who work outside of the home.

3. Yes.　Suggest that Mrs. Andrews spend time with Jenny on a regular basis to help with homework or do something fun. Although adolescents try to establish their own identity, and therefore pull away from their parents, they are also very confused by a need to know that their parents are still available to them. Jenny still needs time with her mother on a regular basis. Remind Mrs. Andrews that adolescence is a time of conflicting emotions for both the child and the parent.

4. Yes.　Discuss with Jenny and her mother that missing school brings only temporary relief from an uncomfortable situation. It is better to discover the underlying issues that cause emotional trauma leading to physiologic discomfort. Suggest a meeting with Jenny's teacher or a school counselor to elicit the school's help for Jenny.

Jenny and her mother seem relieved to have the issues out in the open. When you give them written discharge instructions on abdominal pain, Mrs. Andrews thanks you for your kindness. You emphasize the need to seek medical attention if Jenny's symptoms worsen. Jenny's mother brings the car around to the emergency loading area, and you say good-bye as they leave.

REFERENCES

Case Study 1

1. Seidel, J. S., & Henderson, D. P. (1987). *Prehospital care of pediatric emergencies*. Los Angeles: Los Angeles Pediatric Society.
2. Hazinski, M. J. (1984). Children are different. In M. F. Hazinski (Ed.), *Nursing care of the critically ill child*. St. Louis: C. V. Mosby.
3. Chameides, L. (Ed.). (1988). *Textbook of pediatric advanced life support*. Dallas: American Heart Association & American Academy of Pediatrics.
4. McCarthy, P. L., et al. (1985). Predictive value of abnormal physical examination findings in ill-appearing and well-appearing febrile children. *Pediatrics, 76,*23.
5. Berkowitz, C. D., Vehiyama, N., Tully, S. B., Marble, R. D., Spencer, M., Stein M. T., & Orr, D. P. (1985). Fever in infants less than two months of age: Spectrum of disease and predictors of outcome. *Pediatric Emergency Care, 1*, 3.
6. American College of Surgeons Committee on Trauma and Subcommittee on Advanced Trauma Life Support of the American College of Surgeons Committee on Trauma (1989). *Advanced trauma life support program*. Chicago: American College of Surgeons.
7. Murray, R., et al. (1979). Assessment and health promotion for the infant. In R. Murray & J. Zemmer (Eds.), *Nursing assessment and health promotion through the life span* (2nd ed.). Englewood Cliffs, NJ: Prentice Hall.
8. Thomas, D. (1988). The ABCs of pediatric triage. *Journal of Emergency Nursing, 14*, 3.
9. Tecklenburg, F. (1988). Problems in managing cervical spine injuries. In R. C. Luten (Ed.), *Problems in pediatric emergency medicine*. New York: Churchill Livingstone.
10. AAP & ACEP. (1989). *Advanced pediatric life support* (APLS), (p. 18–19).
11. Committee on Infectious Diseases. (1988). *Report of the Committee on Infectious Diseases*. Elk Grove, IL: American Academy of Pediatrics.

12. Committee on Psychosocial Aspects of Child and Family Health (1985–1988). *Guidelines for health supervision* (Vol. 2). Elk Grove, IL: American Academy of Pediatrics.

Case Study 2

1. Green, M. (1980) Approach to the pediatric physical examination. In M. Green (Ed.), *Pediatric diagnosis, interpretation of symptoms and signs in different age periods,* (3rd ed.). Philadelphia: Saunders.
2. Francis, V., Korsch, B. M., & Morris, M. J. (1969). Gaps in doctor–patient communication. *New England Journal of Medicine, 280,* 535–540.

Case Study 3

1. Barkin, R. & Rose, P. (1987). *Emergency Pediatrics: A guide to ambulatory care* (2nd ed.). St. Louis: Mosby.
2. Cooper, H. E., & Nakashima, I. (1982). Adolescence. In C. H. Kempe, H. K. Siver & D. O'Brian (Eds.), *Current pediatric diagnosis and treatment* (7th ed.). Los Altos: Lange Medical Publications.
3. Nelms, B. C., & Mullins, R. G. (1982). *Growth and development: A primary health care approach.* Englewood Cliffs, NJ: Prentice Hall.
4. Malasanos, L., Barkauskas, V., Moss, M., & Stoltenberg-Allen, K. (1981). *Health assessment* (2nd ed.). St. Louis: Mosby.

RECOMMENDED ROUTINE CHECKUPS AND IMMUNIZATIONS

Exams[1]	DTP[2]	OPV[3]	MMR[4]	Hib[5]	Td[6]	TB Skin Test[7]
2 months 4 months 6 months 15 months* 18 months 4–6 years	2 months 4 months 6 months 15 months* 18 months 4–6 years	2 months 4 months 6 months* optional 15 months* 18 months 4–6 years	15 months	15 months	14–16 years	12–15 months 4–6 years 14–16 years

[1]Normal health care examination recommendations "are designed for children who are receiving competent parenting, have no manifestations of any important health problems and are growing and developing in satisfactory fashion" (Committee on Psychosocial Aspects of Care and Family Health Care, 1988, 155).

[2]*DTP.* Diphtheria and tetanus toxoids with pertussis vaccine.

    (a) Fourth dose should be given 6–12 months after the third dose.

    (b) May be given simultaneously with MMR (see below) and at 15 months (Committee on Infectious Diseases, 1988, p. 15).

[3]*OPV.* Oral poliovirus vaccine containing attenuated poliovirus types 1, 2, and 3.

    (a) May be given simultaneously with MMR at 15 months.

    (b) May be given at any time between 12 and 24 months of age.

    (c) The third dose is optional.

    (d) The fifth dose (4–6 years) should be given at or before school entry, up to the seventh birthday (Committee on Infectious Diseases, 1988, p. 15).

[4]*MMR.* Live measles, mumps, and rubella viruses in a combined vaccine.

[5]*Hib. Haemophilus influenza b* conjugated vaccine (examples: PRP–D, HbOC, PRP–OMP).

[6]*Td.* Adult tetanus toxoid (full dose) and diphtheria toxoid (reduced dose).

[7]*TB skin test.*

    (a) Old tuberculin used in multiple puncture preparations.

    (b) PPD (Purified protein derivative) is used more often than OT because it is purer and more specific.

    (c) Annual testing recommended only for those patients considered high risk (Committee on Infectious Diseases, 1988, p. 15).

Sources:

Committee on Infectious Diseases: Haemophilus influenza type b conjugated vaccines: immunization of children at 15 months of age. Elk Grove, IL, American Academy of Pediatrics, 1989–1990.

Committee in Infectious Diseases: Report of the Committee on Infectious Diseases, Elk Grove, IL. American Academy of Pediatrics, 1988.

Committee on psychosocial Aspects of Child and Family Health, 1985–1988: Guidelines for Health Supervision II, Elk Grove, IL. American Academy of Pediatrics, 1988.

TEMPERATURE CONVERSION TABLE
Centigrade to Fahrenheit (9/5 x C) + 32 = (F)
Fahrenheit to Centigrade 5/9 x (F − 32) = (C)

Fahrenheit	Centigrade	Fahrenheit	Centigrade	Fahrenheit	Centigrade
94.0	34.4	99.0	37.2	104.0	40.0
94.2	34.5	99.2	37.3	104.2	40.1
94.4	34.7	99.4	37.4	104.4	40.2
94.6	34.8	99.6	37.5	104.6	40.3
94.8	34.9	99.8	37.7	104.8	40.4
95.0	35.0	100.0	37.8	105.0	40.5
95.2	35.1	100.2	37.9	105.2	40.7
95.4	35.2	100.4	38.0	105.4	40.8
95.6	35.3	100.6	38.1	105.6	40.9
95.8	35.4	100.8	38.2	105.8	41.0
96.0	35.5	101.0	38.3	106.0	41.1
96.2	35.7	101.2	38.4	106.2	41.2
96.4	35.8	101.4	38.5	106.4	41.3
96.6	35.9	101.6	38.7	106.6	41.4
96.8	36.0	101.8	38.8	106.8	41.5
97.0	36.1	102.0	38.9	107.0	41.7
97.2	36.2	102.2	39.0	107.2	41.8
97.4	36.3	102.4	39.1	107.4	41.9
97.6	36.4	102.6	39.2	107.6	42.0
97.8	36.5	102.8	39.3	107.8	42.1
98.0	36.7	103.0	39.4	108.0	42.2
98.2	36.8	103.2	39.5	108.2	42.3
98.4	36.9	103.4	39.7	108.4	42.4
98.6	37.0	103.6	39.8	108.6	42.5
98.8	37.1	103.8	39.9	108.8	42.7

Chapter Two

Respiratory Assessment and Intervention

Prerequisite Skills

Before beginning this chapter, the learner should have

- Knowledge of the basic anatomy and physiology of the respiratory system
- Understanding of the principles of the respiratory system assessment through auscultation, palpation, and percussion
- Knowledge of the basic pathophysiologic principles associated with respiratory disease in an adult patient
- Basic understanding of blood gas interpretation

PREVIEW

Airway problems occur more frequently in the pediatric age group than in the adult age group for reasons related to both the size of children and their physiological development.[1,2] Respiratory distress and failure is the primary cause of cardiopulmonary arrest in children, unlike in the adult population, where cardiac problems are primary. Early recognition of the respiratory distress and early intervention is therefore the key to preventing the progression of respiratory distress to respiratory failure and cardiopulmonary arrest in children. This chapter reviews the most important issues in assessment of respiratory distress and failure in pediatric patients.

CASE STUDY 1 OBJECTIVES

On completion of this case study the learner will be able to

- List four assessment findings indicating respiratory distress in a pediatric patient
- Differentiate between the signs of upper- and lower-airway obstruction
- Cite differences between the adult and pediatric airway that affect assessment of respiratory status and airway management

- Prioritize interventions for a child in respiratory distress
- List three methods of delivering oxygen to a child in respiratory distress
- Indicate the correct locations for chest auscultation in a pediatric patient
- Identify the most common cause of airway obstruction in the pediatric patient
- Select the appropriate intervention for complete airway obstruction in a child
- Recognize the purpose of pulse oximetry and correctly interpret a pulse oximeter reading
- List three topics that should be included in a teaching plan for the parent of a child with croup

CASE STUDY 1

Spencer Is Having Difficulty Breathing

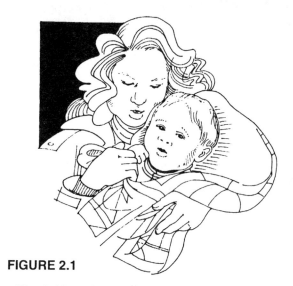

FIGURE 2.1

Spencer Young is an 18-month-old white male child brought to the emergency department by his mother, Mrs. Young (see Figure 2.1). It is early in the morning during the week after Christmas, and Spencer is dressed in a new fire-engine red blanket sleeper and wrapped in a large quilt. Mrs. Young seems frightened and tells you that Spencer is having difficulty with his breathing, "has a funny cough," and "won't eat or drink." She says that Spencer has had a runny nose for 3 or 4 days. She also tells you that he "feels a bit warm" when she feels his forehead, but she did not have a thermometer to take his temperature. When asked whether this has happened before, she says that he has had colds before, but he has never stopped eating. She says she is worried because he seems worse today, and he has had some coughing spells followed by vomiting.

You look at Spencer in the triage area and see that he is pale and drowsy. He is reluctant to lie down on the stretcher when he is placed there by his mother. He does not resist your unwrapping him and unzipping his new sleeper.

TRIAGE DECISION

On the basis of your initial rapid assessment, this patient should be triaged as

Emergent.   A life-threatening situation in need of immediate intervention.

Urgent.   Patient needs care within 1 hour to prevent further deterioration.

Nonurgent.   Patient is able to wait more than 1 hour without further deterioration.

TRIAGE DECISION ANSWER

He should be triaged as emergent. Your rapid assessment indicates that he does not look well. Spencer's breathing is not normal, his skin color is pale, and his lack of resistance all are indications that he may be in respiratory distress and will need immediate intervention.

You take Spencer and his mother into the treatment area for further assessment and intervention. His mother sits down in a chair in the treatment room, with Spencer in her lap. You are most concerned about Spencer's respiratory status. Knowing that airway obstruction is much more common in children than in adults, you want to be very careful in assessing Spencer's airway and breathing.

Question

List four other signs that you might observe in a pediatric patient who is in respiratory distress. (Fill in the blanks.)

1. _____

2. _____

3. _____

4. _____

Answer

Table 2.1 provides a summary of visual assessment guidelines.

TABLE 2.1. Signs and Symptoms of Respiratory Distress and Failure in Children

General Appearance	*Position:* Children in respiratory distress position themselves so as to maximize air movement (ventilation). It is common for children to assume the "tripod" position, in which they sit leaning forward, neck slightly extended, supported by their arms (this allows use of accessory muscles), with their head in the "sniffing" position (which helps to maintain an open airway). Reluctance to lie down may be indicative of a need to maintain an open airway—it is most commonly seen with epiglottitis, but may be seen with other causes of airway obstruction.
Respiratory Effort	*Increased respiratory effort:* This may be shown by the child's anxious look and the obvious concentration on breathing, as well as the use of accessory muscles for breathing. *Presence of retractions:* The effort to draw in air against resistance causes a sinking in of the soft tissues between bones and cartilage in the thoracic area. *Use of accessory muscles in neck and chest:* A child having difficulty breathing will use the intercostal, spinal extensor, and neck muscles to assist in breathing. *Nasal flaring:* The child's nostrils dilate to open the air passages as much as possible. *Seesaw abdominal and chest movement:* Seesawing movement is caused by increased respiratory effort and increased use of the diaphragm as an accessory muscle in respiration.
Rate and depth of breathing	*Tachypnea or bradypnea:* Tachypnea may be an early sign of respiratory distress. As a child progresses to respiratory failure, respiration slows. Bradypnea is therefore a very serious sign in pediatric patients.
Alteration in level of consciousness	*Alteration in level of consciousness:* An important indicator of the adequacy of oxygenation in the brain. Restlessness and anxiety are common signs of hypoxia. When a parent indicates that a child is "not acting normal," this should be taken seriously.

You ask the emergency physician to see Spencer right away, and you review treatment priorities as she comes down the hall to examine him.

Question

What intervention would be of highest priority at this point? (Choose one answer.)

1. To attempt to determine the cause of Spencer's respiratory distress
2. To reposition Spencer to assure maximal airway opening
3. To check the back of Spencer's throat with a tongue blade and penlight to see if there is an obstruction
4. To give Spencer oxygen by mask at 6 to 10 L/min

Answer

The correct answer is (4). Giving Spencer oxygen by mask at 6 to 10 L/min would be the first priority because of his respiratory distress. If Spencer is unable to tolerate the mask, other alternatives should be considered. Improving oxygenation would be more important than determining the cause of his distress. Usually a child in respiratory distress will assume a position affording maximal airway opening, so it is usually unwise to attempt to reposition an awake child. Determining the cause of Spencer's respiratory distress is not as immediately important as intervention in this situation.

Examining Spencer's throat could have serious consequences. Virtually any invasive procedure that might stimulate Spencer and cause him to cry should be avoided becuase of the risk of airway spasm. In the child with stridor and cough, examination with a tongue blade is contraindicated until the possibility of epiglottitis is ruled out. Initiation of the child's gag reflex on insertion of the tongue blade coupled with anxiety caused by the procedure could result in complete airway obstruction.[3]

You place an oxygen mask on Spencer with a flow rate of 6 L/min. He fights the mask a little but does not seem too uncomfortable right now.

Question

What other means might be used to deliver additional oxygen to a pediatric patient who seems uncomfortable with a mask? (Fill in the blanks.)

1. _____

2. _____

3. _____

Answer

Any of the methods in Table 2.2 would be useful.

TABLE 2.2. Suggestions for Pediatric Oxygen Administration

To avoid nasal irritation to the nares from prongs that are too long, cut the prongs off and position the holes in the cannula below the nares.

If a child will not tolerate wearing a mask, hold the oxygen tubing near the nose and mouth. This is called the "blow-by" technique.

A preschool child may tolerate a mask better if you describe it as a "space mask" and integrate it into an astronaut role play.

Cut a hole the size of the oxygen tubing into the bottom of a paper or styrofoam cup. Thread the oxygen tubing through the hole and have the child breathe from the cup.

Do not exceed a flow rate of 6 L/min by nasal cannula to avoid irritation of mucous membranes.

Note. From L. Campbell Upper airway emergencies. In D. Thomas & L. Campbell (Eds.), *Quick reference to pediatric emergency nursing.* © 1991, Rockville, MD: Aspen. Adapted with permission.

You continue your assessment of Spencer's airway and breathing. There are differences in the anatomy and physiology of the respiratory system of children and adults. These may be important considerations when caring for any child in respiratory distress. Several of these are important in Spencer's case.

Question

List three specific differences between the pediatric and adult airway (size, configuration, and location of airway structures, for instance) that should be taken into consideration in assessment and management of a child in respiratory distress. (Fill in the blanks.)

1. _____

2. _____

3. _____

Answer

Any of the answers contained in Table 2.3 (following page) would be appropriate.

When you look at Spencer's chest, you note moderate substernal and intercostal retractions with nasal flaring. You also observe that Spencer is using accessory muscles to assist in breathing. You increase his oxygen flow to 8 L/min.

As you continue to assess Spencer, you ask his mother if he looks pale to her; she tells you he does seem somewhat pale. His capillary refill is normal, however. Continuing your full assessment of Spencer's *ABCs*, you assess his mental status. You have already noticed that Spencer seems quiet and does not resist your assessment, and you suspect that he would normally protest a little more. You ask his mother about this, and she says she is surprised at how quiet he is, too. Using AVPU, you write down that he is alert, but you also note that his mother says he is more subdued than normal.

You completely remove his sleeper, and there are no signs of injury. He feels warm to your touch but does not feel hot. You take his vital signs. His heart rate is 160 beats/min. You count his breaths for 1 minute, and note that his respiratory rate is 40 breaths/min.

TABLE 2.3.   Respiratory Assessment: Differences between Adults and Children

In the infant and young child, the tongue is proportionately larger than in the adult, and it can more easily obstruct the airway.

The radius of the pediatric airway is smaller in proportion to body size than that of the adult, predisposing the child to airway obstruction from mucus or foreign objects.

The child's head is larger in relation to the trunk than the adult's, and neck muscles are less well developed. This results in children having less support and control of the head, predisposing them to compression of the airway from flexion or extension of the neck.

The tracheal rings are soft and more susceptible to compression when the neck is improperly flexed or extended.[1]

The larynx is higher and more anteriorly located in children than in adults; this may make it more difficult to visualize the vocal cords in children.

The narrowest point of a child's airway is at the cricoid cartilage, unlike the adult, where the narrowest point is at the vocal cords. The narrowing at the cricoid helps to stabilize an endotracheal tube and diminishes the need for cuffed tubes in children.

Intercostal muscles and accessory muscles are poorly developed in small children so the rib cage moves easily inward or outward. For these reasons, infants and small children are dependent on effective diaphragmatic function for breathing.[2]

Questions

1. Is Spencer's respiratory rate (40 breaths/min) normal for his age? (Answer Yes or No.)

   (a) Yes   (b) No

2. Is Spencer's heart rate (160 beats/min) normal for his age? (Answer Yes or No.)

   (a) Yes   (b) No

Answer

The correct answer to both questions is (b). Neither the heart nor the respiratory rate is normal for his age. His normal heart rate should be 100 to 120 beats/min, and his respiratory rate should be between 20 to 30 breaths/min. (See Vital Signs Chart, Table 1.4 in Chapter 1.)

Spencer's mother asks you, "Is he all right? I've never seen him so quiet—usually he won't sit in my lap like this at all!" You tell her that you also are concerned, and that she is a great help right now in keeping Spencer calm. You also tell her that Spencer will need careful evaluation to determine what is wrong, and you will let her know what is going on as much as possible. Right now, you are planning to listen to Spencer's chest, so you warm your stethoscope on your arm as you talk to her.

Question

Where do you listen for breath sounds in a pediatric patient? (Fill in the blanks.)

_____

_____

Answer

Auscultation of a child's chest is similar to auscultation of an adult's chest. You should listen anteriorly and posteriorly, in several locations, alternating side to side for comparison. With children, you should listen also in the mid-axillary line on each side. The breath sounds of children are transmitted throughout the chest, and listening at the mid-axillary line allows you to differentiate between the two sides more effectively.

Important points to remember in auscultating a child's chest are

- Infants and children have thin chest walls and relatively small thoracic cavities, so breath sounds may be transmitted throughout the chest. This makes determining the origin of adventitious sounds difficult.
- Always follow the same sequence, as in Figure 2.2, comparing one side to the other, anteriorly and posteriorly. Be sure also to include the extreme lateral fields in the axilla and along the midaxillary line.

Note: To encourage a child to take a deep breath, turn on a penlight, hold it several inches from the child's face, and ask the child to "blow out the candle."[3]

With Spencer sitting up on his mother's lap, you listen to his lung fields. You notice a harsh, high-pitched sound on inspiration.

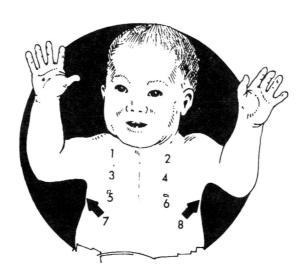

FIGURE 2.2 When listening for breath sounds, alternate side to side anteriorly, then posteriorly. Also listen in the mid-axillary line on each side.

Question

Is this type of high-pitched sound more likely to be an *upper* or *lower* airway sound? (Choose one answer.)

1. Upper airway   2. Lower airway

Answer

The correct answer is (1). You are probably hearing stridor, which is caused by air being forced through a narrow opening, usually in the upper airway—in the trachea or larynx. Table 2.4 gives a list of abnormal breath sounds. Figure 2.3 shows the location of breath sounds.

TABLE 2.4.   Most Common Breath Sounds Associated With Respiratory Distress[3]

Sounds	Description
Nasal congestion	Nasal congestion is usually caused by secretions in the nares, but may also result from anatomic obstruction, trauma, or from obstruction by a foreign body in the nose.
Gurgling	Gurgling is a coarse, bubbling upper-airway sound caused by uncleared secretions in the back of the throat (hypopharynx).
Hoarseness	Hoarseness is roughness of the voice, often with a change in pitch. It may be present with retropharyngeal obstruction and lesions of the vocal cords and subglottic area.
Grunting	Grunting is a brief, pressured vocalization emitted on expiration. The sound is due to expiration against a closed glottis (Valsalva's maneuver). The patient is instinctively creating partial occlusion of the upper airway resulting in positive end expiratory pressure, which helps to keep the smaller airways open.
Stridor	Stridor is a high-pitched crowing sound usually heard on inspiration. It is caused by air passing through the narrowed laryngeal or subglottic area. The classic sound of stridor is a high-pitched crowing or barking sound heard predominantly on inspiration.
Rhonchi	Rhonchi are low-pitched musical rattling sounds resulting from air moving past secretions or narrowing in the larger airways (trachea and mainstem bronchi). Rhonchi can sometimes be cleared by coughing or clearing the throat.
Rales	Rales are fine, high- to medium-pitched crackling sounds heard during middle to late inspiration. The sound of rales is similar to the sound made when several strands of hair are rubbed back and forth between two fingers. These sounds result from air bubbling through fluid present in the small airways and alveoli. Rales are usually described as being either fine, medium, or coarse.
Wheezing	Wheezing is a whistling, musical sound caused by air passing through partially obstructed lower airways. Wheezing can be audible in moderate to severe respiratory distress and can be present on both inspiration and expiration.

Spencer is still awake and maintaining his airway the best he can, and you continue to watch him carefully. If his mental status were to deteriorate, you would have to help him to maintain the airway.

Question

If Spencer's mental status deteriorated so that he could no longer maintain his airway himself, the most likely cause of upper-airway obstruction would be: (Choose one answer.)

1. Aspirated mucus or vomitus
2. His tongue

3. Tissue swelling and edema
4. Bronchospasm

Answer

The answer is (2). The tongue is proportionately larger in children, and can relax back into the posterior pharynx and obstruct the airway, especially in patients who have altered mental status. Mucus and edema may also obstruct the airway, but are less likely causes. Bronchospasm occurs in the lower airways.

Spencer continues to have some stridor, probably from a partial airway obstruction, most likely in the upper airway. You know that the three most likely causes are croup, epiglottitis, and foreign-body obstruction; because of the history you have obtained, you consider croup to be the most likely cause.

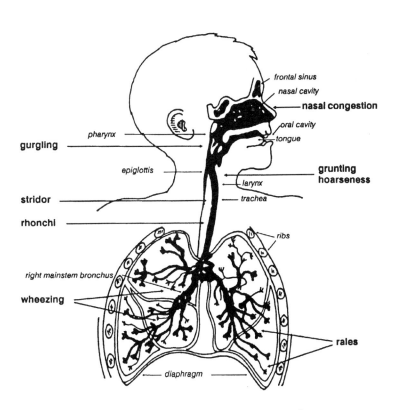

FIGURE 2.3 Location of breath sounds.

Question

Which of the following descriptions are most indicative of a child with croup? (Choose as many answers as are appropriate.)

1. Sudden onset of respiratory distress in an afebrile child
2. Harsh, barking cough
3. Rapid onset of symptoms over a period of hours
4. One to two days of upper-respiratory symptoms before this illness
5. Drooling
6. Age of child between 2 and 6 years old
7. Age of child younger than 2 years old

Answers

The correct answers are (2), (4), and (7). A barking cough, as with Spencer, is a common occurrence in croup. Croup is a viral disease, with onset over 1 to 2 days. It is seen most often in children younger than 2 years, although it can occur in older children.

Answers (1) and (5) are suggestive of foreign body obstruction. Because the obstruction is caused by a mechanical object rather than an infectious process, the child will usually be afebrile. (Remember, though, that children with viral illnesses can also aspirate small objects.)

Answers (3), (5), and (6) may indicate epiglottitis. This bacterial infection is usually seen in children 2 to 6 years old; it may occur at any age, although more rarely. Without intervention, epiglottitis can rapidly progress to total airway obstruction and death (Table 2.5).

TABLE 2.5.   Differentation Between Upper-Airway Obstruction Etiologies

Parameter	Foreign body	Croup	Epiglottitis
Age	Any age—common in 2–3 year olds	6 months to 2 years	3 to 7 years, peaks at 3–4 years
Etiology	Mechanical	Viral (rarely bacterial)	Bacterial
Onset of symptoms	Acute	Over 2–3 days	Over a few hours
Fever	Absent	Low grade	Infant: low Child: high
Cough	Partial obstruction: present Complete obstruction: absent	Barking	Usually absent
Inspiratory stridor	Present	Present	Present (soft)
Upper-respiratory infection signs and symptoms	Absent	Present for several days	None
Drooling	Possible	Absent	Present in 10% of cases

Note.   From Campbell, L. Upper airway emergencies. In D. Thomas & L. Campbell (Eds.), *Quick reference to pediatric emergency nursing.* © 1991, Rockville, MD: Aspen. Adapted with permission.

The emergency physician is preparing to examine Spencer, and you describe your findings to her. As you report the signs and symptoms you have observed, you realize that this will probably turn out to be croup, but you also review emergency interventions for a patient with foreign-body obstruction and epiglottitis.

Question

List three important nursing interventions for a patient with epiglottitis. (Fill in the blanks.)

1. _____

2. _____

3. _____

Answer

A patient with epiglottitis is always at risk for complete airway obstruction. Nursing interventions should include assessment of the child's perfusion status, maintenance of the airway, and preparations for the possibility of emergency airway intervention, such as intubation and tracheostomy. A list of interventions for a patient with epiglottitis are listed in Table 2.6.

TABLE 2.6. Interventions for Epiglottitis

Allow the child to sit in any position that maintains airway patency.[1]
Activate a team capable of providing emergency airway management if necessary.
Pay close attention to the child at all times—the child should not be left alone[3]; parents should be allowed to remain with the child to assist in keeping him or her calm.
Apply oxygen by mask or "blow-by" if mask is not well tolerated.
Avoid situations that might upset the child and increase airway obstruction.[1]
Prepare emergency airway equipment to take with the child when transporting to other departments.[3]
Controlled intubation will be necessary and should be performed in an operating room.[3] Necessary preparations should be made for this.
After the patient has been intubated, assess the need for sedation and make sure the patient is restrained to prevent accidental extubation.
Initiate intravenous lines and antibiotics only after airway is stabilized.

Spencer is continuing to move air in and out, so his airway is not, as yet, fully obstructed. Although he has no history of foreign-body aspiration, you must still consider it a possibility, and you review emergency interventions for this.

Question

If Spencer's airway became **completely** obstructed by a foreign body, what method should be used to try to clear it? (Choose one answer.)

1. Four back blows and four chest thrusts
2. Six-to-ten abdominal thrusts (Heimlich maneuver)
3. Three back blows followed by 6-to-10 abdominal thrusts

Answer

The correct answer is (2). In the older child, however, only the Heimlich maneuver (six-to-ten abdominal thrusts) is recommended.[4] After this, you should check again to see if the airway is cleared and remove any foreign body you can actually see (blind finger sweeps are *not* used). If the airway is still not clear, you should resume the Heimlich maneuver and continue the cycle until the airway is cleared.

Answer (1) would be correct if Spencer were younger than 1 year of age, in which case you would turn the child over, give four firm back blows between the shoulder blades and four chest thrusts, and then check to see if the obstruction cleared. A combination of back blows and Heimlich maneuver is not recommended.

Your emergency department has recently purchased a pulse oximeter. You decide to use it to assess Spencer's respiratory status. You explain to him that you will be putting it on his finger and offer him a chance to hold the sensor you will be using.

Question

When you obtain a reading from the pulse oximeter, what will you be able to determine? (Choose one answer.)

1. How effectively Spencer is ventilating and oxygenating
2. The degree of oxygen saturation of the hemoglobin
3. The arterial carbon dioxide and pH levels in Spencer's blood
4. Readings equivalent to all of the parameters of arterial or capillary blood gases

---

Answer

The correct answer is (2). Pulse oximetry is a rapid, noninvasive procedure that measures the amount of oxygen carried by hemoglobin (oxygen saturation), giving a general indication of the effectiveness of ventilation and gas exchange.[5] It does not, however, give any indication of perfusion—an anemic patient may have a normal pulse oximeter reading, for instance, and still not have adequate perfusion. Assessment of respiratory status should always include observation of the patient's level of consciousness, assessment of the work and quality of breathing, and perfusion status. To obtain a clear picture and precise measurement of respiratory status such as carbon dioxide level and acid-base balance, an arterial blood gas analysis should be performed.

After letting Spencer hold the sensor to lessen his fear of it, you put it on his index finger. You also explain the purpose of the oximeter to Mrs. Young. Spencer is quiet, watching you with an anxious look. You note his saturation on the oximeter is 89%.

Question

This oximeter reading is: (Choose one answer.)

1. Normal for a child   2. Abnormally high for a child   3. Abnormally low for a child

Answer

The answer is (3). Adult and pediatric pulse oximeter values are the same, so a child, like an adult, should be considered sufficiently hypoxic to require administration of oxygen if oxygen saturation is less than 90%. Normal readings on room air should be 99% to 100%, as with an arterial blood gas.

Arterial blood gases or capillary blood gases may also be used to obtain a measure of oxygen saturation. Because both of these are invasive procedures, pulse oximetry, a noninvasive procedure, has significant advantages in measuring this parameter, although it does not provide other information such as acid-base balance and carbon dioxide level.

Spencer is now being given oxygen at 6 L/min by mask. He is beginning to struggle to remove it, and he starts to cry. You notice that the reading on the pulse oximeter has dropped to 86%, an extremely low reading because he is already receiving oxygen. He remains alert, however, despite this low reading.

TABLE 2.7. Pulse Oximetry[5,6]

Pulse oximetry allows for continuous noninvasive monitoring of arterial oxygen saturation: the amount of hemoglobin carrying oxygen in relation to its total carrying capacity.[5] Two types of probes may be used: disposable adhesive sensors or a clip-on reusable type. The disposable sensors are most often used in infants, and the clip-on variety may be used in children older than the age of 4 (see Figure 2.4). The disposable sensor is usually attached to a finger or a toe.
Pulse oximetry has the following limitations:
Pulse oximetry only measures arterial blood oxygen saturation by measuring pulsatile blood flow. The probe must be positioned properly to provide accurate readings. To obtain saturation values, the oscilloscope must reflect a high correlation between the heart rate pulsations on both the electrocardiogram and oximetry tracing. Other sources of light such as overhead lights, warming lights, or surgical lights may interfere with probe readings, so probes should be covered to minimize this problem (see Figure 2.4). Peripheral vasoconstriction may impair the probe's ability to assess capillary flow accurately; care should be taken to ensure that the child's hands are warm, and that the probe is placed on a well-perfused digit (either fingers or toes may be used). If there is trauma to one extremity, another should be used for the probe.[6]

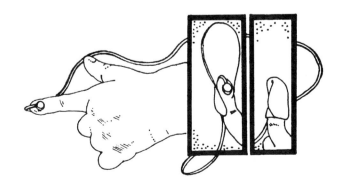

FIGURE 2.4   Pulse oximeter, properly covered.

Question

What methods could you use to improve oxygenation for Spencer? (Choose all that are appropriate.)

1. Use of a nonrebreathing mask
2. Use of a Venturi mask
3. Use of an anesthesia mask
4. Use of blow-by oxygen

Answer

All four methods could be used to improve oxygen delivery for Spencer, although (1), (3), and (4) are the most common. Any means of oxygen delivery that the child is comfortable with would be acceptable. It may be very helpful for parents to assist in oxygen delivery because the child will be more trustful of a familiar person.

You are now using a nonrebreathing mask, and Spencer's oxygen saturation increases to 92%, and you inform the emergency physician of this. She has finished examining Spencer, and orders lab work and acetaminophen for him. A tentative diagnosis of croup (laryngotracheobronchitis) is made. You add a cool mist to the oxygen source. He continues to have some retractions, although his stridor has diminished.

Question

What other interventions do you anticipate the physician ordering at this time? (Mark each answer "Yes" or "No".)

1. _____ Endotracheal intubation

2. _____ Epinephrine 0.01 mL subcutaneously

3. _____ Oral fluids

4. _____ Racemic epinephrine by aerosol

5. _____ Intravenous (IV) access

Answers

1. No. Endotracheal intubation is not necessary at this time—Spencer is not showing signs of deterioration. Preparations should be made for this possibility, however, because Spencer is still at risk for progression from partial to complete airway obstruction.
2. No. Although it is appropriate to direct intervention toward opening the air passages, subcutaneous epinephrine is not as effective as racemic epinephrine for croup.
3. Yes. Oral fluids should be encouraged to help thin secretions in the lungs, preventing thick secretions from narrowing the airway.
4. Yes. An aerosol treatment with racemic epinephrine may help to open narrowed air passages, increasing ventilation.
5. No. IV insertion is an inappropriately invasive intervention at this time; pain and anxiety could agitate Spencer and further compromise his airway.[3] If Spencer were severely dehydrated, the benefit of IV fluids might justify the risk.

The emergency physician now orders a racemic epinephrine aerosol treatment. From experience with this medication, you know that once this choice has been made Spencer will not be discharged immediately, even if he improves rapidly. You explain the use of racemic epinephrine to his mother and the probability of hospitalization.

TABLE 2.8. Use of Racemic Epinephrine

Racemic epinephrine is a medication for aerosolized use; the effects are very similar to epinephrine. Administration of racemic epinephrine may result in a "rebound" effect, and respiratory distress may return within minutes or hours after the treatment. If the child is discharged immediately after receiving racemic epinephrine aerosol treatments, the rebound effect may occur in a setting outside the emergency department and place the child at risk for partial or complete airway obstruction.[1] Children receiving racemic epinephrine treatments should therefore remain in the emergency department for continuous observation for a minimum of 3 to 4 hours after treatment; in many hospitals patients receiving racemic epinephrine are routinely admitted for observation.

You assess Spencer after his racemic epinephrine aerosol treatment and find that his condition has improved markedly. His temperature is down to 38.2°C after receiving acetaminophen. He no longer has retractions, and his respiratory rate is 30 breaths/min. He continues to have mild inspiratory stridor, and his skin is pink and warm.

Mrs. Young is still very anxious about Spencer. She asks you questions about what he has and what she could have done differently. You make a brief assessment of her understanding of croup and decide that it may be helpful to spend some time with her explaining some of the basic issues in the care of a child with croup.

Question

List three educational topics that should receive priority attention in your teaching plan. (Fill in the blanks.)

1. _____

2. _____

3. _____

Answer

Mrs. Young's educational needs include but are not limited to

- Causes of croup
- Rehydration measures
- Home care measures for future croup episodes
- Signs and symptoms of moderate and severe respiratory distress

TABLE 2.9.   Sample Home Care Instructions: Signs, Symptoms, and Treatment of Croup

Croup is a common viral infection of the upper-respiratory tract of infants and children, which usually comes on after several days of a cold or runny nose. The symptoms are hoarseness, a barking cough (seal bark), and a high-pitched noise when breathing in (stridor). It may last during a period of 1 week and is generally worse at night. Croup is usually severest on the first night symptoms appear.
Treatment of croup
Humidity is the most important treatment for croup. For quick relief, take the child into the bathroom, close the door, and turn on all the hot water faucets (shower if available), fogging the entire room. Stay there with the child until his or her condition improves. Use a vaporizer or humidifier in the child's room with the doors and windows closed. A cold mist vaporizer is best because it is safest, but a steam vaporizer may also be used. The more humidity, the better. More than one humidifier may be necessary in a large room.
Encourage your child to drink plenty of liquids such as flat lemon-lime soda, fruit juices, and fruit-flavored drinks. Gelatin desserts and frozen treats are also good sources of fluid.
Over-the-counter medications may make a child's condition worse. Cough suppressants should not be used. Antihistamines dry secretions too much. Check with your physician before giving any over-the-counter drugs. Antibiotics are seldom necessary and should be started only if ordered by your doctor.
For severer croup, especially at night, it may be helpful to take the child outside into the cold air for 10 to 15 minutes.
Call your doctor or come to the Emergency Department *immediately* **if your child** • Develops gray or bluish lips; this is usually caused by not having enough oxygen • Looks very sick or does not appear to be acting normally to you • Has so much difficulty breathing that he or she is restless and can't sleep • Struggles when you lie him or her down, can't swallow, complains of a severe sore throat, or drools excessively • Does not improve or seems worse despite home treatments • Has a temperature over 104°F (40.0°C)
Adapted with permission from Primary Children's Medical Center, Salt Lake City, UT.

You discuss some of Spencer's needs with Mrs. Young while Spencer continues under observation in the emergency department. He will be admitted to the hospital, so you explain admitting procedures to Mrs. Young. She asks you more questions about croup, and you give her a copy of the home care instructions (Table 2.9) for croup so that she can read them while she waits with him for transport to the floor.

When Spencer's room is ready for him, Mrs. Young gives him a hug before she gives him to you and thanks you for your help. Spencer looks much happier now.

CASE STUDY 2 OBJECTIVES

On completion of this case study you will be able to

- Choose the correct initial triage level for a child in mild respiratory distress
- List three common childhood respiratory conditions that have wheezing as a presenting sign
- Determine the level of respiratory distress (mild, moderate, or severe) in a child based on presence or absence of specific physiologic signs
- Identify two areas in a patient's history that would help determine the cause of respiratory distress

- Recognize three signs indicating deterioration of the asthmatic child's condition
- Identify the most common side effects of adrenergic drugs
- Select appropriate oxygen delivery devices for a child in respiratory distress
- Specify the correct sizes of equipment needed for endotracheal intubation of a pediatric patient
- List two indications for transferring a child in respiratory distress from a community hospital to a tertiary care center

CASE STUDY 2

Agnes Kobuk is Having Difficulty Breathing

Agnes Kobuk, a 4-year-old Alaskan Native, is brought to the triage desk by her mother, who says that Agnes has had "difficulty breathing." As Mrs. Kobuk fills out the registration form, Agnes sits in her mother's lap; Agnes has a thumb in her mouth and is clutching a well-worn "Winnie the Pooh" bear. Another child, who Mrs. Kobuk tells you is Agnes's sister, is standing nearby, hanging onto her mother's skirt and watching carefully; you guess that she is about 6 years old. Mrs. Kobuk says Agnes has been ill for 1 week with a cough and some congestion. Agnes began wheezing today, her mother says and has an oral temperature of 39°C.

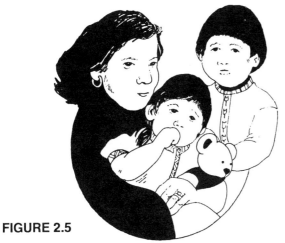

Mrs. Kobuk is concerned that Agnes has not been eating or drinking—she won't even eat frozen fruit popsicles, usually her favorite treat. She also says that Agnes has vomited three times this morning and that she is worried about her "not holding anything down." When you ask about what illnesses Agnes has had in the past, Mrs. Kobuk replies that Agnes has had a few colds during the last 2 years, but otherwise Agnes is healthy and is not taking any medications. Her sister has not had anything other than the normal childhood illnesses either. Mrs. Kobuk pauses for a moment, and then tells you hesitantly that one doctor she saw when Agnes had a cold told her that Agnes might develop asthma, and she is not sure what that meant.

FIGURE 2.5

You rapidly assess Agnes and see that she is quiet and slightly pale. She seems to be breathing rapidly, but she is not audibly wheezing. As you touch her skin, she watches you suspiciously and clings more tightly to her mother and to her bear (see Figure 2.5).

TRIAGE DECISION

On the basis of your brief assessment, you think Agnes's condition should be categorized as

Emergent.   A life-threatening situation in need of immediate intervention.

Urgent.   Patient needs care within 1 hour to prevent further deterioration.

Nonurgent.   Patient is able to wait more than 1 hour without further deterioration.

TRIAGE DECISION ANSWER

You should triage Agnes as urgent. You decide that Agnes needs treatment to prevent deterioration of her respiratory status. You are most concerned about how pale she is, how rapidly she is breathing, and about her mother's statement that Agnes was having difficulty breathing and was wheezing.

You observe Agnes carefully, talking to her gently without touching her to help her become more accustomed to you. Although Agnes has been vomiting, you can see that her mucous membranes are moist and her lips are slightly dry. You touch her little hand; her skin feels warm and dry. You decide she is probably mildly dehydrated and hope there is a fruit popsicle in the freezer that you can offer her when she is breathing more easily.

Question

What else in her history might help to determine the cause of Agnes's respiratory distress? (List two areas to explore.)

1. _____

2. _____

Answer

Some important issues include the following:

- *Onset of symptoms.* This might help to differentiate asthma from foreign-body aspiration.
- *Family history of asthma.* Because asthma often runs in families, it might help to know about whether there have been other family members with asthma.
- *Prior history of wheezing.* Although Agnes may not have been diagnosed with asthma previously, her mother may have noticed wheezing on other occasions.

You take Agnes to an examination room to take vital signs. Mrs. Kobuk tells you she will wait outside with her other daughter, and you let her know that she can ask for you if she wants to come in later. Agnes allows you to take her vital signs, but she is obviously not feeling well. Vital signs are as follows:

Temperature	39.4°C
Pulse	140 beats/min
Respirations	48 breaths/min
Blood pressure	110/80
Estimated weight	18 kg

Agnes's respiratory rate and pulse are definitely faster than normal for her age. As you remove her shirt to listen to her chest, you see some intercostal and substernal retractions. Listening carefully to her chest, you hear very little air movement, and with your stethoscope at the midaxillary line you hear some slight wheezing on each side. You discuss her case with the emergency physician, who examines her quickly and gives a tentative diagnosis of asthma.

Question

What conditions besides asthma might cause wheezing in children? List two of the most common. (Fill in the blanks.)

1. _____

2. _____

Answer

In addition to asthma, two common conditions that cause wheezing are bronchiolitis and foreign-body aspiration (into the lower airway). Both of these cause narrowing of the lower airway, resulting in the wheezing sound.

TABLE 2.10.   All That Wheezes Is Not Asthma[1]

Asthma	Bronchiolitis	Foreign-Body Aspiration
Most commonly seen in children older than 1 year of age; family history of asthma or allergies	Most commonly seen in children younger than 2 years old	Can occur at any age, usually seen in children less than 5 years old
Signs and symptoms vary with severity Expiratory wheezing with prolonged expiration Dyspnea Use of accessory muscles Tachycardia Tachypnea Upper-respiratory symptoms Fever (only if underlying infection) Wheezing (may be absent with severe distress)	*Signs and symptoms* Coryza Cough Gradual onset of respiratory distress May progress to apnea Wheezing (prolonged expiratory time) Tachycardia Tachypnea May or may not have fever	*Signs and symptoms* Choking Coughing Abrupt onset of respiratory distress Unilateral wheezing or decreased breath sounds History of playing with small objects or eating food such as peanuts, hot dog, hard candy, etc. Afebrile (unless there is predating infection)
Other less common causes of wheezing include pneumonia, intraluminal masses, and congestive heart failure with pulmonary edema.		

Note.   From *Handbook of Pediatric Emergencies* (pp. 69–75) by D. Smith and J. Dean (Eds.), © 1989, Boston: Little, Brown. Adapted by permission.

At this point, you consider the seriousness of Agnes's respiratory distress. Assessing the degree of respiratory distress in a child can sometimes be difficult because children are less able to describe their condition, and the signs and symptoms are different from those of adults.

TABLE 2.11.   Evaluating the Degree of Respiratory Distress

Degree of distress	Signs and symptoms
Mild	Wheezing, tachypnea, tachycardia, good air movement on auscultation
Moderate	Anxiety, respiratory grunting, nasal flaring, use of accessory muscles, retractions, breath sounds decreased bilaterally
Severe	Decreasing level of consciousness, restlessness or agitation, somnolence, severe retractions, cyanosis, distant or absent breath sounds, wheezing may be absent

---

Question

Considering Agnes's signs and symptoms, how would you rate her degree of respiratory distress? (Choose one answer.)

    1. Mild   2. Moderate   3. Severe

Answer

Agnes is in moderate respiratory distress right now. She has markedly decreased breath sounds and is using accessory muscles for breathing, with some intercostal retractions. She is not cyanotic, and although she is not very active, you don't feel her mental status is significantly altered. You should worry, however, that her respiratory distress might become severer and progress to respiratory failure. Your nursing diagnosis is ineffective breathing pattern related to bronchial obstruction, with a desired patient outcome of a normal respiratory rate, and diminished or absent use of accessory muscles.

Your nursing diagnosis for Agnes is possible impaired respiration, evidenced by her retractions, use of accessory muscles, and wheezing. Your intervention at this point is to talk to Agnes softly, telling her that you will stay with her, and you want to help her breathe better. Although she seems fairly calm, you know that anxiety may be a factor in increasing her difficulty breathing, and this must be a frightening experience for her. Your emergency department protocol allows you to use oxygen for patients in respiratory distress. Despite your encouraging Mrs. Kobuk to stay in the emergency department, she decides she wants to wait with her other child outside.

Question

Based on your current assessment, which oxygen-delivery devices would you select as most appropriate for Agnes? (Choose all that apply.)

    1. Oxygen mask at 4 L/min

    2. Nasal cannula at 6 L/min

    3. Blow-by technique

Answer

The correct answers are (2) and (3). Either the nasal cannula, with a flow of 6 L/min, or blow-by oxygen would be appropriate for Agnes. Using blow-by oxygen would require assistance of a staff member or a parent, and you have none available. An oxygen mask is also a good choice, but the oxygen flow must be a minimum of 6 L/min to supply an adequate amount of oxygen. Some children, if they are extremely air hungry, will be willing to cooperate by using a mask and may actually hold the mask themselves. Sometimes this is an indication of severe hypoxia (see Table 2.12, facing page).

You explain to Agnes that you are putting on the cannula to help her breathe, and she makes a face but doesn't resist. To further assess Agnes's respiratory status, you use a pulse oximeter and obtain an oxygen saturation measurement of 88%. You add ineffective gas exchange secondary to bronchospasm as a nursing diagnosis. You adjust the initial flow to 6 L/min. You notice that the oxygen saturation on the monitor rises to 90, but then quickly drops back down to 88.

Although Agnes's respiratory status is still being evaluated, you decide to prepare for more advanced airway interventions should her condition suddenly deteriorate. You make sure the bag-valve-mask device and a pediatric-size mask is readily available in case Agnes's condition worsens rapidly.

TABLE 2.12. Airway Adjuncts for Pediatric Patients

Type of equipment	Oxygen flow rate	Major purpose	Limitations
Nasal cannula	4–6 L/min	Provides a modest amount of supplemental oxygen	Cannot be humidified adequately; more than 6 L/min may cause irritation to mucous membranes
Oxygen mask	6–10 L/min	Delivers 35%–60% oxygen; this is a higher percentage than nasal cannula	Mask may not be well tolerated by child; must use minimum of 6 L/min flow because of entrainment of room air
Partial rebreathing mask (face mask with reservoir bag)	10–12 L/min	Delivers higher percentage of oxygen than simple mask, because patient inhales less entrained air	Mask may not be well tolerated by child; unable to determine exact percentage of inhaled oxygen
Venturi mask	12 L/min	Delivers oxygen from 25%–60% in a controlled amount	Not generally used for children
Oropharyngeal airway	Variable by need	Used to maintain airway patency in unconscious patient; can be used with B-V-M device if needed	May obstruct airway if size is incorrect; Not used in conscious patients, or if gag reflex intact
Nasopharyngeal airway	Variable by need	Used to maintain airway patency in conscious patient.	May cause trauma on insertion; uncomfortable for patient
Endotracheal tube	Full flow	Full control of airway, usually in unconscious patient	Requires expertise for insertion; can result in complications
Oxygen hood	10–15 L/min	Used for children under 1 year of age	Limits movement, not useful for children older than 1 year of age

---

Question

Knowing that Agnes's oxygen saturation is 88, what interventions would help improve perfusion? (Fill in the blanks.)

1. _____

2. _____

Answer

There are several interventions you might consider: (a) You could make sure Agnes is still positioned well to assure maximal airway opening; (b) you could discuss the possibility of a breathing treatment or additional medication with the emergency physician; and (c) you could consider changing to an oxygen mask because you would not want to increase the oxygen flow through the cannula because of possible irritation to nasal membranes.

You change to an oxygen mask, letting Agnes hold it on herself at first. As you increase the oxygen flow to 8 L/min, the pulse oximeter reading remains at 88% to 90%. After checking the oximeter probe to be sure it is making good contact, you increase the oxygen flow by mask to 10 L/min. Agnes's oxygen saturation increases to 92%. The physician orders a nebulizer treatment with a beta agonist. When the respiratory therapist comes to assist, Agnes takes a look at the nebulizer.

Question

What side effects might you expect Agnes to experience from the nebulizer treatment?

1. Blurred vision, nausea, weakness
2. Drowsiness, thirst, tachypnea
3. Tachycardia, nausea, vomiting

Answer

The correct answer is (3). Some of the most commonly used adrenergic drugs are the beta-adrenergic stimulants including medications such as albuterol (Proventil) and terbutaline (Brethine, Brethaire, and others). Also included in this category are epinephrine and isuprel. All of these medications usually increase the heart rate, and may cause nausea or vomiting (see Table 2.13, facing page).

After the nebulizer treatment, you listen to Agnes's chest. You hear bilateral high-pitched wheezing. Her respiratory rate has decreased slightly to 36 breaths/min.

Question

The increase in amount of wheezing indicates that Agnes is more hypoxic despite her seemingly increased alertness. (Choose True or False.)

1. True   2. False

Answer

The correct answer is False. The wheezing may indicate improved air movement through the smaller air passages. Absence of wheezing is often a severer sign because it indicates a greater degree of obstruction when combined with other signs and symptoms such as tachypnea and use of accessory muscles.[1]

Although you have seen some slight improvement, Agnes did not respond as well to the albuterol nebulizer treatment as expected, and the physician orders another nebulizer treatment and arterial blood gases. She also asks you to start an IV for fluid and give Agnes prednisolone. You insert a 22-gauge IV catheter in Agnes's hand. She becomes agitated during the procedure but quiets down when you finish.

After the second nebulizer treatment, Agnes's oxygen saturation has decreased to 86%, her respiratory rate increases again, and is now up to 48, with a heart rate of 180. On auscultation, you don't hear wheezing. In fact, you barely hear breath sounds. You ask Agnes to look at you, and she seems confused.

TABLE 2.13. Most Common Drugs Used for Emergency Treatment of Asthma[2–4]

Type/Name	Effect	Comments	Nursing implications
Adrenergic Agents			
Albuterol (Proventil, Ventolin) Metaproterenol (Alupent, Metaprel) Terbutaline (Brethine, Brethaire, Bricanyl)	Bronchodilation	Most common first-line medications; duration: 3–6 hrs. Two or three nebulizer treatments may be given; has selective beta effects; if patient is very ill, usually steroids are given in addition	**Side effects**: tachycardia, dizziness, nausea, headache (rarely); cardiovascular effects potentiated by MAO inhibitors and antidepressants; contra- indicated with use of imipramine (used for bed wetting)
Epinephrine (Adrenaline, Susphrine)	Bronchodilation	Formerly first-line medication, now less used because it has both alpha and beta effects; also, injection is painful; short duration of action: 30–60 min; Susphrine is longer acting: 6 hr.	Explain need for injection, allow child to stay with caretaker **Side effects**: tremor, restlessness, tachycardia, nausea, vomiting, headache
Isuprel	Bronchodilation	Used when other medications are ineffective	**Side effects**: same as epinephrine
Anticholinergics			
Ipratropium (Atrovent)	Bronchodilation	Not recommended for children under 12 years of age; duration of effect: 3–4 hr	Requires training for use of inhaler **Side effects**: dry mouth, cough, gastrointestinal distress, blurred vision, headache, nervousness. and dizziness.
Methylxanthines			
Aminophylline Theophylline	Bronchodilation	Given IV; May be used when other treatments are not effective; has many side effects; theophylline is long acting: 10–12 hr	If patient takes theophylline, draw blood level before administering **Side effects**: nausea, tachycardia, rhythm disturbances, seizures
Steroids			
Prednisolone	Anti-inflammatory	Given after bronchodilators, usually given IV; shows effects in 4–6 hr	**Side effects**: gastrointestinal problems

Question

How would you rate Agnes's degree of distress now? (Choose one answer.)

1. Mild   2. Moderate   3. Severe

Answer

Agnes is experiencing severe hypoxemia and needs further intervention to prevent respiratory failure. Your major concern should be to prevent further deterioration. Impending respiratory failure is usually assessed by sequential assessments combined with the patient's history (Table 2.14).[3]

TABLE 2.14.   **Signs and Symptoms of Impending Respiratory Failure**[3,5]

Decreasing level of consciousness over previous examinations
Increased work of breathing and respiratory rate
Decreased air movement on auscultation
Hypoventilation or apnea
Fatigue
Ashen color, cyanosis, grayness
Acidosis, hypercapnia, or hypoxemia (measured on arterial blood gases)
Failure to respond to therapy

After a third nebulizer treatment, Agnes's condition has not improved. You tell the emergency physician you are very worried about her, and ask the respiratory therapist to stay in the emergency department for the time being. You change to a nonrebreathing mask and increase the flow to 10 L/min to increase the available oxygen. You also place Agnes on a cardiac monitor and ask another nurse to help you prepare for possible intubation. When the emergency physician returns, Agnes's oximeter reading remains at 86%.

Question

Knowing that Agnes weighs 18 kg and is 4 years old, what sizes of equipment should you prepare for Agnes?   (Fill in the blanks.)

Endotracheal tube size? _____

Nasogastric tube size? _____

Laryngoscope blade size? _____

Type of blade (straight or curved) _____

Suction catheter size? _____

Answer

It is usually helpful to keep a list of correct sizes for all of these supplies and equipment ready at hand on the resuscitation cart. Approximate sizes for an 18-kg child are

Endotracheal tube	5.0
Nasogastric tube	10–12 F
Laryngoscope blade size	2 (straight)
Suction catheter size	10 F

In general, a straight blade is preferred for children under 15 kg and a curved blade for older children.

TABLE 2.15.   Average Endotracheal Tube and Suction Catheter Sizes

Age	Weight (kg)	Endotracheal tube size (mm) (2.5–6.0 uncuffed)	Suction catheter size (French)
Newborn–5 months	2–6	2.5–4.0	6–8
6–23 months	6–12	4.0–4.5	8–10
2–6 years	12–25	4.5–5.0	10–12
7–10 years	22–40	5.5–6.0	10–12
> 10 years	40–70	6.0– 8.0	10–14

Note. From *Prehospital Care of Pediatric Emergenices* by J.S. Seidel and D.P. Henderson © 1987, Los Angeles, CA: Los Angeles Pediatric Society. Reprinted by Permission.

Other items that might be needed include medications for paralysis and sedation. Medications and equipment for resuscitation should be readily available.

As you prepare the equipment for possible endotracheal intubation, you also keep an eye on Agnes. The respiratory therapist is assisting Agnes in keeping her airway open and maintaining a high flow of oxygen. A bag-valve-mask device is ready at the head of the bed. The emergency department physician is preparing to intubate and tells you she will use rapid sequence intubation if endotracheal intubation becomes necessary.

Question

Atropine, lidocaine, and succinylcholine are three commonly used medications for intubation of pediatric patients. What is the rationale for using each of these medications?

Medication   **Rationale**

Atropine   _____

Lidocaine   _____

Succyinylcholine   _____

Answer

The usage and effects of pancuronium, atropine, lidocaine, and succinylcholine are described in Table 2.16. These medications are often used in sequence: pancuronium, atropine, lidocaine, and succinylcholine, but the sequence and medications may vary by hospital protocol or physician preference. Two very important points regarding controlled intubation are that

- Children should always be sedated before paralysis. The experience of being paralyzed is very frightening.
- A backup plan should be in place in the event that intubation is not successful. This would include other temporary means of ventilation such as a bag-valve-mask device immediately available, and personnel and equipment available to establish a surgical airway if necessary.

TABLE 2.16. Rapid Sequence Intubation

Rapid controlled anesthesia induction is used to relax muscles and render the child unconscious rapidly, increasing ease of intubation and lessening the child's stress[6]	
Medications that may be used prior to intubation include	
To prevent fasciculation (uncontrolled muscular twitching)	Pancuronium, vecuronium, or atracurium: are nondepolarizing agents. Given in low dosages, they prevent fasciculation.
Adjunctive agents: to block vagal stimulation	Atropine is commonly used to prevent bradycardia and decrease secretions.
	Lidocaine lowers intracranial pressure and suppresses the cough reflex.
To paralyze muscles: to facilitate intubation	Succinylcholine is given for paralysis. It has many side effects that need to be considered.[6]
For sedation	Fentanyl, lorazepam, or other short-acting barbiturates or narcotics are usually given to treat pain and anxiety associated with intubation and paralyzation.
Performing rapid sequence intubation	
• A team approach and proper equipment is necessary. • There should be protocols for IV access, preoxygenation, cardiac monitoring, and use of pulse oximetry.[6] • Nurses and physicians should be familiar with the drugs used, their contraindications, and side effects.	
Ventilation after intubation	
• One of the common errors that occurs after intubation of a child is aggressive ventilation at a rapid rate in an effort to decrease the $PaCO_2$ rapidly. This may result in a tension pneumothorax because of increased lung and airway pressures.[7] The goal is to lower the CO_2 level and increase the PaO_2, but this must be done without overexpansion of the lungs. The best rule to follow is to ventilate with each breath only until the chest begins to rise. Careful attention should also be given to providing time for exhalation to occur. Oxygen-powered ventilators ("Elder valves") are not used on small children, because they are more difficult to control.	

Agnes's blood gases return from the laboratory. The results are as follows:

PaO_2	85
$PaCO_2$	45
pH	7.38
HCO_3	22

Question

Indicate T (True) or F (False) for the following statements:

1. These are normal for an asthmatic—Agnes may simply need a higher flow of oxygen delivered. T F

2. The $PaCO_2$ level is within normal limits. T F

3. Agnes should be given a bolus of sodium bicarbonate to improve her acid-base balance. T F

Answer

Remember that blood gases must always be interpreted on the basis of clinical signs and symptoms.

1. False.   These blood gases combined with her altered level of consciousness and abnormal vital signs indicate impending respiratory failure.

2. True.   The $PaCO_2$ is at the upper limit of normal. This value seen in a tachypneic, wheezing child, however, is a very serious sign of respiratory distress and impending respiratory failure. It indicates that she is incapable of blowing off carbon dioxide to lessen her respiratory acidosis.

3. False.   Sodium bicarbonate is almost never needed in the management of the severely ill asthmatic. Respiratory acidosis is corrected by improving ventilation and oxygenation rather than by giving sodium bicarbonate.[5] Administration of sodium bicarbonate to a child with inadequate ventilation will worsen respiratory acidosis. (The bicarbonate breaks down to water and carbon dioxide.)

Note: The 50–50 rule: A PaO_2 level of 50 or a $PaCO_2$ level of 50 is indicative of respiratory failure. ***This a life-threatening emergency.***

After the aminophylline has infused, Agnes's respiratory rate is slower, and she seems exhausted but more alert. The cardiac monitor shows a normal sinus rhythm, and her pulse oximeter reading rises to 92%. Expiratory wheezes are louder now than before. You set up the continuous aminophylline drip. Your hospital doesn't have a pediatric intensive care unit so you discuss transferring Agnes to the pediatric referral hospital 2 hours away.

Question

List two indications for transfer of this child.

1. _____

2. _____

Answer

1. Agnes needs care not available at your hospital.
2. Agnes's condition does not improve with therapy.

It has been shown that seriously ill and injured children have lower mortality and morbidity when cared for in tertiary centers offering a variety of pediatric subspecialists than they do in mid-level facilities where they are cared for in adult intensive care units. If Agnes's condition did not improve during her emergency department stay, or if she required the more aggressive intervention, it might be advisable to seek additional expertise. This decision is often a difficult one, because transferring a child to a tertiary care facility often means considerable hardship for the family. It is helpful for physicians in smaller hospitals to develop clear transfer guidelines to assist in these difficult decisions. Even when such guidelines exist, each case must be considered carefully.

The physician contacts the pediatric emergency physician at the referral hospital who suggests that you obtain another arterial blood gas.

Blood gases are again obtained; the values are

PaO_2	94
$PaCO_2$	38
pH	7.40

Agnes's respiratory rate is 36, and her pulse is now 140. She appears a little more comfortable and takes a sip of apple juice. You find an orange popsicle to give her, and her eyes light up. She licks it slowly, holding her mother's hand.

Because Agnes has continued to improve in your emergency department she will not need to be transferred to a higher level of care. She is admitted to the pediatric unit in your hospital, and during your lunch break, you go to visit her. Mrs. Kobuk and Agnes's sister are there, and Mrs. Kobuk is reading them a story. Agnes looks sleepy as she sits on her mother's lap (see Figure 2.6) and no longer has the anxious look of a child in respiratory distress. After about 4 hours on aminophylline, she is resting comfortably on 3 to 4 L of oxygen by nasal cannula, with oxygen saturations of 94%. Mrs. Kobuk tells you what a relief it is to see Agnes looking so much better.

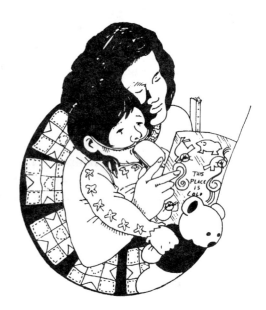

FIGURE 2.6

REFERENCES

Case Study 1

1. Kelley, S. (1988). *Pediatric emergency nursing.* Norwalk, CT: Appleton & Lange.
2. Hazinski, M. (1984). *Nursing care of the critically ill child.* St. Louis: Mosby.
3. Whaley, L., & Wong, D. (1987). *Nursing care of infants and children* (3rd ed.). St. Louis: Mosby.
4. American Academy of Pediatrics and American College of Emergency Physicians (1989). *Pediatric advanced life support.* Elk Grove Village, IL, & Dallas, TX: Authors.
5. Spy, R., & Preach, M. (1990). Pulse oximetry: Understanding the concept, knowing the limits. *RN, 53,* 38–45.
6. Gilboy, N.S., & McGaffegan, P.A. (1989). Noninvasive monitoring of oxygenation with pulse oximetry. *Journal of Emergency Nursing, 15,* 26–31.

Case Study 2

1. Bolte, R. (1986). Nebulized beta-adrenergic agents in the treatment of pediatric asthma. *Pediatric Emergency Care, 2,* 250–253.

2. Chameides, L. (Ed.) (1988). *Textbook of pediatric advanced life support.* Dallas: American Heart Association.

3. Stemple, A., & Mellon, M. (1984). Management of acute, severe asthma. *Pediatric Clinics of North America, 31*, 879–889.

4. Luten, R. (1988). *Problems in pediatric emergency medicine.* New York: Churchill Livingstone.

5. Yamamoto, L., Yim, G., & Britten, A. (1990). Rapid sequence anesthesia induction for emergency intubation. *Pediatric Emergency Care, 6*, 200–213.

6. American Academy of Pediatrics and American College of Emergency Physicians (1989). *Pediatric advanced life support.* Elk Grove Village, IL, & Dallas, TX: Authors.

Chapter Three

Cardiovascular Assessment and Intervention

Prerequisite Skills

Before beginning this chapter, the learner should

Appreciate the differences in cardiovascular hemodynamics between children and adults

Be able to identify major anatomic structures relating to the circulatory system:

- Heart
- Great vessels
- Structures of microcirculation

Be able to describe the following normal physiology:

- Normal sympathetic nervous system response to stress
- Effect of catecholamines on the cardiovascular system
- Anaerobic versus aerobic metabolism

Be able to identify the following physical assessments and parameters:

- Normal variations in skin color, temperature, and turgor
- Normal adult breath sounds
- Normal adult heart sounds
- Normal values for arterial blood gases, complete blood count, coagulation profile, urinalysis, electrolytes, serum glucose, and blood urea nitrogen
- Recognition of adult cardiac rhythms and rhythm disturbances seen in lead II

PREVIEW

The cardiovascular system of the newborn undergoes tremendous changes in a short period. The change from maternal circulation to independent circulation is such a profound change that it seems incredible that neonatal circulatory problems are relatively rare. Despite these amazing changes, the cardiovascular function in the pediatric patient becomes very similar to that of an adult within a few weeks of birth. It is important, however, to be aware of some of the significant differences between children and adults. Keep some of these differences in mind as you progress through this module:

1. Cardiopulmonary arrest is not a sudden event in infants and children, but is most often a result of respiratory failure or volume deficits rather than primary cardiac dysfunction.

2. Cardiopulmonary arrest can often be prevented if the symptoms of impending respiratory failure or shock are recognized immediately and promptly and appropriately treated.[1]

3. Once cardiopulmonary arrest occurs, the outcome of resuscitative attempts is very poor. Respiratory arrest is associated with better survival than cardiac arrest.[1]

These facts emphasize that prompt recognition and rapid intervention are necessary to save the lives of children. When a child with a life-threatening injury arrives in the emergency department, careful triage and accurate assessment will identify those pediatric patients needing special care. Airway and breathing are always the first concern; however, cardiovascular assessment is also essential, and the early recognition of compensated shock can be life saving. In addition, continued reassessment and rapid intervention when needed are crucial to improve outcomes for pedatric patients.

CASE STUDY 1 OBJECTIVES

On completion of this case study, you will be able to

- Identify the normal parameters for pulse, respiratory rate, and blood pressure, urine output, and capillary refill in various pediatric age groups and recognize the importance of monitoring trends

- Identify the clinical manifestations of shock in pediatric patients

- Recognize the components of cardiac output and describe the relationship to perfusion and blood pressure

- Identify, in order, the immediate priorities of care for the pediatric patient in shock

- Calculate appropriate volume replacement and route of administration for a pediatric patient showing signs of compensated shock

- Identify the clinical parameters associated with continuous reevaluation of the cardiovascular system and outcomes of treatment interventions

CASE STUDY 1

Freddie Needs to Be Seen Right Away!

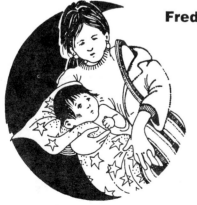

FIGURE 3.1

Freddie Valdez, a 14-month-old male child, is brought into your emergency department late at night by his mother. Mrs. Valdez rushes in with him and tells you in a panicked voice that her son needs to be seen right away. She says he has been having diarrhea for the last 48 hours. She tried giving him apple juice and then tried a cola drink, but he has not been taking either one for the last few hours. You see a very tired-looking, frantic young mother holding a pale toddler in her arms. He is crying weakly, and his lips look dry and wrinkled. She tearfully tells you she and Freddie have not slept in the last 48 hours, and she is very worried about him (see Figure 3.1).

TRIAGE DECISION

On the basis of your initial rapid assessment, this patient should be triaged as

Emergent. A life-threatening situation in need of immediate intervention.

Urgent. Patient needs care within 1 hour to prevent further deterioration.

Nonurgent. Patient is able to wait more than 1 hour without further deterioration.

TRIAGE DECISION ANSWER

You would consider Freddie's condition to be emergent. Your rapid assessment of Freddie's condition took less than 30 seconds. You noted he was crying, moving air well, but he is pale and breathing rapidly. His skin is very warm and dry, and his diaper is dry. You decide he needs immediate care to prevent further deterioration in his condition.

A quick look at Freddie told you that he was very ill. This ability to assess the sick quickly, differentiating between a very ill child and a child who needs less urgent care often comes with experience, but it is often helpful to ask yourself what specific indications contribute to this first impression.

Question

What were the indications that Freddie needed rapid intervention?

1. _____

2. _____

3. _____

Answer

Any of these are correct:

- Pale skin color
- Dry mucous membranes
- Weak cry
- History of 48 hours of diarrhea and lack of fluid
- Mrs. Valdez's panicky behavior

You cannot always be sure that a caretaker's anxiety is directly related to the condition of the child, but in most cases these concerns should be taken seriously—usually the child is very ill.

You bring Freddie in right away and place him on a gurney. Because you are very concerned that you will have to perform invasive procedures, you ask Mrs. Valdez to wait outside momentarily. You assess his *ABCs* to determine his immediate needs and page the emergency physician; he is attending to a patient in the intensive care unit and will be coming down as soon as possible. Because you are concerned about Freddie, you prioritize your interventions.

Question

What is your first priority at this time? (Choose one answer.)

1. Complete your assessment: obtain full vital signs, capillary refill and neurologic status.
2. Start an IV and give him a fluid bolus.
3. Make sure his airway is clear, and give him oxygen.
4. Place him on a cardiac monitor.

Answer

The first priority is *always* assuring an open airway, ventilation, and oxygenation. Whether Freddie is progressing in the downward spiral toward shock, or is actually in shock already, you can assume that his tissues are not receiving adequate oxygen. Whatever the *cause* of his illness, his airway should be assured, and oxygen should be given to increase end-organ perfusion.

You will need to complete his assessment, but his pale skin and history are sufficient evidence for you to intervene immediately. Becuase he is probably hypovolemic, he may require a fluid bolus, but this is not the first priority. Placing him on a cardiac monitor will provide additional information, but this also is not a priority right now.

Note: Oxygen should never be withheld during a pediatric emergency. The highest concentration of oxygen available should always be used until the child is stabilized.[1]

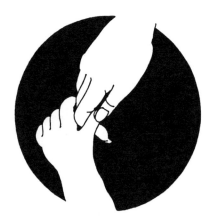

FIGURE 3.2

As you continue to assess the *ABC*s, you note that he is moving air well, although his respiratory rate is rapid. Listening to his anterior and posterior chest and in the mid-axillary lines you hear no unusual breath sounds. The emergency physician arrives, and after a brief look at Freddie, he goes to the waiting room to obtain Mrs. Valdez's history of Freddie's illness. You give Freddie oxygen by mask at 10 L/min and continue your assessment. He does not resist the mask and only cries a little as you reposition him. His heart rate is rapid, and his pedal pulses feel weaker than his radial pulses. You assess Freddie's perfusion status by elevating his hand above the level of his heart and measuring capillary refill in the nail bed of his thumb (see Figure 3.2).

Question

What are two other locations you could use to assess capillary refill in a pediatric patient lying supine on a gurney? (Fill in the blanks.)

1. _____

2. _____

Answer

You can assess capillary refill in any location where you can see the skin blanch as you press on it. Assessment of capillary refill requires compression of tissue against a resistant surface: the nail beds of the hands or feet, the earlobe, gums, forehead, and over the patella are all good locations. After 2 seconds of compression, release pressure and count the seconds until the skin turns pink again.

Elevation above the level of the heart assures that reperfusion is caused by the circulatory system rather than the force of gravity. Also remember that in trauma patients, capillary refill time should be assessed in an uninjured portion of the body, unless you are purposely assessing the circulation only to the injured area.

Freddie's capillary refill time is slightly longer than normal: 3 seconds. Before you assume that the prolonged time is due to hypovolemia, you consider what other factors might be causing this delay in reperfusion.

Question

Which of the following factors, besides fluid volume deficit, might affect capillary refill time? (Choose all that apply.)

1. Body temperature
2. Medication
3. Skin color
4. Age
5. Anxiety

Answer

The correct answers are (1) and (2). A child with a low body temperature may have a slower capillary refill time, as will a child taking any type of medication that causes vasoconstriction. The patient's skin color does not affect the time required for the capillaries to refill. Age has not been shown to alter the length of capillary refill time. Anxiety may have an effect by causing some vasoconstriction, but there is no available research documenting this effect.

Note: If a patient has a very dark skin color, you should choose a location where pigmentation is light for a good assessment of capillary refill—fingertips and mucous membranes would be good choices.

You complete your assessment of Freddie's *ABC*s by assessing his neurologic status. Freddie cries, but his cry is not vigorous, and he responds, although weakly, to loud verbal stimuli by turning his head toward the sound. You undress him to see if there are any injuries contributing to his condition and find no signs of injury. He does not appear to be hypothermic, and because he has a history of dehydration, you attribute Freddie's prolonged capillary refill time to possible fluid volume deficit. You use this as your nursing diagnosis.

You elevate his legs on a pillow to help improve perfusion. Freddie will probably need intravenous fluid or medication for his fluid volume deficit, so you begin to gather the equipment for insertion of an IV, and you ask your nurse-colleague to continue taking Freddie's vital signs. The vital signs he obtains are

Heart rate	165 beats/min
Respiratory rate	34 breaths/min
Blood pressure	No pediatric cuff available
Temperature	38.2°C (100.8°F)

Questions

Circle one answer for each question.

    1. Is Freddie's heart rate within normal limits for his age?

        1.   Yes   2.   No

    2. Is Freddie's respiratory rate within normal limits for his age?

        1.   Yes   2.   No

Answers

The answers are No for both questions. Both Freddie's heart rate and respiratory rate are fast for his age. Although tachycardia may be associated with less life-threatening conditions such as pain, fever, or anxiety, it is also a sensitive indicator of circulatory compromise and may be an indicator of a serious problem.[1] In this case, Freddie's heart rate is well above the normal range, so the possible causes for this elevation should be explored. His respiratory rate is also slightly more rapid than normal and is cause for concern. (See Vital Signs Chart, Table 1.4, in Chapter 1.)

    The emergency physician returns and asks you to start an IV and obtain blood for laboratory tests: glucose, electrolytes, complete blood count, creatinine, blood urea nitrogen, blood cultures, and urinalysis. A respiratory therapist is called to draw blood for blood gas analysis. The house supervisor is trying to locate a child-sized blood pressure cuff so you can obtain a blood pressure reading. Before attempting the IV you make sure your initial impression that Freddie is not perfusing adequately is correct.

Question

What are three ways you can assess end-organ perfusion?

    1. _____

    2. _____

    3. _____

Answer

Any of the means listed in Table 3.1 can be used to assess end-organ perfusion.

    You review Freddie's assessment to determine the seriousness of his condition. He has the following:

1. Tachycardia
2. Pale skin color
3. Dry mucous membranes
4. Difference in strength and quality of pulses
5. Capillary refill > 2 seconds

You compare Freddie's signs with the classifications of the stages of shock in the pediatric patient (Table 3.2). Early recognition of and intervention for shock is important.

TABLE 3.1. Assessment of End-Organ Perfusion

End-organ perfusion can be evaluated best in	
Skin	
Capillary refill time	Capillary refill time is normally < 2 s, and prolongation is a sensitive and early indicator.
	Note: Refill time may be prolonged by hypothermia.
Comparative pulses	Comparing proximal and distal pulses gives a qualitative assessment of perfusion status.
Skin temperature and color	Compromised perfusion may produce color or temperature variation in extremities.
	• Mottling, pallor, and peripheral cyanosis indicate poor skin perfusion.
	• Gray or ashen color in newborns and pallor in older groups indicate severe vasoconstriction and poor perfusion.
Brain	
Alteration in mental status	Lack of adequate perfusion to the brain produces changes in mental status and is therefore a valuable indicator of cerebral hypoxia or ischemia in infants and young children. This can be recognized by
	• A parent's statement that the child is "not acting normally."
	• A child's failure to recognize caretakers.
Kidneys	
Urine output	At least 1 mL/kg/hr indicates adequate kidney function
	A child should have at least one wet diaper every 4 hr and an infant one wet diaper every 2 hr

TABLE 3.2. Classifications of Shock

Compensated shock	Increase in heart rate
	Skin mottling or pallor, but with continued perfusion
	Normal or near-normal blood pressure
	Increased respiratory rate
Decompensated shock	Impaired or compromised end-organ perfusion
Irreversible shock	This diagnosis is retroactive, and means that the processes resulting in and from inadequate tissue perfusion could not be reversed; irreversible shock, by definition, results in death of the patient

---

Question

The clinical signs you have observed indicate that Freddie is in what type of shock? (Choose one answer.)

1. Compensated shock   2. Decompensated shock   3. Irreversible shock

Answer

Freddie is definitely showing the signs of compensated shock. He is compensating for fluid deficit right now by increased heart rate and peripheral vasoconstriction, but his condition could deteriorate rapidly without intervention. Recognition of and intervention in the early stages of shock in children (compensated shock) are essential; once the child is no longer able to compensate, decompensated shock and irreversible shock may develop.[1]

Note: Assessment of end-organ perfusion (skin signs, capillary refill, mental status) is the best way to recognize impending or early shock in children. Hypotension is a very late sign of shock in the pediatric age group.

As you get the equipment together for Freddie's intravenous line, you prioritize interventions for Freddie, because he is in compensated shock.

Question

After review of your clinical findings you decide your next intervention should be: (Choose one answer.)

1. To begin rehydration by giving Freddie some fluid by mouth
2. To increase Freddie's oxygen flow rate
3. To obtain intravenous access and give Freddie a fluid bolus
4. To insert a urinary catheter to determine urinary output

Answer

Freddie's immediate problem is impaired perfusion secondary to volume loss from diarrhea. His most pressing need is fluid replacement. Oral rehydration would not be effective at this point, as he is likely to vomit. Answer (2) is not correct at this point, as his oxygen flow rate is already high. It is important to determine urinary output, but improving his fluid volume is the priority at this point.

You attempt to start an IV in Freddie's left hand, and the emergency physician attempts a line in the right antecubital vein. Because his hand veins are not immediately visible and he is not moving around, you do not tape his hand to the arm board before attempting IV cannulation (see Figure 3.3, facing page).[2]

Both you and the emergency physician are unsuccessful in starting IVs. You stop and take a deep breath. Before attempting another peripheral line, the two of you discuss how to obtain intravenous access.

Question

Which one of the following would be the most rapid and useful method of obtaining intravenous access at this point? (Choose one answer.)

1. Intraosseous catheterization
2. Subclavian catheterization
3. Scalp vein cannulation
4. Femoral vein catheterization

Answer

Intraosseous catheterization would be the best choice. Freddie needs a route for administering fluid established rapidly. In a child younger than 6 years of age, failure to obtain peripheral intravenous access is an indication for intraosseous catheterization. Intraosseous placement is both rapid and safe.[3-6]

Insertion of a subclavian catheter may be useful for older children, but it carries a higher risk of pneumothorax in the pediatric age group. Scalp vein cannulation is most useful for infants (younger than 1 year). Figure 3.4 shows sites for scalp vein cannulation.

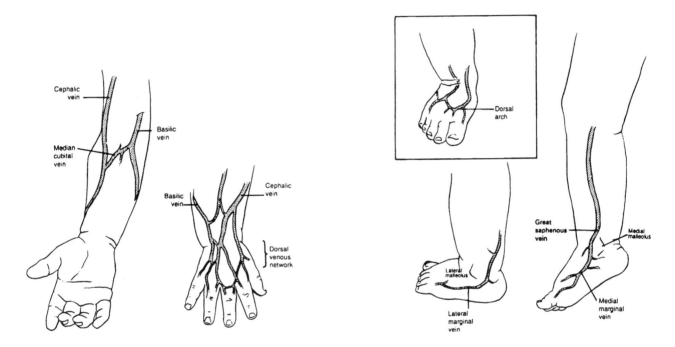

FIGURE 3.3   Locations for venous access. (Courtesy of Utah EMSC Project.)

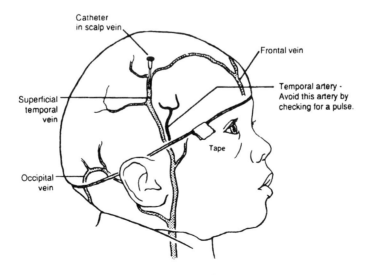

FIGURE 3.4   Scalp vein cannnulation. (Courtesy of Utah EMSC Project.)

Femoral vein catheterization or saphenous vein cutdown are reliable but time-consuming procedures. If immediate access is required, fluid or medications may be given by intraosseous infusion until another more lengthy procedure is completed.

> *Note:* Research has demonstrated that vascular access is obtained more rapidly when a protocol is used.[7] Each emergency department should have clear guidelines for rapid establishment of a route for administering fluid and medication.

INTRAVENOUS ACCESS PROTOCOL

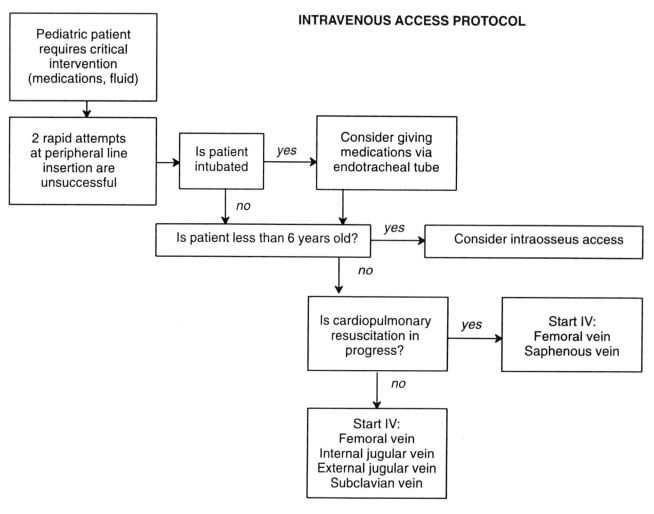

The house supervisor brings a neonatal blood pressure cuff but is still unable to locate a child-sized cuff. However, the neonatal cuff does reach around Freddie's arm, and the other nurse tells you that Freddie's blood pressure is within normal limits: 88/62.

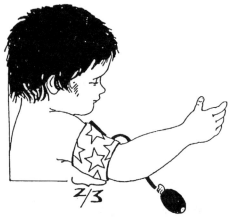

FIGURE 3.5. Freddie wearing a properly sized blood-pressure cuff.

Question

You consider this blood pressure reading to be: (Choose one answer.)

1. About equal to the reading taken with a cuff appropriate for his size.
2. Lower than you would obtain with a cuff appropriate for his size.
3. Higher than you would obtain with a cuff appropriate for his size.

Answer

The correct answer is (3). Using too narrow a cuff for a child's size gives a falsely *elevated* blood-pressure reading.[8]

Note: A correctly sized cuff should have a width equal to about two-thirds the length of the child's arm from shoulder to elbow. Another way of conceptualizing the correct size is that it should be about 20% greater than the diameter of the child's arm.[8]

Freddie has now been in the emergency department for 10 minutes. You manage to find a child-sized cuff (see Figure 3.5) from another area in the hospital, and the blood pressure reading is 70/50; the difference between this pressure reading and the first one is due to the change in cuff size. Because a systolic blood pressure of more than 80 is the normal blood pressure for a child Freddie's age, you know that his systolic pressure is about 10 mmHg below normal.

Question

Is a blood pressure of 10 mmHg systolic below normal indicative of shock in a child? (Choose Yes or No.)

1. Yes   2. No

Answer

Yes. Even a slight drop in blood pressure can be a very ominous sign in children. Children can lose 25% to 50% of their blood volume and still maintain a normal blood pressure through compensatory mechanisms such as increasing peripheral vascular resistance, increasing heart rate, and shifting cardiac output to vital organs.[1] Any drop in blood pressure indicates depletion of all compensatory resources.

Although children have the same per kilogram amount of blood as adults—80 mL/kg, it is important to remember that because of their size, young children have a much smaller *total* blood volume. The loss of the same amount of fluid as an adult therefore represents a much larger *percentage* of a child's total volume (Figure 3.6).[9]

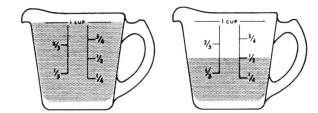

FIGURE 3.6 One-and-one-half cups—one half of an 9-kg child's total blood volume.

Because you may be giving fluid or medication, you estimate Freddie's weight to be about 11 kg. The family's pediatrician has been called and is in the hospital; she will be coming down immediately. The emergency physician briefly considers waiting for her to do a cutdown, but decides instead to go ahead with the intraosseous line to give Freddie some fluid. You prepare the equipment and review the procedure (see Figures 3.7 and 3.8).

TABLE 3.3. Intraosseous Infusion Procedure[3–6]

1. Determine location for infusion, usually the proximal tibia, but the distal femur is also used.

2. Stabilize the child's leg with the knee slightly bent. A sandbag or rolled towel under the leg may be helpful in maintaining this position.

3. Select insertion site for the needle:
   - *Proximal tibia:* The midline of the medial flat surface of the anterior tibia, approximately 1 inch below the tibial tuberosity (depending on the size of the child).
   - *Distal femur:* Midline, 2–3 cm above the external condyles.

4. Prepare site for the procedure by cleaning with iodine or alcohol.

5. Begin inserting needle using a back and forth screwing motion:
   - *Proximal tibia:* The needle should be inserted at an angle of 60°–90° *away from growth plate*.
   - *Distal femur:* After penetrating the skin, the needle should be angled toward the head at slightly less than a right angle (75°– 80°) to the leg.[10]

6. Successful insertion may initially be confirmed by the lowered resistance on penetration into the marrow.

7. When a bone marrow, intraosseous infusion, or spinal needle is used, the trocar or stylet should be removed once the needle is situated in the bone marrow.

8. Bone marrow may be aspirated for confirmation. The aspirated marrow may be used for laboratory analysis.

9. The needle may be flushed with heparinized normal saline solution to prevent clotting before attaching it to IV tubing.

10. Further stabilization may be provided by taping the flanges of the intraosseous needle to the leg. Bone marrow and spinal needles rely on the bone for stabilization.

11. Continue to observe the insertion site for extravasation and watch for dislodgement of the needle.

12. When the intraosseous needle is removed, a sterile dressing should be placed over the insertion site and pressure applied for about five minutes.

Note: If intraosseous needles are not available, a spinal needle or bone marrow needle may be used as a substitute. Intraosseous needles only come in one size.

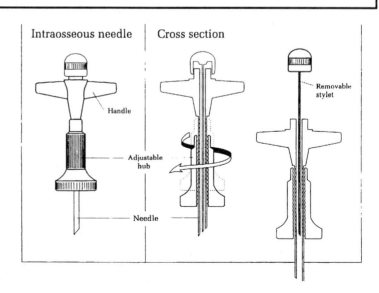

FIGURE 3.7 Intraosseous needle.

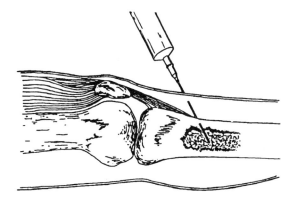

FIGURE 3.8   Intraosseus needle insertion.

Note: If intraosseous needles are not available, a spinal needle or bone marrow needle may be used as a substitute. Intraosseous needles only come in one size.

You aspirate 8 mL of bone marrow and begin a crystalloid infusion through the intraosseous needle using lactated Ringer's solution.

Question

The laboratory technologist asks you whether the marrow withdrawn in this procedure can be used for the laboratory analyses the physician has ordered. What is the answer to this question? (Choose one answer.)

1. Most laboratory studies can be performed on bone marrow.
2. Only hemoglobin and blood gas analyses can be performed on bone marrow.
3. No analyses can be performed on bone marrow.

Answer

Most laboratory studies can be performed on aspirated bone marrow. The aspirated bone marrow may be used for electrolytes, blood chemistries, $PaCO_2$, and hemoglobin.[11] Although this method may not be ideal, it is a rapid method for obtaining results and the results for the tests listed are comparable with results of analyses of venous or arterial blood. The results of blood gas analyses run on bone marrow, fall between arterial and venous results, and are therefore less useful than arterial blood gases.

The site of the intraosseous needle insertion shows no signs of extravasation, and the fluid is flowing well. Based on your estimation that Freddie weighs 11 kg, you calculate the amount of fluid Freddie should be given.

Question

How much fluid should be given for Freddie's first bolus? (Choose one answer.)

1. 300 mL   3. 220 mL
2. 550 mL   4. 440 mL

Answer

The answer is 220 mL. For pediatric patients, fluid boluses are calculated on a per-kilogram basis. A standard bolus is 20 mL/kg, so because Freddie weighs about 11 kg, the correct amount would be $11 \times 20 = 220$ mL.

You begin giving Freddie his first bolus over a 3- to 5-minute period and then reassess Freddie. Freddie's latest vital signs are

Heart rate	175 beats/min
Respiratory rate	30 breaths/min
Blood pressure	76/52
Capillary refill time	3 s

Question

When you complete the fluid bolus, what additional assessment should you make? (Fill in the blank.)

_____

Answer

The correct answer is assessment of Freddie's breath and heart sounds. This is an important assessment to make sure he is absorbing the fluid well and not experiencing fluid overload. Freddie's chest should be clear with no abnormal heart sounds; if you hear rales or abnormal heart sounds, Freddie may have been given too much fluid, and the flow of IV fluid should be slowed to a minimal rate while further assessment is made. Most children can tolerate one fluid bolus without ill effects, and Freddie is probably hypovolemic, so you would not expect fluid overload at this point.

Freddie's lungs are clear, and his heart sounds are normal. The unit secretary comes in to tell you that Freddie's mother is asking about him. You ask her to tell Mrs. Valdez that Freddie's condition is remaining the same and that you will be out to talk with her within the next 5 minutes.

Question

What would the most likely next intervention for Freddie? (Choose one answer.)

1. Change his IV to maintenance rate.
2. Change his intravenous fluid to 5% dextrose-1/2 normal saline.
3. Give him another 20 mL/kg fluid bolus.
4. Use a dopamine drip to increase his blood pressure.

Answer

Give Freddie another 20 mL/kg fluid bolus. He should have another 20 mL/kg bolus of isotonic crystalloid (normal saline or lactated Ringer's) to improve his perfusion status. He is still showing some signs of fluid deficit, so he will need more than a minimal rate, and dopamine is not indicated when hypovolemia is suspected—it definitely is not indicated at this time.

Reassess breath and heart sounds after each intervention (especially fluid boluses) to prevent or minimize risk of fluid overload. At the first sign of moist respirations, fluid bolus administration should be discontinued.

After the second bolus is started you go to the waiting room to talk with Mrs. Valdez. You briefly describe the procedures you are doing, tell her that Freddie's condition has improved slightly, and assure her that you are hoping (as you know she is, too), that his condition will continue to improve. You return to the treatment room.

Freddie has now been given two bolus doses of 20 mL/kg of lactated Ringer's, for a total of 440 mL. You reassess Freddie.

Heart rate	148 beats/ min
Respiratory rate	30 breaths/min
Blood pressure	78/54
Capillary refill time	2+ s

His chest remains clear, and you do not hear any abnormal heart sounds.

Question

At this time the next intervention should probably be to: (Choose one answer.)

1. Administer another bolus of intravenous fluid.
2. Start a dopamine drip.
3. Give him packed red blood cells.
4. Begin maintenance fluids.

Answer

Administer another bolus of intravenous fluid. The most common error in treating hypovolemic shock in children is not providing adequate volume replacement.[1] Freddie's blood pressure is now closer to normal, but he could probably benefit from one more fluid bolus. Vasopressor agents such as dopamine are contraindicated in hypovolemic shock. Blood products should be administered for traumatic shock or when based on specific laboratory data indicating their use.[1]

Now that Freddie's condition is improving, it will be easier to insert an IV line in a peripheral site. The intraosseous line is at best a temporary measure. You gather your supplies and examine his hand for a good site. You decide to immobilize his hand with an armboard and tape before insertion, because the veins now seem very accessible.

Question

Which of the following would you use to start to start an IV line? (Choose one answer.)

1. 24-gauge over-the-needle catheter
2. 16-gauge over-the-needle catheter
3. 25-gauge butterfly
4. 20-gauge over-the-needle catheter

Answer

A 20-gauge over-the-needle catheter would be approximately the correct size for a 14-month-old, 11-kg child, although an 18-gauge over-the-needle catheter could also be used if his veins seem large enough. A 16-gauge catheter would probably be too large for most children this age. Clinicians who rarely care for pediatric patients tend to choose smaller needles than necessary, and some might choose a 22-gauge over-the-needle catheter. Each decrease in diameter of the catheter, however, increases the resistance and slows the flow of the fluid, so the largest needle possible is the best choice. Butterfly needles are not recommended in the emergency setting except to draw blood, because they tend to infiltrate. Other needle sizes are listed in Table 3.4.

TABLE 3.4. Equipment for Venous Cannulation[1]

Age (years)	Weight (kg)	Over-the-needle catheters (gauge)
<1	<10	20, 22, 24
1–12	10–40	16, 18, 20
>12	>40	14, 16, 18

You reassess Freddie.

Heart rate	140 beats/min
Respiratory rate	30 breaths/min
Blood pressure	82/62 mmHg
Capillary refill time	2 s

Freddie's skin color is still pale, but Freddie is now crying more vigorously and fighting the oxygen mask. His peripheral pulses are stronger, as are his central pulses. A maintenance fluid infusion is ordered. You look up at the pediatric maintenance fluid chart on the wall of the treatment room (see Table 3.5).

TABLE 3.5. Maintenance Fluid Requirements[12,13]

Weight	Fluid requirement
For the *first* 0–10 kg	Calculate 100 mL/kg/24 hr Example: 10-kg child = 10 × 100 = 1,000 mL/24 hr = 42 mL/hr
For *each* kg over 10 and up to 20	Start with 1,000 and add 50 mL/kg/24 hr for each kg over 10 kg Example: 15-kg child = 1,000 for 10 kg, *plus* (5 × 50) for kg over 10 = 1,250 mL/24 hr = 52 mL/hr
For *each* kg over 20 and up to 50	Start with 1,500 and add 20 mL/kg for each kg over 20 kg Example: 23-kg child = 1,000 + (10 × 50) = 1,500 for first 20 kg, *plus* (3 × 20) for kg over 20 = 1,560 mL/24 hr = 65 mL/hr

---

Question

At *about* what rate would you expect to set the intravenous flow rate for Freddie's maintenance requirements? (Choose one answer.)

1. 44 mL/hr
2. 110 mL/hr
3. 25 mL/hr
4. 66 mL/hr

Answer

The correct answer is 44 mL/hr. Based on Freddie's weight of 11 kg, maintenance fluid administration would be 1,050 mL over 24 hours, or 44 mL/hr.

Calculation:

1. 10 kg × 100 mL = 1000 mL
2. Add 50 mL/kg for each kg over 10 kg: 1,000 + 50 = 1,050 mL
3. Divide by 24 hr: 1,050/24 = 43.75 mL/hr

You comfort Freddie by talking to him and giving him a small soft toy, and you consider what additional interventions may be needed for him.

Question

Based on your nursing diagnosis of Freddie, which of the following interventions are indicated at this time? (Place an **X** next to each selection.)

_____ Insert a urinary catheter

_____ Oral hydration

_____ Parental involvement

_____ Reevaluation and monitoring of the patient

_____ Repeat vital signs

_____ Weigh patient

Answer

X Insert a urinary catheter

___ Oral hydration

X Parental involvement

X Reevaluation and monitoring of the patient

X Repeat vital signs

X Weigh patient

Oral hydration could increase Freddie's gastrointestinal distress and would not be advisable at this point. The most essential nursing interventions for Freddie are to continue evaluation and maintain cardiovascular perfusion. Repeating vital signs, assessing urinary output, and weighing the patient would be useful. Insertion of a urinary catheter will help to monitor kidney function, a measure of end-organ perfusion. Obtaining an accurate weight will allow monitoring his progress and provision of appropriate dosages of medications. Parental involvement should begin as soon as the patient becomes more responsive. Parental presence plays an important role in the comfort of pediatric patients.

You insert the urinary catheter and measure the initial output: 10 mL of clear, dark yellow urine. You go to the waiting room and ask Mrs. Valdez to come in and stay with Freddie, explaining the various tubes to her. She says Freddie seems "more awake" to her now. Although some physicians might decide to perform a full septic workup for this patient, including a chest X-ray film and a lumbar puncture, the emergency department physician has decided that this will not be necessary in this case. He has diagnosed Freddie with severe viral gastroenteritis and is admitting him to the hospital for further treatment and observation.

Nurses should always teach parents about how to start oral rehydration when a patient with a history of diarrhea is discharged. Although Freddie is being admitted, some of this teaching could be initiated in the emergency department once Freddie is stable. In a less severe case of dehydration, parental teaching of oral rehydration is especially important before discharge to parents' care. Basic elements for parental teaching are included in Table 3.6.

TABLE 3.6. AAP Oral Rehydration Recommendations[14]

Glucose-electrolyte solutions (Rehydrite, Pedialyte, Lytren, Resol) are used for rehydration and maintenance therapy.

Rehydration fluids can be used in combination with water, breast milk or low-carbohydrate juice.

Feeding should be reintroduced in the first 24 hours of the episode.

Initial foods include

- *Infants*. Breast milk, diluted formula, or milk
- *Older infants and children*. Rice cereal, bananas, potatoes, other nonlactose carbohydrate-rich foods

The recommendations listed in Table 3.6 are based on studies of thousands of cases and hundreds of clinical trials. Oral rehydration therapy can help to speed recovery, and improve nutritional outcomes.[14]

As you wait for Freddie's transport to the pediatric ward, you explain some of the signs of dehydration (see Table 3.7) to watch for in children to Mrs. Valdez, and she asks you many questions.

TABLE 3.7. Warning Signs of Dehydration

Decreased desire to take fluids

Increase in frequency and amount of vomiting or diarrhea

Changes in skin color and temperature

Changes in behavior pattern:

- Increased irritability
- Failure to recognize parents

Absence of tears

Mrs. Valdez is relieved to see that Freddie is better, and she appears much calmer than earlier, stroking his head and talking to him softly. The floor nurse comes down to take Freddie upstairs, and Mrs. Valdez thanks you and the emergency physician. She also apologizes for rushing into the emergency department and making such a fuss. You reassure her that her behavior was appropriate—she had reason for concern, and she did the right thing by coming in to have Freddie treated.

CASE STUDY 2 OBJECTIVES

On completion of this case study, you will be able to

- Recognize the characteristics of supraventricular tachycardia (SVT) on a rhythm strip
- Identify the recommended treatment for an unstable patient with SVT
- Prioritize interventions for an unstable pediatric patient with a fast rhythm disturbance
- Explain the use of electrical shock for treatment of cardiac rhythm disturbances to an anxious parent

CASE STUDY 2

Andy's Pulse Is Too Fast to Count!

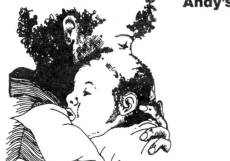

FIGURE 3.9

Andy Hawkins is a 6-week-old African-American male infant brought to your emergency department by his mother at 3:00 P.M. on a weekday afternoon. Andy's mother says that he has been acting strangely, he doesn't seem to be hungry, and he is breathing harder than normal. You see immediately that he has a very fast respiratory rate. His pulse feels weak and is too fast to count. His hands feel cool to touch, and his color is mottled. He responds to painful stimuli with whimpers (see Figure 3.9).

TRIAGE DECISION

On the basis of your initial rapid assessment, this patient should be triaged as

Emergent. A life-threatening situation in need of immediate intervention.

Urgent. Patient needs care within 1 hour to prevent further deterioration.

Nonurgent. Patient is able to wait more than 1 hour without further deterioration.

TRIAGE DECISION ANSWER

This is definitely an emergency. Andy definitely does not look well to you, and you suspect that his condition at this point is critical. Your assessment is based on Andy's young age, his mother's report of his behavior, very rapid heart rate, rapid respiratory rate, mottled coloring, and his mental status.[1]

Although there are no beds available in the emergency department right now, you quickly take Andy and his mother into the treatment room, moving a patient with a finger laceration to a chair in the holding room. You quickly remove his sleeper. Having rapidly assessed his *ABC*s, your initial nursing diagnosis is decreased tissue perfusion related to cardiac rate and rhythm.[2] You immediately place Andy in the sniffing position, give him oxygen by face mask at 10 L/min, and make sure he is kept warm. The emergency department clerk asks Mrs. Hawkins to step outside to give her some information. As she leaves, you place Andy on the cardiac monitor; his heart rate is 300 beats/min. Dr. Butler, the emergency physician, hurries in to examine Andy. Figure 3.10 shows Andy's cardiac rhythm strip at this point.

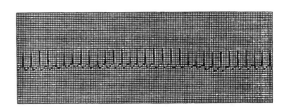

FIGURE 3.10 Andy's cardiac rhythm strip.

Question

Assessing Andy's rhythm strip, you strongly suspect that his cardiac rhythm is: (Choose one.)

1. Sinus tachycardia   2. Ventricular tachycardia   3. SVT

Answer

Because Andy has a rate of more than 220 beats/min with a narrow QRS configuration, you strongly suspect he is in SVT.[1] SVT is an abnormal cardiac rhythm, seen mainly in children. This rhythm disturbance results from the reentry of electrical impulses above the bifurcation of the bundle of His (see Figure 3.11).

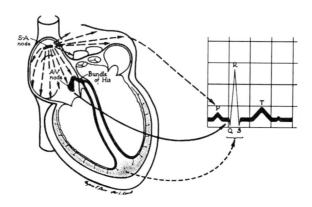

FIGURE 3.11   Heart.

The normal spread of the impulse across the ventricles accounts for the narrow configuration of the ventricular complex (QRS) (see Table 3.8).[3]

TABLE 3.8.   Rapid Heart Rates in Children[3]

	Sinus tachycardia	Supraventricular tachycardia	Ventricular tachycardia
Characteristic	Narrow QRS	Narrow QRS	Wide QRS
Heart rate	< 200/min	> 220/min	Normal to > 400
History	Volume depletion, anxiety, fever, blood loss	Nonspecific: irritability, pallor	Structural hypoxia, acidosis, poison
Physical examination	Consistent with dehydration, blood loss: pallor, poor skin turgor, dry mucous membranes, altered mental status, normal liver	Increased work of breathing, moist crackles, abnormal skin signs, altered mental status, enlarged liver	Dependent on cardiac output: patient may have poor perfusion, altered mental status
Electro-cardiogram	Rarely helpful	Rarely helpful unless wide complexes are evident	Helpful: may see wide complexes without apparent atrial conduction
Chest X-ray film	Normal heart, clear lungs	Enlarged heart, possible pulmonary edema	Depends on structural component

Andy's color is a little better now that he is receiving oxygen, but his rapid heart rate is continuing, and you know that he cannot remain stable with such a rapid rate. You decide to elevate his legs slightly with a towel to improve perfusion of his brain and vital organs.

Question

If Andy's cardiac rhythm is SVT, which answer would best explain why he is not perfusing adequately? (Choose one answer.)

1. Cardiac output of Andy's heart is increased because of his rapid heart rate.
2. Andy's rapid heart rate does not allow adequate filling of the heart and full contraction of the heart muscle.
3. The faulty reentry of the electrical impulse above the bundle of His prevents contraction of the ventricles.

Answer

The correct answer is (2). Cardiac output is the result of several interrelated factors, as shown in Figure 3.12.[4] Cardiac output is decreased rather than increased as a result of the rapid rate. The faulty pattern of electrical conduction does not prevent ventricular contraction; rather it causes the ventricles to contract too rapidly, shortening filling time and compromising cardiac output.[5]

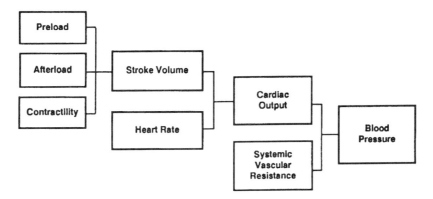

FIGURE 3.12   Factors affecting cardiac output and blood pressure.

Dr. Butler suggests replacement of the oxygen mask being used with a nonrebreathing mask to increase the oxygen concentration being delivered to Andy. She also starts an intraosseous infusion of normal saline to be able to give medications. The cardiac rhythm displayed on the monitor remains the same, and Andy's color improves only slightly. His capillary refill time is 3 seconds.

Realizing Andy's condition is unstable and he will need further critical intervention, you consider what the alternatives are.

Question

What is the standard treatment for a patient with SVT whose condition is unstable? (Choose one answer.)

1. Cardioversion   2. Valsalva's maneuvers   3. Intravenous verapamil

Answer

Because Andy is acutely unstable, he needs immediate intervention, so cardioversion is the best choice.[3] The usual treatment for an unstable patient with SVT is synchronized cardioversion. If a patient is tolerating the rapid rate, that is, if perfusion is adequate, Valsalva's maneuvers would be considered. The use of verapamil is not recommended in infancy because of reports of cardiovascular collapse.[3] Another alternative is adenosine, but because the use of adenosine is questionable in infants, cardioversion will be the most likely choice.

Note: The decision to cardiovert SVT as an emergency measure is based on a patient's ability to tolerate the rapid heart rate and maintain perfusion.[3]

Dr. Butler decides to cardiovert. You switch the defibrillator to synchronized mode and set the dosage. You estimate Andy's weight at 5 kg.[6]

Question

Because you have estimated Andy's weight at 5 kg, what would be the correct dosage for cardioversion in this case? (Choose one answer.)

1. 10–20 joules
2. 100–110 joules
3. 2.5–5 joules
4. 55–60 joules

Answer

Dosage for cardioversion in children is 0.5 to 1.0 joules/kg (5 kg × 0.5 or 1 joule = 2.5–5 joules).[3] This is given with pediatric paddles if available. If pediatric paddles are not available, the front-to-back position may be used (see Figure 3.13). With the child lying on his or her side, the paddles are placed anteriorly and posteriorly in such a way that the current generated by the defibrillator will pass through the heart.

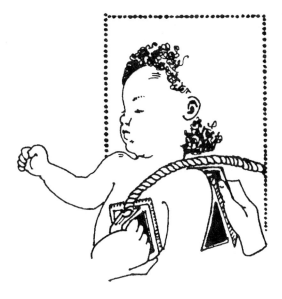

FIGURE 3.13 Front-to-back defibrillator position.

TABLE 3.9. Cardioversion[3]

Dose	Joules/Kg
Initial	0.5–1.0
Second	2.0
Note: Joules = Watts/Second.	

You reassess Andy's respiratory rate and heart rate. There is no change in either one or in Andy's general condition after synchronized cardioversion.

Question

The next intervention for Andy should be: (Choose one answer.)

1. Initiate pharmacologic agents
2. Cardioversion at 10 joules
3. Repeat cardioversion at 5 joules
4. Defibrillate at 5 joules

Answer

If SVT persists the dosage is increased to a maximum of 2 joules/kg. If cardioversion still does not convert, the diagnosis of SVT may be incorrect, and the rhythm may be a sinus tachycardia.

After the second synchronized cardioversion, Andy's cardiac rhythm immediately converts to sinus tachycardia. Your reassessment of his vital signs is

Heart rate	180 beats/min
Respiratory rate	50 breaths/min
Temperature	37.5°C (99.6°F), rectal
Capillary refill	< 2 s
Skin signs	Mottling has decreased

Andy is now crying more vigorously. His perfusion status has improved, and there is sufficient time to evaluate him thoroughly to determine the possible underlying cause of these events. Dr. Butler orders laboratory analyses and a portable chest X-ray film. She also telephones the on-call cardiologist. Andy's mother is brought into the room, and you obtain a history from her while Dr. Butler completes a detailed assessment on Andy. Dr. Butler explains to her what has been done for Andy.

Dr. Thomas, the cardiologist, arrives and evaluates Andy. He leaves to talk with Dr. Butler. Andy is fussing a little, and you suggest that Mrs. Hawkins hold him. You show her how to handle him with the oxygen mask and IV line. Andy calms down immediately. Mrs. Hawkins seems very upset, and wants more information about Andy's condition. She says that Dr. Butler told her that Andy was given an electrical shock to slow down his heart rate. She seems very concerned about this procedure.

Question

Mrs. Hawkins says that she is very worried that Andy will have to be given another shock if his heart starts beating rapidly again. You should tell her that: (Fill in the blanks.)

_____

_____

Answer

You should tell Mrs. Hawkins that you can understand her concern and explain to her that when cardioversion is used, the patient is only given a very small shock, much less than you would receive from touching an electrical outlet. Usually only one dose is needed, and if a patient's rhythm reverts to SVT after initial successful cardioversion, electrical shock is usually not repeated—medication is given to maintain control. If Andy's heart started beating rapidly again, medications would probably be used. The major concern in SVT is to determine and treat the underlying cause of the rapid rate, which may require extensive testing and possible surgical intervention.[7]

Dr. Thomas recommends immediate transfer to a pediatric specialty facility 20 miles from your location. Arrangements are made for Andy to be transported via an ambulance sent by the receiving hospital. Mrs. Hawkins seems a little overwhelmed, and you talk with her as you prepare Andy for transfer. The transport team arrives, and you give one of the attendants Andy's X-ray films, lab reports, and a copy of his chart with your nursing notes.

Mrs. Hawkins is permitted to remain with Andy during transport. As she gets into the ambulance, you reassure her that the facility Andy is being transferred to is well equipped to handle his special needs. The ambulance leaves, and you hope everything will turn out well for Andy.

CASE STUDY 3 OBJECTIVES

On completion of this case study, you will be able to

- Prioritize interventions for cardiopulmonary arrest in a pediatric patient.
- Identify the correct rate and depth of compression for cardiopulmonary resuscitation of a 2-year-old child.
- Identify the correct sequence of medications given in cardiopulmonary arrest.

CASE STUDY 3

Cindy Is Gasping for Breath!

You are the only nurse working with an emergency physician in a small community hospital. It is about 6 P.M. on a Friday evening, and you receive a call from Mrs. Lang who says her 2-year-old daughter Cindy has had a cold for several days. Mrs. Lang is very upset; she tells you that she saw her physician 2 days ago, and he prescribed medication for Cindy's cold. "I gave Cindy her medicine today and put her down for her nap. Now I can't get her to wake up and she's gasping for breath, what should I do?" You tell her to call 9-1-1 immediately, and you ask for her address and telephone number.

You hang up the telephone and call 9-1-1 yourself to make sure Mrs. Lang received assistance. It is now 6:05 P.M. You tell the emergency department physician about your conversation with Mrs. Lang.

At 6:20 P.M. the dispatcher contacts you to let you know that an ambulance is en route to your hospital with a 2-year-old female child in full arrest. Cardiopulmonary resuscitation is in progress and they should be there in 2 minutes.

At 6:22 P.M. the ambulance arrives. The emergency medical technicians are ventilating with a bag-valve-mask device with 100% oxygen, an oropharyngeal airway is in place, and cardiac compressions are creating a carotid pulse.

As the emergency medical technicians (EMTs) are placing Cindy on the bed, they tell you that Mrs. Lang says she has no known allergies. They show you the medication bottle Mrs. Lang gave them; the medication Cindy was taking was an antibiotic.

You realize Mrs. Lang has followed the EMTs into the room. As you show her to the waiting area, she tells you "I thought I did everything right—I was using a vaporizer, and taking her temperature, and she seemed to be getting better."

You tell her that you are sure she did her very best, and that you need to take care of Cindy, but that you will be back to talk to her as soon as you can. You return to the treatment room.

Question

In what order should the following procedures be performed? (Place a **1** next to the first priority procedure, a **2** next to the second, etc.)

____ Endotracheal intubation

____ Assessment of adequacy of ventilation

____ Placement of pulse oximeter

____ Insertion of an IV or intraosseous line

Answer

The answers are (3), (1), (2), and (4), respectively.

You should first determine whether Cindy's airway is open and whether she is being adequately ventilated.[1] If not, you should try to correct the problem, starting with checking the oropharyngeal airway size and assuring correct airway positioning. If available, a pulse oximeter can be quickly placed on her finger to aid in this assessment.[2] It may be necessary to intubate Cindy if you are unable to ventilate her adequately with the bag-valve-mask device, but this may not have to be a crash procedure if she is being adequately ventilated with a bag-valve-mask device. Insertion of an intravenous line is essential, but does not take priority over airway management and ventilation.

As you auscultate Cindy's chest you hear equal breath sounds bilaterally, with some crackles as her lungs are inflated. Her chest expansion appears equal. The pulse oximeter reading is 78; you increase the rate of bag-valve-mask ventilation and prepare for intubation.

The EMTs are staying to help with cardiopulmonary resuscitation, and you continue to palpate a pulse with compressions. The EMTs tell you that Cindy was in full arrest when they arrived and their dispatcher was attempting to give CPR instructions to the mother on the telephone. Mrs. Lang reported that Cindy had taken two doses of medicine today and drank one half glass of juice before taking her nap at 3:00 P.M.

As the EMTs give you this information, you notice that the rate of compressions has slowed slightly and you suggest that the rate be increased.

Question

What rate and depth of compression is correct for a 2-year old child? (Choose one answer.)

1. A rate of 80–100 and a depth of 1 to 1-1/2 inches.
2. A rate of 110–130 and a depth of 1-1/2 to 2 inches.
3. A rate of 80–100 and a depth of 3/4 to 1-1/2 inches.
4. A rate of 120–140 and a depth of 1 to 1-1/2 inches.

Answer

Cardiac compressions should be performed at rate of 80 to 100 times per minute, and a depth of 1 to 1-1/2 inches. For a child 2 years of age, it would be advisable to perform compressions at 100 per minute, because this would most closely approximate the child's normal rate.[1]

Chest compressions are now being performed adequately. The emergency physician has intubated Cindy without difficulty, and you have started an intraosseous line in Cindy's left leg.[3] You connect leads to a cardiac monitor and observe asystole in Lead II.

Question

The next action now should be: (Choose one answer.)

1. Defibrillation at 2 joules/kg
2. Assuring that the monitor leads are correctly attached
3. Synchronized cardioversion at 1 to 1.5 joules/kg
4. Administration of intracardiac epinephrine

Answer

The answer is (2). Asystole should also be confirmed in two leads. The most common rhythm disturbances in the pediatric age group are asystole and abnormally slow rhythms, so the need for defibrillation is unlikely. Although very fine ventricular fibrillation sometimes appears as asystole on a monitor, this rhythm is seen in less than 10% of pediatric cardiac arrests. Cardioversion is only appropriate when there is a rapid rhythm, because it requires a QRS complex for activation. Intracardiac epinephrine would be given only as the very last resort and would not be considered at this point.[1]

Asystole is confirmed in the second lead; cardiopulmonary resuscitation continues. You prepare to give Cindy medication.

Question

Which medication should be given first and via what route? (Choose one answer.)

1. Atropine via intraosseous line
2. Epinephrine via intraosseous line
3. Epinephrine via endotracheal tube
4. Sodium bicarbonate via intraosseous line

Answer

Epinephrine is the first medication given in asystole. If you had been unable to initiate an intraosseous line immediately, epinephrine could also have been given via the endotracheal tube, but this is not necessary in this case. The simplest way to remember what medications may be given via endotracheal tube is the use of the acronym LEAN (see Table 3.10).[4]

L   Lidocaine
E   Epinephrine
A   Atropine
N   Naloxone

Sodium bicarbonate is not routinely recommended, because the cause of acidosis is usually respiratory in etiology. Sodium bicarbonate would therefore be given only after careful review of arterial blood gases, when metabolic acidosis is confirmed. Atropine is routinely used as the first medication for bradycardia but not for asystole.

TABLE 3.10. Administration of Medications During Cardiac Arrest[1,5]

Medication	Route	Indications
Epinephrine	I.V. Push I.V. Infusion Endotracheal tube	Can create a spontaneous impulse electrically and mechanically in the heart Most useful drug in cardiac arrest management
Atropine	I.V. Push Endotracheal tube	Used to treat bradycardia that is hemodynamically unstable Useful in asystole to initiate an impulse in epinephrine refractory rhythms
Naloxone	I.V. Push Endotracheal tube	Useful if etiology of cardiac arrest is unknown or there is suspicion of narcotic drug ingestion Creates an increase in cerebral perfusion through vasodilation
Dextrose	I.V. Push	Pediatric patients have limited glycogen stores that are rapidly depleted with stress Should be administered based on fingerstick glucose test or to patients who fail to respond to usual resuscitative measures
Sodium bicarbonate	I.V. Push	Cardiac arrest is secondary to respiratory arrest in most pediatric patients Useful for treatment of metabolic acidosis Preferably given in accordance with arterial blood gas analysis

Note: For pediatric patients, medications are always given by weight in kilograms.

You note that there is no response to the epinephrine; Cindy remains in asystole on support ventilation. You have 5 minutes before the next dose of epinephrine, so you go quickly to the waiting room to talk to Mrs. Lang. You tell her that Cindy is not breathing on her own and has no heartbeat. She looks at you blankly, trying to assimilate this information. You encourage her to call her family or a close friend to come in and be with her, but she does not seem able to do this right now. You tell her you will be back very soon to talk to her again.

Question

Cindy should be reassessed or her condition reevaluated: (Choose one answer.)

1. Every 5 to 10 min
2. After every intervention
3. Once a perfusing rhythm is established

Answer

The effect of every intervention requires documentation of its effects or evoked changes.[6] The evaluation must include evaluation of the patient's pulse. ***Never rely on the cardiac monitor alone.***

You return to the treatment room. The time is now 6:30 P.M.; resuscitation has been in progress for 8 minutes in the emergency department, and there has been no positive change in the clinical picture.

Question

The order of the medications to be given is: (Place **1** next to the first, **2** next to the second, etc.)

____   Atropine   ____   Epinephrine

____   Dextrose   ____   Naloxone

Answer

The answers are: (2), atropine; (3), dextrose; (1), epinephrine; and (4), naloxone.

Epinephrine should be given again. There is currently considerable controversy about using low dosages versus high dosages of epinephrine. Atropine may be used as a second choice when epinephrine has not proved effective. Dextrose is given if the patient is hypoglycemic, and naloxone is given in case there has been a narcotic ingestion.

You have now given epinephrine for the third time, 5 minutes between each administration, and each time you have reassessed and found no improvement. Atropine was given once. A fingerstick for dextrose showed 40 mg%, so dextrose 50% was given.

Question

When dextrose is ordered to be given via intraosseous line, you should: (Choose one answer.)

1. Give the dextrose 50% rapidly through the intraosseous line.
2. Start an IV line rather than giving the dextrose 50% through the intraosseous line.
3. Dilute the dextrose 50% with normal saline, and give it through the intraosseous line.
4. Give the dextrose 50% via slow infusion (over 10 min).

Answer

The 50% dextrose solution should be diluted and given through the intraosseous line. Almost all medications that can be given through an IV line may be given via intraosseous line, but strongly hypertonic or hypotonic solutions should be diluted. The dextrose solution should therefore be diluted with an equal amount of normal saline, producing a 25% solution, which may be given safely into the bone marrow.[7] Because this solution may be given safely, another IV line would not be needed for this purpose, although one should be started when feasible. Giving the dextrose 50% by slow infusion would not be appropriate in this case.

Naloxone is given in case narcotic ingestion is the cause of Cindy's arrest. The nursing supervisor has arrived and is now serving as liaison between Cindy's mother and the emergency department staff during this period. The supervisor has contacted Mr. Lang (Cindy's father) at work. She tells you that Mrs. Lang wants to come in to see Cindy. You suggest that this would be a good moment, because you have a few minutes before the next medication will be given. The nursing supervisor brings in Mrs. Lang, who hesitantly touches Cindy's foot. The nursing supervisor guides her out almost immediately, comforting her. You think of your own daughter, probably having supper at home right now.

Arterial blood gases have been drawn, and blood has been sent for electrolytes and complete blood count. Despite all interventions, Cindy remains pulseless, apneic, and in asystolic cardiac rhythm. Her pupils are fixed and dilated, and her extremities are pale and cool to touch.

> **Question**
>
> Would a temporary pacemaker be indicated for Cindy's condition? (Choose Yes or No.)
>
> 1. Yes 2. No

Answer

The correct answer is No. Pacemakers are rarely indicated in pediatric patients because the etiology of cardiopulmonary arrest is usually respiratory rather than cardiac failure.[1] Children's hearts are young and strong, and rarely have rhythms that can be improved with insertion of a pacemaker. There is no indication that this would be helpful in Cindy's case.

It is now 7:05 P.M. and resuscitation has been attempted for 43 minutes without positive response to any intervention. The emergency department physician decides to terminate resuscitation based on lack of cardiopulmonary response. The cause of death is unknown and will have to be determined by an autopsy.

The emergency department physician leaves to tell Mr. and Mrs. Lang about Cindy's death. Knowing that the nursing supervisor will ask the Langs if they want to hold Cindy, you quickly tidy the room a little, and although you have to leave the IV tubes as they are, you tie them off to prevent leakage. You clean Cindy's face and wrap her in a little blanket to make her look as normal as possible for the Langs.

Once they have been told of Cindy's death, Cindy's parents ask to go into the treatment room to see her. You stay with them to explain the various tubes, and why these must remain in place. They want to hold Cindy, so you place her in their arms and tell them you will be available right outside if they need you. After leaving the family alone for a few minutes you knock and enter quietly to ask if they need any assistance. They ask you what happens after this, and you discuss the final procedures with them.

After staying with Cindy for about an hour, the Langs decide it is time to leave. You stay with Cindy while another nurse helps them to the car. Once they have left, the emergency physician, the EMTs, and the nursing staff discuss Cindy's death. You wonder aloud what might have been done differently, even though you know the chances of a child surviving an out-of-hospital arrest are less than 10%. Although you all acknowledge that there was nothing more you could have done, you also know that it is impossible not to hope for survival even against all odds.

You thank the EMTs for their help and reassure them that they did everything they could. You talk with them for a brief moment, each of you trying to understand and cope with the pain of this experience. When they leave for their station a few minutes later, you return to the other patients waiting for your care.

REFERENCES

Case Study 1

1. American Heart Association and American Academy of Pediatrics. (1988). *Textbook of pediatric advanced life support* (1st ed.). Dallas, TX: AHA/AAP.
2. Campbell, L. S., & Jackson, K. (1991). Starting intravenous lines in children: Tips for success. *Journal of Emergency Nursing, 17,* 177–178.
3. Fiser, D. H. (1990). Intraosseous infusion. *New England Journal of Medicine, 322,* 1579–1581.
4. Hodge, D., III. (1984). Intraosseous infusions: A review. *Pediatric Emergency Care, 1,* 215–218.
5. Wagner, M. B., & McCabe, J. B. (1988). A comparison of four techniques to establish intraosseous infusion. *Pediatric Emergency Care, 4,* 87–91.
6. Brickman, K. R., Rega, P., Koltz, M., & Guinness, M. (1988). Analysis of growth plate abnormalities following intraosseous infusion through the proximal tibial epiphysis in pigs. *Annals of Emergency Medicine, 17,* 121–122.
7. Utah EMSC Program (1991). *Pediatric vascular access.* Salt Lake City, UT: Utah Department of Health, Bureau of Emergency Medical Services.

8. Chaney, P. S., (Ed.). (1978). *Nursing skillbook: Assessing vital functions accurately.* Horsham, PA: Intermed Communications, Inc.

9. Mayer, T. (1985). *Emergency management of pediatric trauma,* (1st ed.). Philadelphia: Saunders.

10. Fleischer, G., & Ludwig, S. (1988). *Textbook of pediatric emergency medicine* (2nd ed.). Baltimore: Williams & Wilkins.

11. Orlowski, J. P., Porembka, D. T., Gallagher, J. M., & VanLente, F. (1989, December). The bone marrow as a source of laboratory studies. *Annals of Emergency Medicine, 18,* 12.

12. Hazinski, M. F. (1984). *Nursing care of the critically ill child.* St. Louis: Mosby.

13. Barkin, R. M., & Rosen, P. (1987). *Emergency pediatrics: Guide to ambulatory care* (2nd ed.). St. Louis: Mosby.

14. American Academy of Pediatrics, Committee on Nutrition (1985). Use of oral fluid therapy and post-treatment feeding following enteritis in children in a developed country. *Pediatrics, 75,* 358–361.

15. Snyder, J. D. (1991, January). Use and misuse of oral therapy for diarrhea: Comparison of US practices with American Academy of Pediatrics recommendations. *Pediatrics, 87,* 28–33.

Case Study 2

1. Kitt, S., & Kaiser, J. (1990). *Emergency nursing: A physiologic and clinical perspective.* Philadelphia: Saunders.

2. Carpenito, L. J. (1989). *Nursing diagnosis: Application to clinical practice.* (3d ed.). Philadelphia: JB Lippincott.

3. American Heart Association and American Academy of Pediatrics (1988). *Textbook of pediatric advanced life support* (1st ed.). Dallas, TX: AHA/AAP.

4. Henderson, D. P. & Seidel, J. S. (Eds.). (1989). *Pediatric cardiovascular assessment.* Robert Wood Johnson Foundation Grant #12964.

5. Kelley, S. J. (1988). *Pediatric Emergency Nursing.* Norwalk CT: Appleton and Lange.

6. Seidel, J. S. & Henderson, D. P. (1987). *Prehospital care of pediatric emergencies.* Los Angeles: Los Angeles Pediatric Society.

7. Hazinski, M. F. (1984). *Nursing care of the critically ill child.* St. Louis: Mosby.

Case Study 3

1. American Heart Association and American Academy of Pediatrics (1988). *Textbook of pediatric advanced life support* (1st ed.). Dallas, TX: AHA/AAP.

2. Foster, R. L., Hunsberger, M. M., & Anderson, J. J. (1989). *Family-centered nursing care of children.* Philadelphia: Saunders.

3. Fiser, D. H. (1990). Intraosseous infusion. *New England Journal of Medicine, 322,* 1579–1581.

4. Seidel, J. S., & Henderson, D. P. (1988). *Prehospital care of pediatric emergencies.* Los Angeles: Los Angeles Pediatric Society.

5. American Heart Association (1987). *Textbook of advanced cardiac life support.* Dallas, TX: Author.

6. Budassi, S., & Barber, J. M. (1981). *Emergency nursing: Principles and practice.* St. Louis: Mosby.

7. Hodge, D., III. (1984). Intraosseous infusions: A review. *Pediatric Emergency Care, 1,* 215–218.

Chapter Four

Assessment and Management of Neurologic Emergencies

Prerequisite Skills

Before beginning this chapter, the learner should have

- Knowledge of the basic anatomy and physiology of the neurologic system
- Knowledge of the principles of rapid primary and secondary assessments
- Ability to assess vital signs in the pediatric patient
- Ability to perform a basic neurologic assessment including

  - Mental status
  - Pupillary response
  - Eye movement
  - Sensory and motor response

- Ability to plan, prioritize, and evaluate nursing interventions based on history and physical findings

PREVIEW

The child presenting to the emergency department with a neurologic emergency offers a unique assessment challenge. The brain of a young child may withstand a traumatic insult better than the brain of an adult. Still, it remains a very complex organ with its function being highly sensitive to changes in its milieu.[1]

Pediatric neurologic emergencies result from a wide variety of diseases and injuries.[2] The presenting signs and symptoms can be related to primary central nervous system disorders or secondary to other diseases.[3] They may range from very subtle changes in the child's activity level to comatose states. Despite the nature of the initial neurologic event, most brain damage is the end result of tissue hypoxia or ischemia.

Preservation of pediatric neurologic function depends on health care providers having the knowledge and foresight to anticipate and react quickly to changes affecting the central nervous system. This self-learning module will help you to recognize common presentation patterns, refine your assessment skills, and review the basic management principles for pediatric neurologic emergencies.

CASE STUDY 1 OBJECTIVES

On completion of this case study, you will be able to

- Prioritize assessment tasks for the pediatric patient with altered mental status
- Identify possible causes of altered mental status in pediatric patients presenting with neurologic emergencies
- Calculate the modified Glasgow Coma Scale for a pediatric patient with altered mental status
- State three factors in the child's history and clinical presentation that would alert the emergency department nurse to suspect poisoning as a probable cause of altered mental status
- Describe at least two methods for assessing altered mental status in the pediatric patient
- Select an appropriate nursing diagnosis for the child presenting with a neurologic emergency
- Prioritize emergency nursing interventions for a child with an altered mental status
- Describe the procedure for identification of the type and amount of suspected toxic ingestions
- Describe procedures appropriate for the administration of charcoal following gastric lavage
- Identify the nursing responsibilities associated with gastric decontamination of the pediatric poisoning victim
- List three appropriate topics for discharge instructions regarding prevention of pediatric poisonings

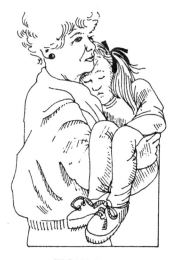

FIGURE 4.1

CASE STUDY 1

Nancy and Grandmother's Medicine

Mrs. White arrives at the emergency department at 12:45 P.M. carrying Nancy, her 3-year-old granddaughter (see Figure 4.1). Mrs. White is frantic and blurts out, "Someone help me, please! She was singing and playing in the living room earlier this morning. Then I found her lying on the floor with all my medicines and the other stuff from my purse poured out everywhere. Now she doesn't even recognize me, and she isn't talking at all."

Nancy, who is clean and neatly dressed, opens her eyes only momentarily as you call her name and take her from her grandmother's arms. She does not resist your efforts to take her but cries softly. Her body feels warm, her face is flushed, and her arms and legs are limp. You note that her breathing is unlabored and regular. Capillary refill is less than 2 seconds.

TRIAGE DECISION

Based on your rapid initial assessment, you would triage Nancy as

Emergent.   A life-threatening situation in need of immediate intervention.

Urgent.   Patient needs care within 1 hour to prevent further deterioration.

Nonurgent.   Patient is able to wait more than 1 hour without further deterioration.

TRIAGE DECISION ANSWER

Your initial rapid assessment coupled with her history as told by her grandmother indicate that Nancy's condition is emergent. Any child presenting with altered mental status of unknown etiology has potential for rapid deterioration and should be triaged as emergent.[2,4]

Question

The *first* priority in Nancy's initial assessment and emergency care would be: (Choose one answer.)

1. Obtaining a complete history from Nancy's grandmother regarding any history of fever, injuries, or the possibility of ingestions or exposure to toxic substances.

2. Obtaining a set of initial baseline vital signs including the child's weight and pupillary reactions.

3. Assuring the adequacy of Nancy's airway, breathing, and circulation before performing a more complete neurologic assessment.

4. Obtaining baseline lab work including a complete blood count, arterial blood gases, and a serum toxicology screen.

Answer

The correct answer is (3). Assuring the adequacy of the airway, breathing, and circulation is always the first and most important step in the management of pediatric neurologic emergencies.[2] The signs and symptoms of pediatric neurologic emergencies can be both caused by or aggravated by unstable *ABC*s. In addition, the underlying causes for neurologic emergencies can also contribute to life-threatening hypoxia or shock.[5]

You take Nancy into an examination room immediately. Because her *ABC*s appear to be stable, you continue with assessment of neurologic status. You know that Nancy's behavior and response is not normal, and you assess her mental status rapidly. The mnemonic **AVPU** is a simple scale for describing neurologic status. This is especially helpful in the initial rapid assessment of preverbal children (Table 4.1).

You tell Nancy to open her eyes, but she remains unresponsive. When you give this command a little more loudly, however, she opens her eyes slowly and closes them again. You make a note that she is responsive to loud verbal stimuli. You take her vital signs, which are

TABLE 4.1.   Rapid Assessment of Mental Status[5]

A	*A*lert
V	*R*esponds to *v*erbal stimuli
P	*R*esponds to *p*ainful stimuli
U	*U*nresponsive

Blood pressure	80/60
Pulse	160 and regular
Respiratory rate	20 and unlabored
Temperature	37.6°C (rectal)
Weight	15 kg

Question

Are Nancy's vital signs appropriate for her age? (Choose Yes or No.)

_____ Yes   _____ No

Answer

The correct answer is No. Nancy's temperature is slightly elevated, and her pulse is elevated. See Table 1.4 (Chapter 1), which shows normal vital signs by age.

After you tell the emergency physician about Nancy, you talk with her grandmother, who tells you that Nancy has not been ill or sustained any kind of injury within the last few days. At about 11:30 A.M. this morning Mrs. White noticed Nancy was "too quiet" and went to check on her. She thought Nancy had just fallen asleep on the floor and then realized "she was too hard to wake up and acted like she didn't know who I was."

Question

Possible causes for the sudden change in Nancy's mental status could include hypoxia, a postic-tal state, a central nervous system (CNS) infection, an ingestion or exposure to a toxic substance, or a closed head injury. (Choose True or False.)

_____ True   _____ False

Answer

The correct answer is True. All of the causes listed are commonly associated with altered mental status in children. A useful tool in considering possible causes of pediatric neurologic emergencies is the mnemonic AEIOU-TIPS (see Table 4.2).

TABLE 4.2. AEIOU–TIPS[6]

A =	Alcohol:	Alcohol abuse is relatively rare in young children, but caretakers may attempt to cool a fever with alcohol; a child can absorb sufficient alcohol through the skin to affect mental status. Alcohol ingestion should be considered a possibility in older children and adolescents.
E =	Epilepsy:	Postictal state is a common cause of altered mental status. Pediatric seizures may result from several causes including epilepsy, fever, and head injuries.
I =	Insulin:	Hypoglycemia–hyperglycemia may be involved.
O =	Overdose:	Ingestion, inhalation, or skin absorption of toxic substances may be accidents in the young child or suicide gestures in older children.
U =	Uremia:	Multiple metabolic causes for altered mental status in children include electrolyte disorders, renal, hepatic, or adrenal insufficiency, and congenital enzyme defects.
T =	Trauma:	Head injuries are the most common injuries in children, but any injury that results in hypoxia or shock can result in altered mental status.
I =	Infection:	Infections (meningitis, encephalitis, sepsis, postinfectious encephalitis, Reye's syndrome, etc.) are more common causes of altered mental status in children than in adults.
P =	Psychological cause:	Factitious coma is possible but very rare in children.
S =	Shock, stroke, or syncope:	Inadequate brain perfusion owing to hypovolemia or congenital cardiovascular abnormalities such as arteriovenous anomalies may alter level of consciousness.

Note: From Prehospital Care of Pediatric Emergencies by J. S. Seidel & D. P. Henderson, © 1987, Los Angeles, CA: Los Angeles Pediatric Society. Reprinted by permission.

> **Question**
>
> Now that you have completed your initial assessment and assured that Nancy's *ABCs* are temporarily stable, what would be the next priority? (Choose one answer.)
>
> 1. obtain serum glucose level
> 2. assess pupillary response
> 3. assess mental status
> 4. obtain a complete health history from grandmother

Answer

Answer (3) is the correct answer. Pediatric neurologic dysfunction is frequently progressive in nature. Serial observations of the child's mental status are the single most important parameters in identifying a child's deteriorating neurologic status.[2] These observations and documentation should include the child's general activity level, and his or her response to the environment and his or her caretakers.

> *Note:* As a general rule, failure of a child to recognize primary caretakers is an ominous sign![5]

Besides AVPU, which is best for the rapid initial assessment, another useful pediatric neurologic assessment tool, especially for documenting changes in serial assessments, is the Modified Glasgow Coma Scale. It quantifies mental status by evaluating eyeopening, motor responses, and verbal responses in infants and young children (see Table 4.3, following page). *A score of less than 10 points on the Modified Glasgow Coma Scale is considered a very serious sign.*[2]

When you repeat your assessment of Nancy's mental status, you think she is becoming less responsive. Her eyes remain closed unless she is directly spoken to or physically touched. She pulls her leg away in response to tactile stimulation, but does not respond to questions or commands. She is no longer crying but moans in response to painful stimuli.

> **Question**
>
> Based on these assessment findings, what is Nancy's Modified Glasgow Coma Scale score? (Fill in the blank.)
>
> Nancy's current Modified Glasgow Coma Scale score = _____

Answer

The correct point score for the current assessment findings would be 10 points, calculated as follows:

Opens eyes to speech and sounds	3
Withdraws to touch	5
Moans in response to pain	2
Total score	**10 points**

You remove Nancy's clothing with her grandmother's assistance and cover her with a light sheet. Nancy's most recent vital signs are:

Blood pressure	80/54
Pulse	150
Respiratory rate	22 breaths/min

A colleague tells you the emergency department physician will be coming in to see Nancy right away. You start oxygen and attach the cardiac monitor, and repeat your assessment. You find Nancy's status unchanged.

TABLE 4.3.   Modified Glasgow Coma Scale[7]

Child	Infant
Eyes	
4 Opens eyes spontaneously	Opens eyes spontaneously
3 Opens eyes to speech	Opens eyes to speech
2 Opens eyes to pain	Opens eyes to pain
1 **No response**	**No response**
_____ = Score* (Eyes)	
Motor	
6 Obeys commands	Spontaneous movements
5 Localizes	Withdraws to touch
4 Withdraws	Withdraws to pain
3 Flexion	Flexion (decorticate)
2 Extension	Extension (decerebrate)
1 **No response**	**No response**
_____ = Score* (Motor)	
Verbal	
5 Oriented	Coos and babbles
4 Confused	Irritable cry
3 Inappropriate words	Cries to pain
2 Incomprehensible words	Moans to pain
1 **No response**	**No response**
_____ = Score* (Verbal)	
_____ = **Total score (eyes, motor, verbal)**	
Scores will range from 3–15	

* All scores reflect *best* response in each category. Possible total scores range from 3 to 15 points. Having parents assist in eliciting responses may be helpful with young children in unfamiliar environments.[8]

> **Question**
>
> Indicate your priorities for Nancy's immediate emergency care by matching the following interventions to the order in which you would perform them. (Mark "1" for first priority, etc.)
>
> | PRIORITY | NURSING INTERVENTIONS |
> |---|---|
> | _4_ | Assess blood glucose level with a dextrostix |
> | _3_ | Start an IV line of normal saline at a maintenance rate |
> | _1_ | Initiate O₂ at 6 L/min via nasal cannula |
> | _2_ | Initiate cardiac monitoring and serial assessments of mental status |
> | _5_ | Obtain an in-depth history from Nancy's grandmother |

Answer

The correct priorities would be as follows: (4), (3), (1), (2), and (5), respectively.

Initial priorities for Nancy's care at this time should include the use of supplemental oxygen to correct or prevent cerebral hypoxia; hypoxia could be contributing to Nancy's altered mental status. In addition, you should continue careful monitoring of the circulatory and neurologic status. Other initial interventions should include initiating vascular access, and assessing for and treating hypoglycemia. (Hypoglycemia may also be a possible underlying cause of Nancy's altered mental status.) Finally, a more in-depth history is indicated. Table 4.4 summarizes the initial management priorities for children presenting with altered mental status.

TABLE 4.4. Management Priorities for the Child With Altered Mental Status[4]

1. Assess and stabilize *ABCs*
• Secure airway • Support ventilation to avoid or correct hypoxia • Monitor cardiovascular status and initiate support
2. Recognize and prevent progressive neurologic deterioration
• Supplement oxygen to avoid or treat cerebral hypoxia • Initiate intravenous fluid therapy (normal saline or lactated Ringer's) to have a route for medications for seizure control and treatment of fluid electrolyte disturbances • Assess for and manage signs of increasing intracranial pressure • Administer naloxone 0.01–0.1 mg/kg • Administer glucose (dextrose 25%) 250–500 mg/kg for any child presenting in coma from unknown causes if either hypoglycemia or overdose is a possibility
3. Establish and treat underlying cause of neurologic dysfunction including
• Decontamination of toxic exposures • Antibiotics as necessary for central nervous system (CNS) infections • Anticonvulsants as necessary for seizure disorders • Treatment of metabolic disorders • Surgical management of cerebral edema, hemorrhage and obstruction as necessary

A colleague assists you in starting Nancy's IV line and blood is drawn for the laboratory. While awaiting the physician, you review the history and physical signs you have assessed so far.

Question

List three factors in Nancy's history or presenting symptoms that might suggest the possibility of toxic ingestion. (Fill in the blanks.)

1. _____

2. _____

3. _____

Answer

Any of the following would be correct:

- History of sudden onset of altered mental status with no history of preceding trauma or illness
- Physical findings of altered mental status without obvious injury or illness
- Persistent tachycardia without respiratory distress
- Age and developmental level of the child
- History of being found with grandmother's medications (see Table 4.5)

TABLE 4.5.   **Common Initial Findings in Pediatric Ingestions and Toxic Exposures**[3,9–11]

Historical findings
Age and developmental level of child: • Accidental ingestions most common in toddler and preschool ages • Suicide gestures more common in older children and teens
Accessibility to medications, drugs, alcohol, or toxic substances
History of suspected ingestion, chemical exposure, or previous substance abuse
Negative history for preceding trauma, illness, or known central nervous system disorders

Physical findings
Altered mental status, ranging from lethargy and stupor to hyperexcitability
Abrupt change of behavior or personality
Odor of alcohol or other chemicals on breath or clothing
Pupils pinpoint or dilated
Respiratory depression and failure
Cardiac dysrhythmia or chest pain
Acute pulmonary edema
New onset of seizures
Nausea and vomiting

This certainly seems be a case of toxic ingestion, but you decide to obtain some more information about Mrs. White having found Nancy "asleep on the floor" and what type of ingestion might be involved.

Question

Because of your suspicions of an accidental ingestion, the most important information to obtain from Nancy's grandmother at this time would include all of the following *except:* (Choose the exception.)

1. The likelihood that Nancy could have accidentally ingested some of the grandmother's medications
2. The type and amount of medication that Nancy may have ingested
3. The probable length of time that has elapsed since the ingestion
4. Why Nancy had been left unsupervised with access to medications
5. Any emergency treatment or other medications Nancy may have received since the probable ingestion

Answer

The exception is (4). The assessment of children with suspected poisonings must be thorough but rapid. The focus is on gaining as much information as possible on the type and amount of toxic exposure, and any subsequent changes in the patient's clinical status. *The emergency management of the child's presenting symptoms, however, always takes precedence over identification of the poison!*[3]

If possible, obtain the remainder of the suspected toxic substance and its container to help identify the type and amount ingested. When estimating the amount of ingested poison, it is safer to assume that the child has ingested the largest possible amount unless there is definite evidence to the contrary.[3]

TABLE 4.6. Initial Questions in Suspected Pediatric Poisonings[3]

Type of exposure (ingestion, inhalation, absorption)?
What is the identity of the agent?
What amount of the agent was ingested?
How much time has elapsed since the exposure?
Has any treatment been initiated since the exposure?
Have any changes been noted in the child's clinical status?

Question

The additional history you obtain may help to identify the underlying cause of Nancy's problem and how to proceed with her emergency management. (Choose True or False.)

_____ True   _____ False

Answer

The statement is True. Immediate emergency care for children presenting with altered mental status, regardless of the underlying cause, requires stabilizing the *ABCs* and preventing further neurologic deterioration. Definitive care will vary with the underlying cause and the extent of the problem, however. Many underlying causes can contribute to altered mental status in children, and these may be interrelated. Table 4.7 summarizes the major types of pediatric neurologic dysfunctions and their common underlying causes.

TABLE 4.7. Types of Neurologic Emergencies[2]

Dysfunction	Cause(s)	
Increased intracranial pressure	Trauma Obstruction to central nervous system outflow (Hydrocephalic shunt malfunction)	Nontraumatic hemorrhage tumors
Metabolic imbalance	Ingestion Electrolyte imbalance Endocrine disturbance Hypoglycemia Hyperglycemia	Water intoxication Hepatic disease Reye's syndrome Acidosis Uremia
Infectious process	Meningitis Brain abscess Encephalitis	Parasitic infection Sepsis
Seizure disorders	Febrile Epileptic Ingestion	Trauma Neonatal
Congenital problems	Cerebral palsy Down's syndrome Phenylketonuria Neurofibromatosis	Tuberosclerosis Arnold-Chiari syndrome anomaly Dandy-Walker deformity anomaly

Nancy's grandmother tells you that she is currently taking propranolol (Inderal), hydrochlorothiazide (Hydrodiuril), and amitriptyline (Elavil), and normally keeps all of the medications in her purse. She quickly checks the pill bottles and says that she thinks all of the propranolol and hydrochlorothiazide are there but that some of the amitriptyline seems to be missing. You check the prescription label and find that the bottle of pills was recently refilled. By your calculations, you think that five amitriptyline 50-mg tablets are unaccounted for.

Dr. Martin arrives, and you quickly relay the information about the probable ingestion and Nancy's current clinical status. He begins his initial examination, simultaneously ordering a 12-lead electrocardiogram, chest X-ray film, and laboratory analyses (arterial blood gases, complete blood count, blood urea nitrogen, glucose, electrolytes, liver functions, ammonia, toxicology screen, and urinalysis). He also consults the Poison Control Index regarding tricyclic antidepressants (TCA). He finds that a dose of 10 to 20 mg/kg of a TCA can cause serious side effects and that a dose of 35 to 50 mg/kg can cause fatal toxicity.

Question

If Nancy ingested five amitriptyline 50 mg tablets, did she have a sufficient ingestion to cause any serious side effects? (Choose Yes or No.)

____ Yes   ____ No

Answer

The correct answer is Yes. Because Nancy weighs 15 kg, a dose of 150 to 300 mg could cause serious side effects, (10–20 mg/kg × 15 kg = 150 × 300 mg). Nancy may have ingested 250 mg of amitriptyline, which is within this dangerous drug level (5 tablets × 50 mg/tablet = 250 mg).

Nancy's mother arrives and is shown into the examining room. She walks to Nancy's side, takes her hand, and begins comforting her. Nancy barely opens her eyes to her mother's voice, her hand appears limp when touched, and she makes no sound. Fifteen minutes have now elapsed since Nancy's arrival in the emergency department.

Question

Would you reassess Nancy's level of consciousness based on this observation? (Choose Yes or No.)

_____ Yes _____ No

Why or Why not? _____

Answer

The correct answer is Yes. There has been an apparent change in Nancy's motor response since your last assessment; it would be important to reassess the child's neurologic status immediately.

You explain to Nancy's mother what you are doing and then you gently shake Nancy's shoulders and call out her name. Nancy does not open her eyes so you apply pressure to the nailbed on Nancy's middle finger. She pulls her arm away and moans softly. You assign Nancy a Modified Glasgow Coma Scale score of 7 and decide to monitor her neurologic status even more carefully. Your primary nursing diagnosis is potential ineffective airway clearance related to altered mental status, secondary to drug ingestion. You assess her perfusion.

Question

In cases of toxic ingestion, the first priority is always to: (Choose one answer.)

1. Assess neurologic status
2. Prevent or minimize absorption of the toxic substance
3. Determine the amount of toxic substance ingested
4. Assess oxygenation and ventilation

Answer

The correct answer is (4). When there is toxic ingestion, the focus is often on the toxic substance rather than on the patient. When a patient has come in bodily contact with toxins, it is important to remove or detoxify them as quickly as possible, but this should be done simultaneously with assessment and continued attention to the *ABC*s, initiating rapid intervention when necessary (see Table 4.8).

TABLE 4.8.   Emergency Treatment of Pediatric Poisonings[4]

1.   Provide supportive care
• Stabilize *ABCs*. • Avoid further neurologic deterioration.
2.   Prevent or minimize absorption of the toxic substance
• For contact toxins, flush skin, hair, and eye exposures with large volumes of water. • 100% oxygen administered as soon as possible for inhalation toxins. • Prompt gastric emptying for ingestions (***except*** for caustics and most hydrocarbons) via induced vomiting or gastric lavage. When ipecac is used, additional fluid should be given. Water is the *best* fluid to use with ipecac. Koolade or apple juice can be used if necessary, but milk or carbonated beverages may delay the action of ipecac and increase the risk of toxic exposure and absorption.[11,12] • Dilution of caustic or corrosive ingestions.[9,10] • Administration of charcoal for absorption of the toxic substance.
3.   Enhance excretion of the toxin
• Cathartic use to shorten gastrointestinal transmit time. • Diuresis via kidneys achieved with fluid therapy. • Hemodialysis may be helpful for removal of drugs from the blood stream, especially with pulmonary edema, cerebral edema, or renal failure.
4.   Administer antagonists as indicated
• Only available in about 10% of all cases. • If available, can produce dramatic effects especially if given intravenously. • Must be specific to the involved toxin and therefore should be based on most current data from Poison Control Centers.

Because of Nancy's deteriorating mental status, Dr. Martin has decided to intubate Nancy and proceed with gastrointestinal decontamination. He reassures the mother and grandmother, explains what he is going to do, then requests that they wait outside until the procedure is completed. Although they are somewhat reluctant, you show them to a nearby waiting room and assure them that they can come in again once she has been intubated.

Question

Which of the following would affect the type of intervention indicated for suspected poisonings? (Mark all that are appropriate with an **X**.)

_____   Identity and characteristics of the suspected poison

_____   Quantity ingested and amount of exposure

_____   Predicted rapidity of absorption of poison

_____   Rapidity of onset of toxic symptoms

_____   Availability and anticipated effectiveness of proposed interventions

Answer

__X__	Identity and characteristics of the suspected poison
__X__	Quantity ingested and amount of exposure
__X__	Predicted rapidity of absorption of poison
__X__	Rapidity of onset of toxic symptoms
__X__	Availability and anticipated effectiveness of proposed interventions

The correct answer includes all of the factors listed. Once the toxic substance has been identified, the type and pace of the response can be determined (see Table 4.9). Using a poison control reference (such as a toxicology test, Poison Control Center, or computer program), responses can then be prioritized. Factors affecting priorities include the identity and quantity of ingested material, the rapidity of absorption and onset of toxicity, and the availability and effectiveness of proposed intervention.

TABLE 4.9. Key Points in Managing Pediatric Poisonings

Identity and characteristics of the poison
• Attempt to identify the poison; however, focus on treating the patient, ***not*** the poison.[4]
• Assume multiple drug ingestion until identification of all substances is confirmed. *This is particularly important in suicide attempts by adolescents!*
Absorption and onset of toxicity
• Toxic symptoms occur within 2–4 hr postingestion for most substances.
• Caustic materials cause immediate damage during ingestion.
• With medication ingestions, expect to see toxic symptoms about the same time you would expect to note the usual pharmacologic effects.[10]
• Time-release medications have a marked delay in release and absorption.
Availability and effectiveness of proposed interventions
Evaluate potential treatment approaches against
• Appropriateness for child's age and clinical situation
• Risk of delay in removing toxin
• Risk of further injury or complications

The emergency physician inserts an endotracheal tube with little difficulty. With this tube in place Nancy's airway is protected from aspiration. He asks you to begin gastric lavage.

Question

Because you estimate it has been from 2 to 2-1/2 hr since Nancy has ingested the amitriptyline, it is probably not worthwhile to attempt to empty her stomach. (Choose True or False.)

_____ True _____ False

Answer

The correct answer is False. It is generally recommended that gastric emptying be achieved within 2 hours of ingestion.[9,10] However, the onset of symptoms for tricyclic antidepressants is variable, and the drug's anticholinergic effect may result in a delayed gastric emptying time.[3,9] Because of the extremely toxic nature of this drug ingestion, it would be important to attempt to minimize the duration of exposure and reduce the absorption of any remaining drug via gastric decontamination.[4] Table 4.10 (facing page) summarizes these decontamination procedures.

Nancy is still breathing on her own, although you have asked for a respiratory technician to stay with you and assure correct placement of the endotracheal tube while you lavage her. You select your equipment for lavaging. As you do this, you make a mental note to check back with Nancy's mother and grandmother as soon as you can. Because you have children yourself, you know how difficult it is to be waiting outside when a procedure is being performed on your child.

Question

Which of the following would be the best type and size tube to choose for Nancy? (Choose one answer.)

1. 14-French nasogastric tube
2. 8-French feeding tube
3. 28-French orogastric tube

Answer

The correct answer is (3); the use of a large bore orogastric tube is recommended because it increases the return of pill fragments, decreases the likelihood of tube occlusions, and increases the rapidity of the gastric lavage.[15]

Nasogastric tubes and feeding tubes may be too small because they are generally smaller than orogastric tubes.[16] Tubes smaller than a 24 French are usually not helpful unless the toxin is a liquid.[17] It is generally recommended that a 28- to 36-French orogastric tube or a 18- to 24-French nasogastric be used for children.[3,4,18]

Before you begin lavaging, you reassess Nancy's breathing and mental status, which remain stable. You position Nancy for lavage, assuring the patency of her airway. You go to the medication room to obtain fluid for lavage.

Question

Which of the following solutions would you use for Nancy's lavage? (Choose one answer.)

1. 5% dextrose solution
2. Normal saline
3. Water

Answer

Normal saline is correct. Normal saline is isotonic and will not disrupt the child's electrolyte balance.[15] Large quantities of fluid are used for gastric lavage, so the danger of electrolyte imbalance in small children is increased.

Although water is safely used for lavage in adults, it is hypotonic and could cause fluid and electrolyte imbalances in children.[14]

TABLE 4.10. Decontamination Methods

Method	Indications/Contraindications	Comments
Dilution	Used for caustic or corrosive ingestions; also indicated for topical or ocular exposures, and low toxicity ingestions[10]	Use water or milk to dilute ingested caustic: flush ocular areas with sterile water and wash dermal surfaces with soap and water[13]
Induced vomiting	Used for the removal of many ingestions in the alert child with intact gag reflex **Contraindicated if the child** • Is younger than 9 months of age • Has a compromised gag reflex • Is experiencing seizures, coma, and rapidly deteriorating mental status, or respiratory distress • Has ingested a caustic substance, petroleum product, strychnine, or a sharp object[9,10,14]	Method of choice is syrup of ipecac given orally: 10 mL 9–12 months 15 mL 1–12 years 30 mL > 12 years [3,4] Follow ipecac with 100–500 mL clear fluids (water, Koolade, or apple juice) Repeat dose and fluids if emesis has not occurred in 20 min
Gastric lavage	Indicated for • Infants < 9 months of age[3] • Unresponsive patients or those with rapidly declining mental status • Patients with a depressed gag reflex or a predisposition to seizures • Where two doses of ipecac have failed to produce emesis[3] • Where the need for prompt charcoal administration is urgent[9] **Contraindicated in ingestions of** • Caustics • Most hydrocarbons[3]	Use a large catheter–tipped syringe to alternately instill and then aspirate aliquot of 50–100 mL/wash of an isotonic solution via a large bore nasogastric/orogastric tube[3] Continue to lavage until aspirate is clear (may require 1–2 L)[3] Lavage with an additional 1–2 L of wash after aspirate is clear
Enteric detoxification (Activated charcoal)	Indicated for most ingested toxins after gastric emptying to prevent systemic absorption of poisons from the gastrointestinal tract **Contraindicated in ingestions of** • Acetaminophen • Alcohols • Caustics and hydrocarbons • Cyanide • Iron[3]	Usual dose is 5–10 × amount of ingested poison; because amount ingested is rarely known, use minimum pediatric dose of 20 g for a child, 50–100 g for adolescents[14] Repeated dosing every 2–4 hr indicated with drug ingestions of • Hepatic clearance • Prolonged action or absorption • Multiple drugs[14]
Cathartic (sorbitol, sodium citrate)	Of questionable value, but generally used following charcoal administration to speed evacuation of the charcoal-bound toxin Most useful in ingestions of • Solid materials • Enteric-coated tablets • Delay-release and long-acting medications[15] **Contraindicated in children with known renal failure.**	Oil and stimulant cathartics are generally not used because of the increased risk of aspiration and prolonged stooling

Question

During the gastric lavage, the ideal position for Nancy would be: (Choose one answer.)

1. Prone, in a head-down position to avoid aspiration
2. A left lateral decubitus Trendelenburg position to facilitate gastric emptying and protect against aspiration
3. The position of comfort of her choice to facilitate her cooperation with the procedure
4. A supine position with the head of the bed slightly elevated

Answer

The correct answer is (2); the left lateral decubitus Trendelenburg position maximizes the exposure of the gastric contents to the tube and decreases the risk of aspiration if the patient should vomit (see Figure 4.2). The left lateral position also minimizes passive gastric emptying into the duodenum.[9,15] However, the actual position in which a child is maintained will probably be determined by several factors including the cooperativeness of the child, the severity of the poison, the degree of mental alertness, and the presence of respiratory distress.

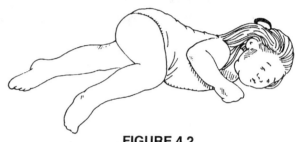

FIGURE 4.2

When you have lavaged Nancy for a few minutes, you reassess her vital signs and note the following:

Blood pressure	86/54 mmHg
Pulse	162 beats/min with irregularities
Respiratory rate	20/min

The cardiac monitor is showing sinus tachycardia. Nancy remains unresponsive to verbal stimulation at this time but does moan in response to the procedure.

Question

Assign a number from **1** to **4** to prioritize the following nursing interventions during the lavage procedure. (Mark the first priority **1**, etc.)

_____   Accurate measurement of intake and output

_____   Assure that properly functioning airway suctioning equipment is immediately available

_____   Monitor Nancy for signs of gastric distention

_____   Monitor Nancy for increasing cardiac dysrhythmias or changes in mental status

Answer

The correct priority for your nursing interventions would be as follows: (4), (1), (3), and (2), respectively.

The most important nursing responsibility during the lavage is to protect the airway to assure that Nancy does not aspirate. Suction equipment should always be readily available for immediate use as necessary.

Once the patency of the airway and adequacy of ventilation are assured, the next most important responsibility would be to monitor for increasing cardiac rhythm disturbances, especially of concern with tricyclic antidepressant ingestions, and to continue to evaluate for changes in Nancy's mental status.

Gastric distention can affect respiratory tidal volume in small children, so the size of the child's abdomen should be carefully observed, along with serial evaluation of the *ABCs*, to prevent hypoxemia.

Accurately measuring intake and output is always important with critically ill infants and small children. In this case, however, it is the least important among the interventions listed.

Nancy tolerates the gastric lavage procedure well and the solution returns clear after a total of 1600 mL. You continue the lavage with an additional 100 mL of saline, and then clamp the orogastric tube and reassess Nancy's vital signs.

Blood pressure	84/50
Respiratory rate	22 breaths/min and regular
Heart rate	Sinus tachycardia, 160–180 beats/min

Though she is not fully awake or alert, Nancy seems to be somewhat more responsive to verbal stimulation than she was earlier. Dr. Martin decides he will proceed with administering activated charcoal.

Remembering Nancy's family in the waiting room, you stop by there briefly. Nancy's mother and grandmother both seem very subdued, but they thank you for updating them on Nancy's progress. You tell them you'll come for them as soon as they can see Nancy.

Question

Indicate whether the following statements regarding the use of activated charcoal are True or False.

_____ The charcoal should be administered rapidly to Nancy to prevent her from vomiting.

_____ In pediatric ingestions, it will only be necessary to administer a single dose of the charcoal.

_____ You would never insert a nasogastric tube to administer charcoal in an alert but resistive child.

_____ If an alert child is resistant to taking the charcoal orally, you may need to restrain him or her to get them to drink the solutions.

_____ Placing the charcoal in an opaque-covered container and having the child drink it through a straw may facilitate administration to an alert child.

Answer

The correct answers are False for all except the last statement, which is True.

Refer to Table 4.11 (following page) for tips on the administration of charcoal to the pediatric patient.

Question

Mark each of the following substances as acceptable (**A**) or unacceptable, (**U**) to disguise activated charcoal's taste.

_____ Jam, jelly, or cocoa powder

_____ Chocolate or cherry syrup

_____ Milk, ice cream, or sherbet

_____ Sucrose, sorbitol, or cola

Answer

The correct answers are **U, A, U,** and **A,** respectively.

Jam, jelly, cocoa powder, milk, ice cream, and sherbet should not be used because they decrease the absorption of the charcoal.[10,15] The other substances (chocolate or cherry syrup, sucrose, sorbitol, or cola) are acceptable to help disguise the taste of activated charcoal.

Nancy is given a 20-g dose of activated charcoal through the orogastric tube, and the tube is then re-clamped. You reassess her vital signs and find that she is less tachypneic, and her heart rate has decreased to 150 beats/min.

Nancy appears to be more alert, and when you bring her mother and grandmother into the room, she opens her eyes at the sound of her mother's voice. Dr. Martin informs them that Nancy will receive a dose of magnesium citrate and then be transferred to the intensive care unit to be observed for complications.

TABLE 4.11. Administration of Charcoal to Pediatric Patients

Activated charcoal may be administered in a single dose (following gastric emptying) for many ingested poisons *or* in repeated doses every 2–4 hr ("pulse dosing") for sustained-release drugs and those excreted by the liver.[4]
Administer charcoal orally or per nasogastric/orogastric tube if the child is not fully alert or is extremely uncooperative.[12]
If used following induced emesis, wait 30–60 min before administering charcoal.[8]
Always administer charcoal slowly, either orally or per nasogastric/orogastric tube, to reduce the risk of vomiting associated with rapid administration.[12]
Never restrain a resistant child to administer charcoal orally because of the increased risk of aspiration.[12]
Place the charcoal mixture in an opaque container with a lid and administer through a straw to facilitate cooperation from an alert child.[11]
When attempting to administer charcoal orally to an alert child, set a definite period for the child to finish drinking the solution.[14]
For oral administration, flavorings can be used to disguise the charcoal's taste and texture, but care must be taken not to use substances that will delay absorption.[15]
Use of new, premixed preparations of charcoal and sorbitol eliminate the need for cathartics but are **not** recommended in pediatric patients if multiple doses of charcoal are indicated.[4,14]

Question

The magnesium citrate is being given to: (Choose one answer.)

1. Ensure that the activated charcoal does not cause Nancy a gastrointestinal obstruction
2. Correct Nancy's fluid and electrolyte status
3. Decrease gastrointestinal transit time and speed evacuation of the charcoal and bound toxin
4. Decrease gastrointestinal irritation secondary to the lavage and charcoal administration

Answer

The correct answer is (3). Cathartics are of questionable value but are generally used following charcoal administration to shorten gastrointestinal transit time for the charcoal-bound toxin and enhance elimination of ingested poisons.[3,4] Irritant or oil cathartics are not recommended for use in children because of the increased risk of aspiration. They may also decrease the effectiveness of the charcoal or result in prolonged stooling.[3,14,15] Commonly used cathartics are listed in Table 4.12.

TABLE 4.12. Common Pediatric Cathartics and Usual Dosages[3,4,14,15]

Cathartic	Dosage
Magnesium citrate	4–5 mL/kg
Magnesium sulfate	250 mg/kg
Sodium sulfate	250 mg/kg
Sorbital	1 mg/kg–75% solution

Nancy's vital signs and neurologic status have now been stabilized, and she is ready to be discharged from the emergency department to the intensive care unit for 48 hours of cardiac monitoring. As the family prepares to accompany Nancy, the grandmother begins crying and says, "I feel so bad about what happened. It has been a long time since I have had young children around, and I forgot how they get into things." Nancy's mother tries to reassure her, and you decide to take a moment to talk with them.

Question

Would this be an appropriate moment to discuss safety issues with Nancy's grandmother and her mother? (Choose one answer.)

_____ Yes _____ No

Answer

The correct answer is Yes. Although some consideration must be given to the amount of guilt and anxiety being experienced, an accidental ingestion usually makes family members receptive to counseling in poison prevention. This is particularly true in incidents where the children have suffered only mild to moderate symptoms.[19]

Appropriate topics for Nancy's grandmother might include but are not limited to[8]

- Child-proof containers and safe keeping of all medicines
- Use of child-resistant locks on cupboards, especially on lower cabinets
- Safe storage of toxic household products: cleaning agents, pesticides, chemicals, and veterinary medications
- Posting of numbers and location of nearest Poison Control Center near all household phones
- Toxic plants hung or placed on high surfaces
- More careful supervision of young children in "high-risk" environments such as farm buildings, homes of elderly persons, sites with accessible alcohol and recreational drugs

Because of the highly stressful nature of Nancy's accidental poisoning, you include written information about poison prevention with the verbal discharge instructions. You encourage Nancy's family to call if they have any questions. Nancy's grandmother thanks you and joins her daughter as Nancy is taken to the intensive care unit.

CASE STUDY 2 OBJECTIVES

On completion of this case study, you will be able to

- Recognize the significance of pediatric temperature variations as a triage parameter in children
- Recognize three common characteristics of a febrile seizure
- Select at least one appropriate nursing diagnosis for a child experiencing a febrile seizure
- Identify the proper dose, route, and infusion time for administration of diazepam to the pediatric patient
- List two pertinent nursing assessments during a seizure
- State the risk factors for a child's developing epilepsy after experiencing febrile seizures
- Discuss nursing interventions for parental anxiety and knowledge deficits regarding acute pediatric seizure activity

CASE STUDY 2

Timmy Feels Really Warm

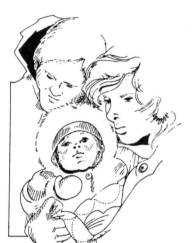

On a cold autumn evening at about 8:00 P.M., a young couple suddenly enters the emergency department (see Figure 4.3). The woman is carrying a sleeping toddler wearing a snowsuit and wrapped snugly in a woolen blanket. As you approach the couple and the baby, the mother implores, "Please check our baby. He's been sick with a cold since yesterday, and he feels so hot tonight. He doesn't want to eat anything and is so sleepy. This just isn't like Timmy!" You introduce yourself, and you find out that the child is 18-month-old Timmy Lee. He is the young couple's only child.

As soon as you touch Timmy, you feel how hot he is. You remove the blanket and snowsuit. Timmy arouses slightly, whimpers, and opens his eyes for a few seconds while you are undressing him. He appears uninterested in his surroundings and does not resist you handling him. When you ask about his weight, the mother answers

FIGURE 4.3

that Timmy weighs 24 lb. As you remove his snowsuit, you see that his skin color is flushed. His respirations are 28/min, but his breathing is not labored. His brachial pulse is strong and regular at about 124 beats/min, and his capillary refill is less than 2 seconds.

Question

What additional information do you need to triage Timmy properly? (Choose one answer.)

1. Complete history
2. Temperature
3. Blood pressure
4. Immunization status

Answer

The correct answer is (2); Timmy feels hot to touch, but this initial impression needs to be validated by core temperature measurement. Significant temperature variations, either hypothermia or hyperthermia, should be taken into consideration during pediatric triage. Either fever or hypothermia may be indicative of illness.

Timmy's *ABC*s appear stable, and you have made a general assessment of his neurologic status. You take his temperature rectally and find that it is 103°F (39.4°C). His mother didn't have a thermometer at home, but Mr. Lee says he gave Timmy a dose of Tylenol Drops (120 mg of acetaminophen) about 2 hours ago because "he felt hot and was so irritable." Mrs. Lee also states that "the Tylenol doesn't seem to have had any effect at all."

TRIAGE DECISION

Based on this additional information and your initial assessment, how would you triage Timmy?

Emergent. A life-threatening situation in need of immediate intervention.

Urgent. Patient needs care within 1 hour to prevent further deterioration.

Nonurgent. Patient is able to wait more than 1 hour without further deterioration.

TRIAGE DECISION ANSWER

The correct answer is urgent. Timmy's airway is clear, and his breathing and pulse are within the normal range for his age. His temperature, however, is significantly elevated despite his having received antipyretic medication. His mental status may be altered, indicated by his irritability and lack of responsiveness to a strange environment. While not in an immediately life-threatening condition, he should be evaluated promptly.

You take Timmy and his mother and father to a treatment room, and notify the emergency physician. You direct Mr. Lee to the registration area and tell him he can join you when he has completed Timmy's registration. You obtain a thorough history from Timmy's mother while she undresses the toddler for his physical examination. You note that Timmy's diaper is dry when removed. Mrs. Lee worries that Timmy will become chilled if he is completely undressed.

Question

How would you answer Timmy's mother regarding her concerns about "chilling"? (Choose one answer.)

1. "We always undress our patients completely so that the physician can examine them."
2. "You're correct. Here is a warm blanket to put on him."
3. "Timmy's temperature is 103 degrees. We need to begin cooling him off a little and removing his clothes is a good first step."
4. "We need to cool Timmy off because this high a fever is very dangerous."

Answer

Answer (3) is correct. Explain to Timmy's mother what you are doing but make sure you monitor her reaction—it will not help to alarm her unnecessarily. Although parents should be aware that fevers may indicate serious illness, they also should know that high fevers in young children are common and learn how to care for them.[1,2]

You begin your secondary survey on Timmy and complete a more in-depth history using the mnemonic **AMPLE**.

The information you obtain includes:

Allergies. Timmy has no known allergies.

Medications. He takes no regular medications. Timmy received one appropriate dose of children's Tylenol approximately 2 hours before arrival.

Previous history of illness. Timmy was a healthy full-term infant, and his growth and development are normal for his age. He has been healthy, with no previous hospitalizations and only one upper-respiratory infection at age 5 months. He sees his pediatrician for regular checkups, and his immunizations are up to date.

Last meal (time and contents). Timmy ate fairly well yesterday with normal fluid intake. He ate some cereal this morning, a few bites of banana in the early afternoon, but has taken only apple juice and a fruit-flavored drink since approximately 4 P.M.

Events preceding incident. Timmy's runny nose started yesterday. Today he has been lethargic and irritable when awake. He has "felt warm" for about 12 hours, but hasn't had vomiting or diarrhea. His last wet diaper was at 5 P.M. today.

Dr. James enters the room, quickly reviews the history and begins to examine Timmy. Once Dr. James completes auscultation of Timmy's heart and lungs he begins to look in the child's ears with an otoscope. Timmy's body suddenly stiffens, his eyes appear glazed, and his extremities begin to twitch and shake.

Question

The most likely explanation for the sudden changes in Timmy's immediate status is: (Choose one answer.)

1. He doesn't like a speculum in his ear.
2. He is having a febrile seizure.
3. He has meningeal irritability causing this motor movement.
4. He has become chilled and is now cold and shivering.

Answer

Because Timmy has had an acute onset of fever with a negative history for previous seizures or neurologic problems, a febrile seizure may be what he is having. However, a thorough clinical evaluation must still be performed by the physician to rule out meningitis as an etiology for the fever and the seizure. Common causes of seizures in children are listed in Table 4.13.

TABLE 4.13.   Etiology of Pediatric Seizures[3,4]

Simple febrile seizures
Traumatic head injuries
Nontraumatic increased intracranial pressure
Central nervous system infections, congenital disorders, or tumors
Ingestions or toxic exposures
Anoxia
Fluid and electrolyte imbalances
Metabolic disorders
Idiopathic epilepsy

Question

Which of the following characteristics make Timmy's seizure likely to be febrile in nature? (Choose one answer.)

1. His age
2. Fever of less than 12 hr of duration
3. Prior medical history negative for neurologic disease or injury
4. All of the above

Answer

The correct answer is (4); Timmy's age, onset of fever, and previous medical history are all suggestive of a febrile seizure. The common characteristics associated with febrile seizures are summarized in Table 4.14.

TABLE 4.14. Characteristics of Simple Febrile Seizures[3]

Seizures usually occur between 3 months and 5 years of age.
Seizures are associated with acute fever of less than 24 hr of duration
There is no history of neurologic problems or nonfebrile seizures.
There is no evidence of intracranial injury or central nervous system disease.
The seizures are usually nonfocal in nature.
Seizure activity is typically less than 15 min of duration.
The family history is positive for febrile seizures but negative for nonfebrile seizures.

You glance at the treatment room clock and note that it has been less than 45 seconds since the onset of Timmy's seizure activity. At present, his neck appears hyperextended, and he is continuing to have twitching in all of his extremities. His skin color is no longer flushed, and his face appears pale. His respirations are regular but shallow.

Question

The most appropriate nursing diagnosis for Timmy at this time is: (Choose one answer.)

1. Noncompliance with medical regimen, related to seizure medications
2. Neurologic status, impaired, related to increased intracranial pressure
3. Fluid volume deficit, related to hyperthermia
4. Potential for injury, related to seizure activity

Answer

The most appropriate nursing diagnosis at this time is (4); your immediate interventions need to be directed toward protecting Timmy from injury during the seizure (see Table 4.15, following page).

You make sure his airway is open and put blankets on the side rails to protect him from injury. You realize you will have to document his condition, and you watch him carefully.

Question

List any three points about Timmy's seizure you need to carefully observe and describe in your nursing assessment. (Fill in the blanks.)

1. _____

2. _____

3. _____

TABLE 4.15.   Nursing Care Priorities: The Seizing Child[5]

1. Ensure a patent airway
    a. Position on side, if possible, for airway protection
    b. Prepare to suction if necessary
    c. Insert oropharyngeal airway if possible but avoid placing potentially occlusive objects into the mouth (i.e., padded tongue blades)

2. Provide supplemental oxygen

3. Protect from physical injury
    a. Do **not** restrain
    b. If necessary, remove patient from immediately dangerous environment (i.e., away from striking furniture, etc.)
    c. Loosen restrictive clothing

4. Continuous monitoring during seizure and postictal phases
    a. Observation of seizure activity
    b. Mental status
    c. Vital signs
    d. Injuries secondary to seizure

5. Prepare to administer anticonvulsant drugs if seizure duration is greater than 15 min or if airway becomes compromised
    a. Prepare to start an IV line
    b. Determine accurate pediatric dose of anticonvulsants
    c. Administer anticonvulsants if required

Answer

Correct answers could include any of the points listed in Table 4.16 (facing page).

As you glance up from monitoring Timmy, you realize that his parents have stayed in the room. They are clinging to each other as they watch their child. They appear shocked at what they are witnessing as Dr. James advises them that Timmy is having a febrile seizure. Mrs. Lee says, "It's all my fault, I should have taken him to the doctor this morning. Is he going to die?" You and Dr. James reassure her that Timmy is not going to die.

Question

As Timmy's parents are obviously very frightened by the seizure activity, should they be told to leave the room immediately? (Choose Yes or No.)

_____ Yes   _____ No

Answer

The correct answer is No. Although this depends on the policy in your hospital, if the parents do not physically interfere with the care of the child and do not appear anxious to leave, they may be allowed to stay in the room.

If the emergency department physician and nurse work well as a team and can explain what is happening, the parents' anxiety will be decreased. Ideally another emergency department staff member, such as a social worker, could be called in to stay close to the parents and offer support. The parents may also need to be reassured that the child is not in pain. Talking to the parents calmly while the seizure is running its course can help decrease their anxiety, but you should be careful not to overwhelm them with extensive explanations at this time.[8,9]

The physician tells you he would like an intravenous line started right away, and that he will stay with Timmy while you set up. As you gather your equipment you also sign out some diazepam because you know that it is on your seizure protocol, and it is what is usually ordered for seizures.

TABLE 4.16. Assessment Parameters for Seizure Activity[6,7]

Time	Initial onset of seizure activity	Mental status	Total loss of consciousness.
	Duration of each phase of seizure		Other changes in mental status
	Total duration of seizure		Duration of changes
			Postictal status
Movement	Part of body affected first	Pupils	Size
	Progression to other body parts	Behavior	Equality
	Type	Elimination	Automatisms
	Spastic		Bizarre behavior
	Tonic		Postictal status
	Tremors		Incontinence
	Postseizure tone		Bowel
	Flaccid		Bladder
	Hypertonic		
	Lack of movement in any body part		
Respiratory status	Airway patency	Oral condition	Presence of loose teeth or dentures
	Respiratory effort		Postictal condition
	Apnea		Tongue
	Presence		Mucous membranes
	Duration		Presence of bloody saliva or sputum
	Secretions		
	Amount		
	Color		
	Need for suctioning		

Question

What two other medications are often ordered for seizures in children? (Fill in the blanks.)

1._____   2._____

Answer

Lorazepam, phenytoin, and phenobarbital are some of the most commonly ordered medications. Lorazepam is often recommended because it has a much longer half-life than diazepam. Phenytoin and phenobarbital have a longer onset of action (20 minutes), so they are most often used to prevent recurrence or for status epilepticus.

TABLE 4.17.   Pediatric Anticonvulsant Therapy[10]

Drug	Recommended Dose (mg/kg)	Administration Route and Rate	Comments
Diazepam (Valium)	0.25 mg/kg	IV push: 1 mg/min	Onset of action within seconds; half-life = 20 min; may repeat dose every 5–15 min to a maximum initial dose of 10 mg
Lorazepam (Ativan)	0.05–0.1 mg/kg	IV push: 1 mg/min	Onset of action within seconds; half-life = 9 hr; may repeat dose every 5–15 min to a maximum initial dose of 4 mg
Phenobarbital	10–20 mg/kg	**SLOW** IV push: *not to exceed 1 mg/kg/min*	Onset in 20 min; half-life = 48 hr; may repeat low initial dose in 20 min; maximum initial dose = 300 mg
Phenytoin (Dilantin)	10–20 mg/kg	**SLOW** IV push: *not to exceed 1 mg/kg/min or 50 mg/min*	Onset in 20 min; half-life = 48 hr; may repeat low initial dose in 20 min; maximum initial dose = 1,000 mg

Caution: Large doses of any of these medications, as well as combinations of any of them, may precipitate respiratory distress.

As you quickly bring the intravenous setup and the medication into the room, Dr. James advises you that the seizure has stopped, and he does not want to give any medication right now. You observe that Timmy appears more relaxed in muscle tone and is asleep. Dr. James tells the parents that the seizure activity appears to have subsided spontaneously for now. He asks you to keep the anticonvulsant therapy nearby in case it is needed later and to monitor Timmy closely during this postictal stage. He also orders an acetaminophen suppository to lower Timmy's temperature.

Timmy's parents move closer to the child's bedside and begin to stroke his hair. Both appear a little less anxious now that Timmy is sleeping, but they are still obviously shaken by what has happened. Mr. Lee hesitantly asks you, "Aren't you going to give him any medication to keep him from having another seizure?" You reinforce Dr. James's message that Timmy's seizure was probably from his fever and that febrile seizures rarely require pharmacologic treatment.

Question

It seems apparent that the seizure is a febrile seizure, so Timmy will probably be discharged without further examination. (Choose True or False.)

_____ True   _____ False

Answer

The answer is False; there are still two questions that should be asked about all children presenting with seizures.

1. Does the child have a central nervous system infection or other severe underlying disease that must be promptly diagnosed and treated?
2. Is the child at risk for recurrent seizures or epilepsy? If so, what diagnosis and therapeutic interventions must be done before the child leaves the emergency department?[11]

TABLE 4.18. Risk Factors for Epilepsy[8]

Neurologic or developmental abnormality before seizure
Initial febrile seizure is focal or multiple in nature or greater than 15 min of duration
History of nonfebrile seizures in one or both parents

After 2 more hours of monitoring in the emergency department, Timmy has not experienced any further seizure activity, and is awake and fully alert. His fever has decreased to 100.8°F (38.2°C), and he appears less irritable. Timmy is appropriately fearful when strangers approach him, although he is enjoying the popsicle you gave him.

On completion of Timmy's physical examination and diagnostic tests, Dr. James has determined that Timmy has bilateral otitis media. You give Timmy his first dose of antibiotics, and Dr. James gives the parents a prescription for home antibiotics. Dr. James does not order any seizure prophylaxis and is ready to discharge Timmy. You start the discharge paperwork and get ready to begin your discharge teaching.

Question

Timmy's parents should be instructed that febrile seizures will occur only once in the lifetime of a child who does not have epilepsy. (Choose True or False.)

_____ True _____ False

Answer

The correct answer is False; approximately 30% of children experiencing a simple febrile seizure will have recurrent febrile seizures. However, febrile seizures are generally benign and are not associated with deleterious educational or behavioral effects.[4]

Question

Even though his febrile seizure is probably benign, Timmy's parents should be taught first aid for a seizure and how to seek emergency assistance if necessary. (Choose True or False.)

_____ True _____ False

Answer

The correct answer is True; counseling the anxious parent is an important aspect in the management of simple febrile seizures. Parents need to know how to react calmly to seizure activity to

1. Protect the airway
2. Protect the child from physical injury
3. Observe the onset, duration, and postictal states
4. Obtain emergency assistance if necessary[12]

In addition, your discharge instructions will need to include proper fever control measures and information about antibiotic therapy and follow-up care for Timmy's ear infection.

The Lees look tired but seem very relieved to be able to take their child home with them. A very wide-awake Timmy is actively trying to get out of his father's arms, and Mrs. Lee carefully carries the instructions you have given her. The Lees thank you and ask you to thank Dr. James for them.

CASE STUDY 3 OBJECTIVES

On completion of this case study, you will be able to

- Identify appropriate activities for conducting the neurologic assessment of the pediatric patient with a given type of head injury
- Evaluate the significance of changes in the Glasgow Coma Scale for a pediatric patient with a head injury
- List five neurologic signs for continuing assessment in a head-injured child
- Describe the clinical significance of two types of skull fractures commonly associated with pediatric head injuries
- Differentiate pediatric clinical manifestations as early or late signs of increased intracranial pressure
- Identify an appropriate nursing diagnosis based on the assessment of the head-injured child
- Discuss the rationale for hyperventilation in the management of increased intracranial pressure in children
- Identify desired metabolic and respiratory parameters for patients treated with hyperventilation
- Prioritize three nursing interventions associated with the care of a head-injured child
- Identify appropriate nursing responsibilities in administering osmotic diuretics to a head-injured child
- Identify appropriate nursing interventions for dealing with parental concerns and educational needs with respect to their child's health

CASE STUDY 3

Danny's Baseball Game

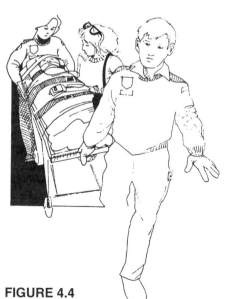

The voice on your emergency department base radio crackles, "We are en route to your facility with an 8-year-old male child who was hit on the right side of the head with a baseball bat. He was unconscious when we arrived, but he is now awake, crying, and restless. His vital signs are blood pressure, 106 (palpated); pulse, 108 and regular; respiratory rate, 16 with no apparent distress. He is immobilized on a backboard, and there is no bleeding. We have started an IV in his left antecubital fossa. Our estimated time of arrival is about 5 minutes."

On arrival of the ambulance, you observe a dark-haired, well-developed white male child dressed in blue jeans and a red T-shirt. His mother, who tells you his name is Danny Coffey, is walking beside the stretcher saying, "It's OK, Danny. You're going to be all right now." In your initial rapid assessment you see that Danny's eyes are closed, his breathing appears adequate, and his color is pink. He flinches occasionally, is moving both legs restlessly, and

FIGURE 4.4

does not seem to be comforted by his mother's efforts to calm him. He is getting oxygen by nasal cannula at 3 L/min, and his IV line is running at a keep-open rate (see Figure 4.4).

TRIAGE DECISION

Based on your initial observations, how would you triage Danny?

Emergent.   A life-threatening situation in need of immediate intervention.

Urgent.   Patient needs care within 1 hour to prevent further deterioration.

Nonurgent.   Patient is able to wait more than 1 hour without further deterioration.

TRIAGE DECISION ANSWER

Emergent is the correct answer. Danny has experienced, by reliable history, a significant head injury with a period of unconsciousness. He continues to show altered mental status. Danny should not wait for further assessment and treatment as he needs to be promptly evaluated and continuously monitored.

A child with head trauma may have received a variety of brain insults, in a variety of locations and with varying degrees of severity. These include contusions, lacerations, damage to the meninges, scalp and skull, and even brain stem infarcts. In addition to these "primary" injuries, further neurologic damage can occur secondary to hypoxia, ischemia from either hypotension or increased intracranial pressure, or metabolic derangements. One of the most significant roles in the initial care of pediatric head injury victims, is to be aware of the risks and prevent these secondary insults.[1]

Danny is moved to the trauma room where he can receive constant monitoring. You enter the room, reattach the oxygen, increasing the flow to 4 L/min and begin your more thorough, systematic trauma assessment.

Question

The initial approach for assessing pediatric trauma victims differs significantly from that used for adults. (Choose True or False.)

_____ True   _____ False

Answer

The correct answer is False. The same method of primary and secondary examination used for adults can be systematically thorough and effective in assessing pediatric trauma victims. An excellent, easy-to-follow method is the *ABCDE* Primary Assessment (see Table 4.19).

TABLE 4.19.   *ABCDE* Primary Assessment[2]

Airway	Airway patency with cervical spine control
Breathing	Adequacy of ventilation
Circulation	Adequacy of perfusion
Disability	Initial neurologic screening
Exposure	Environmental screening Hypothermia control

Question

From the data you have already obtained, have you completed Danny's primary assessment? (Choose Yes or No.)

_____ Yes   _____ No

Answer

The correct answer is No. Danny's *ABC*s appear adequate. For *D* (disability), a brief neurologic assessment needs to be completed. Because of the witnessed isolated head injury without any other obvious injury, it is not necessary to cut off Danny's clothes for further exposure (*E*) at this time.

You continue to monitor Danny's *ABC*s and quickly initiate the neurologic examination with the AVPU assessment. You note that he is not alert but responds by opening his eyes slightly and moving restlessly when you call his name loudly.

Question

Which of the following would be most useful as part of Danny's primary neurologic assessment? (Choose one answer.)

1. Deep tendon reflexes

2. Glasgow Coma Scale

3. Cranial nerve assessment

4. Radiologic evaluation for skull fractures

Answer

The correct answer is (2); the Glasgow Coma Scale is a more precise method for assessing mental status used in many trauma centers. The Glasgow Coma Scale has been widely used in adults with a high degree of consistency among different examiners. Therefore, it is valuable in establishing baseline neurologic status and then for serial monitoring of the patient.[3] Because Danny is 8 years old and has good cognitive and verbal skills, the Glasgow Coma Scale can be used to evaluate him (see Table 4.3).

As you continue to assess Danny you note that he opens his eyes when his mother speaks to him loudly but does not move his arm when you ask him to do so. When his mother asks him to move his leg, however, he moves it back and forth. He will only give you his name after being asked several times, even with his mother's prodding.

Question

What is Danny's current Glasgow Coma Scale Score? (Fill in the blank.)

_____ Glasgow Coma Scale Score

Answer

The correct score is 13, calculated as follows:

Eye opening	Opens eyes to speech	= 3
Best verbal response	Confused (can't give name)	= 4
Best motor response	Obeys commands (he moves his legs for his mother)	= 6
Total score		**13**

When scoring the Glasgow Coma Scale, factors such as fear, anxiety, a strange environment, and guilt must be considered. This is especially true in children whose behavioral responses reflect their emotions. They may keep their eyes closed because they are frightened or retreat from stressful situations by sleeping. Children who are sound asleep may be difficult to arouse and may appear confused, irritable, and disoriented. Many times they will fall back to sleep quickly if awakened from a sound sleep.[5]

Danny's mother continues to comfort him as you complete your initial assessment. You find that Danny's pupils are normal size, equal, and both react to light and accommodation. Dr. Clark enters the room as you complete Danny's latest set of vital signs.

Blood Pressure	96/68
Pulse	120 beats/min
Respiratory rate	20 breaths/min

Dr. Clark completes his secondary survey and determines that there are no other obvious injuries except for the head injury. He orders a complete blood count, electrolytes, arterial blood gases, and serum glucose level. Dr. Clark also points out the large contusion in the right temporal area of Danny's scalp. Danny cries out and attempts to push away the physician's hand when this area is palpated. Dr. Clark tells Danny's mother that he suspects Danny may have a possible skull fracture. He asks you to call radiology and prepare Danny for X-ray films.

The first radiologic examination Dr. Clark orders is a cross-table lateral cervical spine X-ray film to rule out cervical spine injury. Because Danny had such a forceful injury to his head, it is possible he has a cervical spine injury, even though this type of injury is seen much less frequently in children than in adults.[2] Once this has been cleared by the radiologist, Danny will have skull X-ray films.

Question

Which type of skull fracture would be most likely in a child with Danny's history of a forceful blow to the temporal region of the head? (Choose one answer.)

1. Depressed
2. Linear
3. Diastatic
4. Compound

Answer

A linear skull fracture would be most likely in a child with this presenting history. Approximately 75% of all skull fractures seen in pediatric patients are linear skull fractures.[6] The location of the linear fracture is of particular importance. Fractures across vascular arterial grooves under the surface of the skull have significance because of potential bleeding from the associated blood vessels.[6,7] Table 4.20 summarizes the major types of skull fractures seen in pediatric patients.

TABLE 4.20. Pediatric Skull Fractures

Type and Description	Significance
Linear Resembles a simple crack in the skull and usually extends over the cranial vault	• Most common pediatric skull fracture • May be asymptomatic or present with swelling or tenderness over the site • Most heal spontaneously, but management must include treatment of underlying hemorrhage or brain injury
Depressed May be open or closed; usually palpable; significant if the skull is depressed more than 5 mm[6]	• Relatively uncommon in children < 3 years because of soft, malleable skull bones • Concern is for damage to underlying tissue especially with depressions > 5 mm or the thickness of the skull[2]
Diastatic Traumatic separations of the cranial bones at suture sites, usually the lambdoid	• Most common in children < 4 years • Usual cause is sizable blunt trauma; no specific therapy except monitoring for epidural hemorrhage[6]
Compound Direct communication between the scalp and the cerebral contents; (usually involves a scalp laceration with depressed fracture)	• Requires immediate surgical intervention and antibiotic and tetanus prophylaxis[6]

Basilar
Occurs at the base of the skull, especially anterior and middle fossae
May include fractures of the nasal and aural passages (frontal, ethmoid, sphenoid, temporal, or occipital bones)
	• Diagnosis usually per clinical signs
	  – "Raccoon eyes" (periorbital bruising)
	  – Cranial nerve palsies
	  – Hemotympanum
	  – "Battle's sign" (postauricular bruises)
	  – Cerebrospinal fluid
	  – Bloody rhinorrhea or otorrhea
	• May result in meningeal tears and associated meningitis[6]

Dr. Clark completes Danny's physical examination. He finds no evidence of a palpable skull fracture, no tenderness of the neck or spine, no cerebrospinal fluid or bloody drainage from Danny's nose or ears, and no postauricular or periorbital bruising. In addition he notes that Danny appears to have full sensory and motor function in all four extremities. Radiology reports that the cervical spine X-ray films are negative. Dr. Clark states that you may now remove the cervical immobilization device and reposition Danny.

Question

With cervical spine injury ruled out and diagnosis of a traumatic head injury, how would Danny be best positioned? (Choose one answer.)

1. Slight Trendelenburg
2. Flat on his back
3. On his left side with his head lower than his body
4. Head elevated 30° and positioned midline

Answer

The correct answer is (4); Danny would be best positioned with his head elevated 30° and positioned midline (see Figure 4.5). Maintaining the head and neck in a midline position facilitates venous drainage thus decreasing intracranial pressure.[8] Turning the neck too far to one side may compromise the jugular venous drainage causing increases in intracranial pressure.[7]

Keeping Danny flat on his back or in Trendelenburg position could result in increased intracranial pressure as a result of venous flow by gravity, so these answers are not correct.

Keeping a patient on his left side is often recommended when there is danger of vomiting but is not appropriate in this case.

Patient-initiated activities such as flexion of the extremities, flexion/rotation of the neck, and coughing have all been found to result in elevation of the intracranial pressure. Minimizing these as much as possible is also important with head-injured patients.[9]

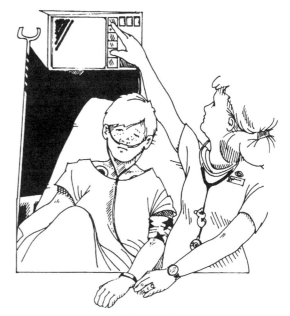

FIGURE 4.5

Dr. Clark orders a computed tomographic (CT) scan of the head to be completed as soon as possible. The radiology department indicates that there will be a wait of 20 to 30 minutes before the CT scan can be completed.

Question

Since the CT scan is not immediately available for Danny, would a skull film series be sufficient? (Choose Yes or No.)

_____ Yes　　　　　_____ No

Answer

The correct answer is No. Pediatric skull fractures are usually associated with significant traumatic force, but diagnosis of the bone fracture itself through radiographs does not necessarily correlate with the presence or absence of intracranial injury.

When intracranial injuries are suspected, the diagnostic study of choice is a CT scan. Because the results of skull films do not influence the initial resuscitation of severe head injuries, routine films are generally postponed until these patients are stabilized, and the CT is completed.[1,2]

In instances in which significant intracranial injury is suspected and CT scan is not available, consideration should be given to transferring the patient to a definitive care facility as soon as possible after stabilization. Table 4.21 (see following page) lists the indications for CT scans versus skull films in pediatric head injuries.

While waiting for the CT scan, you notice that Danny seems less responsive to his mother and his surroundings. You now find that Danny will not open his eyes to anything except painful stimuli. He withdraws his extremities from a painful stimulus but mumbles the word "no" at random. This is the only sound he makes. He does not respond at all to either his mother's voice or her touch. His latest vital signs are

Blood Pressure   98/70
Pulse   124 beats/min
Respiratory rate   22 breaths/min

You recalculate Danny's Glasgow Coma Score and note that it has decreased from 13 to 9 points.

TABLE 4.21. Clinical Indications for Radiologic Studies in Pediatric Head Injuries

Indications for CT Scan[2]
Altered level of consciousness
Seizures
Focal neurologic deficits
Depressed skull fractures
Compound skull fractures
Progressively worsening vomiting
Full fontanelle

Indications for skull film[1]
Obvious skull defects
Possible intracranial foreign body
Significant soft-tissue injury
Significant history of severe trauma
Sign of basilar skull fracture
Presence of cerebrospinal fluid leak

Question

Is this change in Danny's Glascow Coma Scale score significant? (Choose Yes or No.)

_____ Yes   _____ No

Answer

The correct answer is Yes; this score change demonstrates that Danny's condition is deteriorating, and he needs immediate critical intervention. Scores on the Glasgow Coma Scale ranging from 13 to 15 points are generally indicative of mild head injury, scores of 8 to 12 points are indicative of moderate injury, and scores of < 7 points are associated with severe disability.[1]

Note: A drop of 3 or more points from the baseline Glasgow Coma Score is usually an indication for immediate neurosurgical intervention if shock is not the cause of the decreased level of consciousness.[7]

You are concerned about his decrease in level of consciousness. Danny shows no evidence of an alteration in cardiac output, and his vital signs and capillary refill have remained within normal limits. If he were hypotensive, however, you would have to look for a source of hemorrhage, because a child cannot lose sufficient blood into the subgaleal or epidural space to become hypotensive.[1,2]

Question

Danny's deteriorating mental status following a head injury may be related to increased intracranial pressure. In addition to the Glasgow Coma Score, list three other parameters of a neurologic assessment that should be evaluated in Danny. (Fill in the blanks.)

1. _____

2. _____

3. _____

Answer

Additional neurologic parameters that should be assessed are[10]

1. Pupillary response
2. Ocular movements
3. Sensory function
4. Vital signs, particularly the respiratory pattern

It is important to remember that in young children, epicanthal folds are more prominent, and may give the impression that one eye is deviating inward or outward, so eyes should be assessed while the child is looking directly at you with eyes in midline (see Figure 4.6 and Table 4.22).

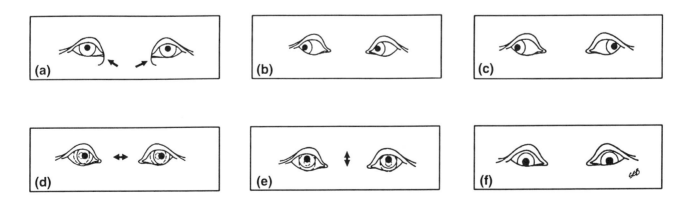

Figure 4.6 (a) Epicanthal folds—normal pupillary response. (b) Tonic gaze. (c) Dysconjugate gaze. (d) Horizontal nystagmus. (e) Vertical nystagmus. (f) Setting sun sign. (Courtesy of PRESEP, Robert Wood Johnson Foundation.)

TABLE 4.22. Abnormal Eye Movements

Tonic gaze	Eyes will deviate from the side where there is an irritating cerebral lesion, and when the lesion is in the pons or below. If the lesion has destroyed brain tissue, however, the eyes may deviate toward the side of the lesion.
Dysconjugate gaze	When the child's eyes move independently, it is more likely there is damage to the neural pathways involving vision than a metabolic problem.
Horizontal and vertical nystagmus	Rhythmic eye movement, usually rapid in one direction with a slower return, may indicate drug toxicity, inflammation of the inner ear, blindness in infancy, or central nervous system injury.
Setting sun sign	This is an ominous sign, indicating obstructive lesion or hydrocephalus.

PUPILLARY RESPONSE IN NEUROLOGIC INJURY

Question

Indicate whether each of the following clinical manifestations are an early (*E*) or late (*L*) sign of increased intracranial pressure. (Mark each answer either *E* or *L*.)

_____ Alterations in mental status

_____ Increased systolic blood pressure

_____ Bradycardia

_____ Confusion, restlessness, lethargy

_____ Progressively severe headache

_____ Irregular respirations

_____ Ipsilateral (side of injury) pupillary dilation

_____ Flaccid posturing

_____ Widening pulse pressure

_____ Contralateral pupillary dilation

Answer

The correct answers are *E,L,L,E,* and *E,* (1st row), *L,L,L,L,* and *L* (2nd row), respectively.[11]

The cranial cavity is filled with three components: brain tissue, blood, and cerebrospinal fluid. Because the cranium is an unyielding container, any increase in the volume of one component must be offset by a decrease in one or both of the remaining components, or pressure inside the cranium will build up very rapidly. This increasing pressure eventually causes compression, and then injury and resulting dysfunction of the brain cells.[12]

Brain cell dysfunction is manifested by abnormal reactions and reflexes. A decreasing level of consciousness is the result of dysfunction of the reticular activating system responsible for arousal and wakefulness.[10] As the pressure continues to mount, distortion and displacement of the brain occur. Later additional clinical signs of increasing intracranial pressure manifest themselves as different areas of the brain (midbrain, brainstem) are affected.[12] Early and later signs of increased intracranial pressure are summarized in Table 4.23 (facing page).

Danny's condition is not improving. On reassessment, he no longer opens his eyes to loud commands, and he is moving around less. Because secondary injury from increased intracranial pressure is a serious concern, you review your alternative interventions to decrease intracranial pressure. As you think about this, Danny's arterial blood gas results return.

TABLE 4.23. Signs of Increased Intracranial Pressure[10-12]

Early	Late
Progressively severe headaches	Respiratory pattern irregularities
Mental status deterioration	Stupor, coma
Confusion, restlessness, lethargy	Hemiplegic, decorticate, decerebrate positioning
Ipsilateral pupillary dilation	Contralateral/bilateral pupillary dilation

Motor weakness (e.g., monoparesis or hemiparesis)	Cushing's syndrome
	    Increased systolic blood pressure
	    Widening pulse pressure
	    Bradycardia
	  Flaccid posturing

pO_2	85 mmHg
pCO_2	42 mmHg
pH	7.32

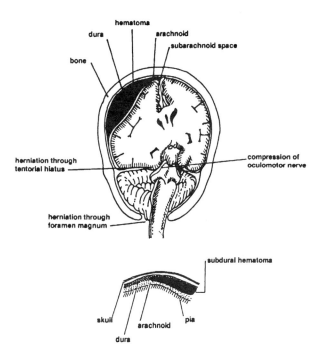

FIGURE 4.7 Increased pressure on cerebrum from enlarging hematoma causes herniation through lower structures.

Dr. Clark responds to Danny's changing status by asking you to assist him in placing an endotracheal tube. You begin hyperventilating Danny with 100% oxygen via bag-valve-mask device in preparation for intubation. Dr. Clark asks for arterial blood gases to be drawn every 15 minutes.

Question

The most important purpose for hyperventilating Danny is to: (Choose one answer.)

1. Correct his severe hypoxia
2. Reduce the hypercarbia
3. Increase his respiratory drive
4. Induce respiratory acidosis

Answer

The correct answer is (2). Hypercarbia (increased pCO_2) causes vasodilation of the cerebral blood vessels. This in turn increases blood flow, which increases intracranial pressure. Hyperventilation will decrease the pCO_2, thus decreasing blood flow and intracranial pressure.[13,14] A decrease in the pCO_2 pressure from 40 to 20 mmHg will decrease the cerebral blood flow to nearly 60% of normal.[15]

Question

What are the desired pO_2 and pCO_2 levels for Danny? (Fill in the blanks.)

Desired pO_2 _____   Desired pCO_2 _____

Answer

The desired pO_2 level is above 90 mmHg. The desired pCO_2 level is 25 to 30 mmHg. Animal studies indicate that cerebral ischemia is not produced until the pCO_2 drops to 15 to 20 mmHg.[7,8] The pCO_2 level should not be brought below 20 mmHg, because this could put Danny at risk for cerebral ischemia.[16]

Danny's mother is waiting for news, and as his condition has become more serious, you need to let her know. You ask the physician to ventilate Danny for a moment and go out to find Mrs. Coffey. You tell her that Danny is not doing well and that the physician has put in a breathing tube to make sure he gets plenty of oxygen. She asks you if she can come in to see him. You return to the treatment room to discuss this with Dr. Clark, who is ventilating Danny.

Question

When assisting with the hyperventilation on Danny, which one of the following ventilatory rates would you choose? (Choose one answer.)

1. 20 breaths/min
2. 30 breaths/min
3. 45 breaths/min
4. 60 breaths/min

Answer

The correct answer is (2). The normal respiratory rate for an 8-year-old ranges from 18 to 25 breaths/min. To maintain a pCO_2 between 25 to 30 mmHg requires a rate of five-to-seven ventilations per minute greater than the normal rate.[7]

Dr. Clark agrees with you that Mrs. Coffey should come in for a moment to see Danny. You quickly bring her in to see Danny, and she touches his foot and talks to him for a few seconds. You take over ventilation after she leaves. After ventilating Danny for 15 minutes, arterial blood gases are drawn and show the following results:

pO_2	98 mmHg
pCO_2	28 mmHg
pH	7.48

Dr. Clark is satisfied that Danny's airway and ventilation are well controlled at this point. He asks you to change the IV line to D_5 0.45 normal saline.

Question

In all pediatric cases of suspected increasing intracranial pressure, intravenous fluid administration is restricted to a minimal volume. (Choose True or False.)

_____ True   _____ False

Answer

The correct answer is False. Appropriate volumes of isotonic intravenous fluids must be given to maintain blood pressure and cerebral perfusion, especially in situations of hypovolemic shock.[1] Once the cardiovascular system is stabilized, an intravenous rate of two-thirds maintenance is recommended for head-injured patients.[2] For increased safety, it is generally advisable to use a volume pump or controller device for pediatric patients with delicate fluid balance.

It has been 35 minutes since Danny was admitted. Radiology calls and tells you that the CT scan is now ready for Danny. You and Dr. Clark accompany him to maintain his hyperventilation and continue your close monitoring.

A repeat Glasgow Coma Scale Score remains at 9. The CT scan shows a linear skull fracture of the right temporal bone with blood in the right temporal epidural area.

Question

Which blood vessel would most commonly be injured with a fracture like Danny's? (Choose one answer.)

1. External carotid artery
2. Middle cerebral artery
3. Anterior communicating artery
4. Middle meningeal artery

Answer

Answer (4) is correct. A blow to the parietal-temporal area of the skull often causes a laceration of a branch of the middle meningeal artery, which in turn frequently results in an epidural hematoma. This type of arterial bleed produces a rapidly expanding clot, and death may ensue in as little as 2 to 6 hours.[8] This also explains Danny's rapidly declining level of consciousness.

Intracranial hemorrhages may be epidural, subdural, or subarachnoid. All will be of primary concern in the head-injured child because of their significant risk for pediatric morbidity and mortality.[2] Table 4.24 compares the clinical features of intracranial hemorrhages.

Dr. Clark summons the neurosurgeon immediately because Danny needs urgent evacuation of the hematoma. As the two physicians make the necessary arrangements for Danny's emergency surgery, you ask if Danny should receive a stat dose of mannitol.

TABLE 4.24. Characteristics of Intracranial Hemorrhages [2,6,15]

Characteristics	Epidural hematoma	Subdural hematoma	Subarachnoid hematoma
Description	Bleeding between the skull and the dura	Bleeding between the dura (outer meninges) and the arachnoid layer of meninges in the subdural space	Bleeding between the pia mater and the arachnoid membrane or beneath the pia mater into the brain
Frequency	Relatively rare but more common in children than adults	5–10 times more common than epidural hematoma	Most common type of bleeding in massive head injuries
Patient age range	Usually > 2 years	Usually < 1 year	Usually > 1 year; associated with severe head trauma, cerebral artery aneurysms, tumors and arteriovenous malformations
Associated skull fracture	Present in 75%; commonly fracture in parietotemporal region	Present in 30%	Common in severe head trauma
Source of hemorrhage	Arterial bleed	Usually venous arterial	May be either venous or arterial
Laterality	Usually unilateral	Usually bilateral	Usually bilateral
Mortality	25%	Less than 25%	High
Morbidity	Low	High	High
Onset of symptoms	Usually acute	Because of venous bleeding, will be slower than epidural; may be acute or slow dependent on cause	Usually acute

Associated signs and symptoms
  Seizures
  Retinal hemorrhages
  Increased intracranial pressure
  CT findings
	< 25%
	< 25%
	Present
	Usually Lenticular
		75%
		75%
		Present
		Usually Curvilinear
			Common
			Present

Question

Mannitol may be indicated in severe head injuries with associated increased intracranial pressure for the purpose of: (Choose one answer.)

1. Expanding intravascular volume
2. Increasing renal output
3. Temporarily decreasing intracranial pressure
4. All of the above

Answer

The correct answer is (1). Mannitol is a hyperosmotic agent that is used to decrease intracranial pressure, thus "buying time" for the patient while arrangements are being made for definitive care.[8] The usual dosage is 0.25 to 1.0 g/kg administered IV bolus.[2] However, because mannitol may cause dehydration and can increase intracranial bleeding, its use is controversial.

Furosemide (Lasix) is often recommended as a suitable diuretic for the first 24 hours after injury, because it can reduce both intravascular volume and cerebral blood volume.[2] The usual dosage is 0.5 to 1.0 mg/kg and reduced intracranial pressure can be expected in 15 minutes.[7,15]

Question

Place an **X** by any of the following that are priority nursing responsibilities when administering an osmotic diuretic to a pediatric head injury victim.

_____ 1. Monitor accurate fluid intake and output at frequent intervals (i.e., every 15–30 minutes).

_____ 2. Insert foley catheter (if not already done).

_____ 3. Monitor urine and specific gravity.

_____ 4. Continuous monitoring of vital signs and neurologic status.

_____ 5. Monitor complete blood count and serum electrolytes.

_____ 6. Assess for signs and symptoms of dehydration and impending shock.

Answer

All of the above are correct answers.[17] Because of the many dramatic side effects of osmotic diuretics, particularly mannitol, it is important to carefully monitor vital signs, serial neurologic status, and hydration status in pediatric patients.

Because Danny is going directly to the operating room and has an active bleed, the physicians state that mannitol is not going to be administered at this time. You complete another set of vital signs and neurologic assessment, finish the necessary charting, and prepare to accompany Danny to the operating room suite.

Danny's father has arrived in the emergency department and is waiting anxiously with his wife who has not seen Danny since he was intubated and taken to CT scan. The physicians and a social worker speak with the parents and obtain the necessary consents for surgery. Danny's mother is trembling and softly crying. His father is also visibly upset. Suddenly they ask if they can see their child briefly before the surgery.

Question

In view of the parents' heightened anxiety, and the child's serious injury and deteriorating condition, should you delay taking him to the operating room so that the parents can see him? (Choose Yes or No.)

_____ Yes   _____ No

Answer

The correct answer is Yes; it is important to consider the sense of helplessness and crisis the parents must be feeling at this time. In a very short time their healthy happy little boy has become seriously injured and is on his way to surgery.

Allow the parents a brief visit with Danny and encourage them to touch him and to talk to him before he goes to surgery. Explain briefly any mechanical devices and the basics about Danny's current care. Have someone escort them to the surgical waiting room, orient them to the area, assist with necessary physical needs such as telephone calls to relatives or a cup of coffee, and make them as comfortable as possible during their wait for Danny. It is also helpful if a staff person can periodically check on the parents and update them on the progress of the surgery.

After allowing the Coffeys a few minutes to visit with Danny, you escort him to the operating room and give the report to the operating room staff. On the way back to the emergency department, you stop in the waiting room to tell Danny's parents that his surgery is about to begin. Both parents now seem more in control and thank you for your care of Danny. The mother begins to apologize for her earlier tearful outburst, and states, "I just can't believe that anything this serious can happen from a baseball game. I wish we had known how to protect him!"

Question

Should you now provide the mother with complete head injury discharge instructions and include information on the use of helmets to prevent pediatric head injuries? (Choose Yes or No.)

_____ Yes   _____ No

Answer

In this instance, the correct answer is No. Danny is seriously injured, the medical management is still in a critical stage, and the prognosis is uncertain. At this time, the parents are likely to be feeling very vulnerable. Discussing how this injury could have been prevented may increase their guilt.

The majority of pediatric head injuries seen in the emergency department are minor. Although it is probably not appropriate in Danny's case to discuss the use of helmets, it is important to talk about prevention of head injuries with most older children, and adolescents and their families. Safety helmets are now relatively inexpensive and were designed to prevent pediatric head injuries. Their use should be encouraged in everyday play activities such as bicycling, skateboarding, and baseball.[8]

Another consideration in the management of minor pediatric head injuries is the necessity of very thorough discharge instructions.

> *Note:* Because these children may be at risk for subsequent complications from their head injuries, it is extremely important that parents thoroughly understand the signs and symptoms of deteriorating neurologic status.

Table 4.25 is a sample discharge instruction sheet for pediatric head injury patients.

TABLE 4.25. Discharge Instructions: Post-Head Injury[8,18]

Activities	Limit activity as directed by physician.
Diet	Give only clear liquids until not vomiting for at least 6 hr and then light meals. *No* alcoholic beverages for 24 hr.
Medications	Acetaminophen for headache. Avoid other over-the-counter medications unless approved by physician.
Monitoring	Check pupil reaction every four hours for 48 hours. (*Check twice during the night.*)

Seek medical attention if any of the following occurs:	
Oral temperature over 101 °F	Severe or worsening headache
Headache that interferes with sleep	Vomiting three or more times
Difficulty arousing from sleep	Blurred vision or double vision
Neck pain or stiff neck	Unsteady gait, stumbling
Weakness in arms or legs	Memory loss
Dilated pupils	Seizures
Confusion or abnormal behavior or personality	

As Danny goes into surgery, you hope he will do well. If the hematoma can be successfully drained, the intracranial pressure will decrease, and he will be carefully monitored in the intensive care unit. You also know that pediatric patients often do better than adults with head injuries, and you talk with the Coffeys about this. Although it is difficult to care for a patient like Danny, you are confident that your emergency department gave him the best care possible.

REFERENCES

Case Study 1

1. Bruce, D. A., Schut, L., & Sutton, L. N. (1988). Neurosurgical emergencies. In G. Fleisher & S. Ludwig (Eds.), *Textbook of pediatric emergency medicine,* (2nd ed., pp. 1112–1126). Baltimore: Williams & Wilkins.
2. Henderson, D. P., & Seidel, J. S. (Eds.). (1990). *Assessment of the pediatric patient.* Torrance, CA: Pediatric Rural Emergency Systems and Education Project.
3. Ferry, F. T., & Yeager, A. M. (1987). Poisonings and ingestions. In F. E. Ehrlich, F. J. Heldrich, & J. J. Tepas (Eds.), *Pediatric emergency medicine* (pp. 239–266). Rockville, MD: Aspen.
4. American Academy of Pediatrics & American College of Emergency Physicians. (1989). *Advanced pediatric life support.* Dallas, TX: Author.
5. American Academy of Pediatrics & American College of Emergency Physicians. (1989). *Pediatric advanced life support.* Elk Grove Village, IL, & Dallas, TX: Author.
6. Seidel, J. S., & Henderson, D. P. (1987). *Prehospital care of pediatric emergencies.* Los Angeles, CA: Los Angeles Pediatric Society.

7. James, H. E., Anas, N. G., & Perkin, R. M. (1985). *Brain insults in infants and children*. Orlando, FL: Grune & Stratton.

8. Whaley, L., & Wong, D. (1987). *Nursing care of infants and children* (3rd ed., pp. 669–681). St Louis: Mosby.

9. Zull, D. N. (1990). Poisoning and drug overdose. In S. Kitt & J. Kaiser (Eds.), *Emergency nursing: A physiological and clinical perspective* (pp. 631–654). Philadelphia: Saunders.

10. Temple, A. R. (1985). Poisoning. In T. E. Thayer (Ed.), *Emergency management of pediatric trauma.* (pp. 444–458). Philadelphia: Saunders.

11. Hopkins-Lotz, E. (1988). Poisonings and ingestions. In S. J. Kelley (Ed.), *Pediatric emergency nursing.* (pp. 164–176). Norwalk, CT: Appleton & Lange.

12. Scherer, J. C. (1985). (Ed.). *Lippincott nurses' drug manual*. Philadelphia: Lippincott.

13. Henretig, F. M., Cupit, G. C., Temple, A. R., & Collins, M. (1988). Toxicologic emergencies. In G. Fleisher & S. Ludwig (Eds.), *Textbook of pediatric emergency medicine* (2nd ed., pp. 548–597). Baltimore, MD: Williams & Wilkins.

14. Gill, F. T. (1989). Pediatric poisoning. In C. E. Joy (Ed.), *Pediatric trauma nursing* (pp. 173–192). Rockville, MD: Aspen.

15. Rodgers, G. C. Jr., & Matunyas, N. T. (1986). Gastrointestinal decontamination for acute poisoning. *Pediatric Clinics of North America, 33*, 261–285.

16. Greensher, J. & Mofenson, H. (1980). Emergency room care of the poisoned child. *Comprehensive Pediatric Nursing, 4*(3),1–21.

17. Kitt, S. & Kaiser, J. (1990). *Emergency nursing—a physiologic and clinical perspective* (pp. 534–535). Philadelphia: Saunders.

18. Rumack, B. H. (1976). Poisonings. In H. C. Kempe, H. K. Silver, & D. O'Brien (Eds.), *Current pediatric diagnosis & treatment* (pp. 862–890). Los Altos, CA: Lange .

19. American Academy of Pediatrics, Committee on Accident and Poison Prevention. (1983). In R. Aranow (Ed.), *Handbook of common poisonings in children* (2nd ed.). Evanston, IL: Author.

Case Study 2

1. Kimmel, S., & Gemmill, D. (1988). The young child with fever. *American Family Physician, 37*,196–206.

2. Kitt, S., & Kaiser, J. (1990). *Emergency nursing—a physiologic and clinical perspective* (pp. 534–535). Philadelphia: Saund.

3. Henderson, D. P., & Seidel, J. S. (Eds.). (1990). *Assessment of the pediatric patient*. Torrance, CA: Pediatric Rural Emergency System and Education Project (Robert Wood Johnson Grant No. 11804).

4. Packer, R. J., & Berman, P. H. (1988). Neurological Emergencies. In G. Fleisher & S. Ludwig (Eds.), *Textbook of pediatric emergency medicine.* (2nd ed., pp. 391–399). Baltimore: Williams & Wilkins.

5. Whaley, L., & Wong, D. (1987). *Nursing care of infants and children* (3rd ed., pp. 1657–1671). St. Louis: Mosby.

6. Hudak, C., Gallo, B., & Lohr, T. (1986). *Critical care nursing* (4th ed., pp. 534–535). Philadelphia: Lippincott.

7. Dejong, A. R. (1983). *The neurologic patient: A nursing perspective* (p. 168). Engelwood Cliffs, NJ: Prentice Hall.

8. Mott, S., Fazekas, N., & James, S. (1985). *Nursing care of children and families* (pp. 1560–1569). Reading, MA: Addison-Wesley.

9. Nelson, D., & Ellenberg, J. (1978). Prognosis in children with febrile seizures. *Pediatrics, 61*,720–727.

10. American Academy of Pediatrics & American College of Emergency Physicians. (1989). *Advanced pediatric life support*. Dallas, TX: Author.

11. Felter, R., & Asch, S. (1986). Febrile seizures: A protocol for emergency management. *Pediatric emergency care, 2*, 93–96.

12. Hirtz, D. (1989). Generalized tonic-clonic and febrile seizures in seizure disorders. *Pediatric Clinics of North America, 36*,365–382.

Case Study 3

1. Ward, J. D. (1987). Central nervous system injuries. In F. E. Ehrlich, F. J. Heldrich, & J. T. Tepas (Eds.), *Pediatric Emergency Medicine* (pp. 169–175). Rockville, MD: Aspen.

2. American Academy of Pediatrics & American College of Emergency Physicians. (1989). *Advanced pediatric life support*. Dallas, TX: Author.

3. Kitt, S., & Kaiser, J. (Eds.). (1990). *Emergency nursing: A physiological and clinical perspective* (pp. 631–654). Philadelphia: Saunders.

4. James, H. E., Anas, N. G., & Perkin, R. M. (1985). Brain insults in infants and children. Orlando, FL: Grune & Stratton.

5. Reeves, K. (1989). Assessment of pediatric head injury: The basics. *Journal of Emergency Nursing, 15,* 329–332.

6. Flint, N. S. (1988). Head trauma and spinal cord injuries. In S. J. Kelley (Ed.), *Pediatric emergency nursing* (pp. 177–217). Norwalk, CT: Appleton & Lange.

7. Walker, M., Storrs, B., & Mayer, T. A. (1985). Head injuries. In T. Mayer (Ed.), *Emergency management of pediatric trauma* (pp. 21, 272–286). Philadelphia: Saunders.

8. Zoellner-Hunter, J. (1990). Head trauma. In S. Kitt & J. Kaiser (Eds.), *Emergency nursing: a physiological and clinical perspective* (pp. 427–444). Philadelphia: Saunders.

9. Boortz-Marx, R. Factors affecting intracranial pressure: A descriptive study. *Journal of Neuroscience Nursing, 17,* 89-94.

10. Hickey, J. V. (1986). *The clinical practice of neurological and neurosurgical nursing* (2nd ed.). Philadelphia: Lippincott.

11. Bruce, D. A., Schut, L., & Sutton, L. N. (1988). Neurosurgical emergencies. In G. Fleisher & S. Ludwig (Eds.), *Textbook of pediatric emergency medicine* (pp. 1112–1126). Baltimore: Williams & Wilkins.

12. McGinnis, G. S. (1988). Central nervous system injury: Head injuries. In V. D. Cardona, P. D. Hurn, P. J. Bastnagel-Mason, A. M. Scanlon-Schilpp, & S. N. Viese-Berry. (1988). *Trauma nursing from resuscitation through rehabilitation* (pp. 368–418). Philadelphia: Saunders.

13. Jennet, B. & Teasdale, G. (1981). *Management of head injuries.* Philadelphia: Davis.

14. Widner-Kolberg, M. & Moloney-Harmon, P. (1988). Pediatric trauma. In V. D. Cardona, P. D. Hurn, P. J. Bastnagel-Mason, A. M. Scanlon-Schilpp, & S. N. Viese-Berry. *Trauma nursing from resuscitation through rehabilitation* (pp. 664–691). Philadelphia: Saunders.

15. DeLong, S. B. (1989). Traumatic head injury. In J. Connie (Ed.), *Pediatric trauma nursing* (pp. 36–67). Rockville, MD: Aspen.

16. Rosman, N. P., Oppenheimer, E. Y. & O'Connor, J. F. (1983). Emergency management of pediatric head injuries. *Emergency Medicine Clinics of North America, 1,* 141–174.

17. Scherer, J. C. (Ed.). (1985). *Lippincott nurses' drug manual* (pp. 655–656). Philadelphia: Lippincott.

18. Whaley, L. F., & Wong, D. L. (1987). *Nursing care of infants and children* (pp. 1642–1648). St. Louis: Mosby.

Chapter Five

Medical Emergencies

Prerequisite Skills

Before beginning this chapter, you should be able to

- Identify typical manifestations of sepsis in an adult
- Identify high-risk groups for sepsis
- Describe the typical manifestations of meningitis in an adult
- Describe typical treatment for fever in the emergency setting
- Outline general management of adults with serious infections such as sepsis and meningitis
- Understand the physiology of normal hemoglobin
- Understand general pathophysiology of thrombotic episodes
- Identify the signs and symptoms of shock in adults
- Identify the general complications of:
  — Near-drowning episode
  — Profound hypothermia
- Identify rewarming techniques available for use in your own hospital
- Describe components of pain management in adults
- Identify adult patient groups requiring transport to an acute care facility after initial stabilization

FEVER/SEPSIS/MENINGITIS

PREVIEW

Fever is defined as a core body temperature above 38.0°C (100.5°F).[1] It is one of the most common medical complaints of children presenting to emergency departments for evaluation.[2] A viral or bacterial infection present somewhere in the body causes a rise in temperature as part of the immune response.[1] Although fever is a general sign of illness, height of fever does not necessarily correlate with degree of illness and must always be interpreted in the context of the child's overall clinical assessment.[3,4] An elevated temperature is not, in itself, harmful unless it reaches levels in excess of 41.7°C (107°F), at which point brain damage may occur.[1,5]

Bacteremia is an invasion of the blood stream by bacterial organisms. It may resolve spontaneously without medical intervention or may result in:

- *Septicemia.* Bacteria develop pathogenic activity in the blood stream, causing the individual to become acutely ill.[6,7]
- *Infection at other sites in the body.* Examples include the lungs (pneumonia), the central nervous system (meningitis), the soft tissues surrounding the eye (periorbital cellulitis).[7,8]

High-risk groups for infection exist within the pediatric population. These children require special consideration and management.

CASE STUDY 1 OBJECTIVES

Once you have completed this case study you will be able to

- Name the two most common causes of fever in children
- Identify why neonates do not always respond to infection with a fever
- Name clinical indicators other than fever that can be used as a triage tool to assess the severity of illness in a child
- List specific contraindications for taking a rectal temperature in some children
- List three components of fever control in children
- Identify high-risk groups for serious infection such as sepsis and meningitis in children
- Identify clinical manifestations of meningitis in infants and children
- Identify general components of a diagnostic workup for an infant with possible sepsis or meningitis
- Identify equipment and materials needed to manage a child with possible sepsis or meningitis
- Calculate maintenance IV fluid requirements for infants and children
- Recognize significant lab values in
  — Meningitis
  — Sepsis
  — Urinary tract infection
- Identify complications of sepsis
- Identify complications of meningitis

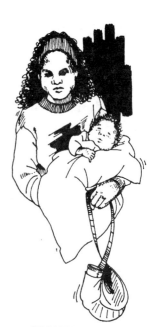

CASE STUDY 1

Tiffany Is Unusually Sleepy

Tiffany Daniels, a 7-week-old female infant, is brought to your emergency department by her mother at 11:45 A.M. on a sunny day in April. Mrs. Daniels tells you that she is worried because Tiffany has been unusually sleepy this morning (see Figure 5.1).

Tiffany is wrapped in blankets and appears to be sleeping. You ask Mrs. Daniels to sit down in the triage area and remove the blankets. When she does this, Tiffany wakes up, cries weakly, and then quickly falls back to sleep. You notice that Tiffany is breathing rapidly, and her face looks pale.

FIGURE 5.1

TRIAGE DECISION

On the basis of your initial rapid assessment, how would you classify this infant?

Emergent. A life-threatening situation in need of immediate intervention.

Urgent. Patient needs care within 1 hour to prevent further deterioration.

Nonurgent. Patient is able to wait more than 1 hour without further deterioration.

TRIAGE DECISION ANSWER

Tiffany should be triaged as urgent. On the basis of the infant's age, rapid breathing, weak cry and pale face, Tiffany warrants intervention within the next hour.

Infants have a limited behavioral repertoire, so the early signs and symptoms of illness may be subtle. Also, because they do not always develop a fever with an infection because of their immature thermoregulatory responses,[9] special indicators must be used to assess for severity of illness and toxicity. In infants less than 3 months of age, manifestations of serious infection may be limited to a change in skin color, irritability, poor feeding, and excessive sleeping.[2] Table 5.1 shows the indicators that should trigger concern about serious underlying illness.

TABLE 5.1. Indicators of Illness in Infants and Young Children[2,8,9]

Item/status	Normal	Moderately ill	Severely ill
Color	Pink	Pale	Mottled Cyanotic
Hydration status	Moist mucous membranes Good skin turgor Flat fontanel Light-colored urine	Sticky mucous membranes Slightly doughy skin turgor Fontanel slightly sunken Dark-colored urine	Dry mucous membranes Tenting skin turgor Very sunken fontanel and eyes No urine
Response to stimulation	Arouses easily, then stays awake and alert	Arouses with repeated gentle stimulation, then falls back to sleep quickly if unstimulated	Arouses only with noxious stimulation or does not arouse at all
Behavior	Unchanged	Fussy but can be comforted	Irritable and inconsolable, if awake
Cry	Unchanged	Whimpers, sobs, or whines	High-pitched and screeching or weak and moaning

Assessing the *ABC*s, you find that Tiffany has rapid but unlabored respirations and cool, somewhat mottled extremities. When you assess her neurologic status you see that she cries when aroused, and becomes irritable when her mother gently rocks her in a calming manner. When Mrs. Daniels stops rocking Tiffany, the infant stops crying and falls back to sleep. Mrs. Daniels tells you Tiffany is not normally irritable. You see some cause for concern, but Tiffany does not seem to be in severe distress. You take her vital signs

Heart rate	190 beats/min
Respiratory rate	68 breaths/min
Blood pressure	68/palpated

Question

Match Tiffany's heart rate, respiratory rate, and blood pressure to the correct descriptions. (Answers may be used more than once.)

_____ Heart rate	1. Abnormally fast (high)
_____ Respiratory rate	2. Abnormally slow (low)
_____ Blood pressure	3. Within normal range

Answer

The correct answers are (1), (1), and (3). Tiffany's heart rate and respiratory rate are abnormally fast. Several factors, including fever, volume depletion, and pain can cause tachycardia. Effortless tachypnea can be caused by fever or by the body's attempt to compensate for metabolic acidosis. Tachypnea helps normalize blood pH by producing respiratory alkalosis.[10] Although Tiffany's blood pressure is within the normal range for her age, she is demonstrating signs of compensated shock: tachycardia, peripheral vasoconstriction, and irritability.[11]

Tiffany demonstrates "paradoxic irritability" when she becomes fussy and inconsolable with rocking, an activity that usually calms an infant. Paradoxic irritability is another clue of serious illness in infants.[2] Table 1.4 (Chapter 1) lists the normal vital signs for children of different ages.

As you listen to Tiffany's apical pulse, you notice that her body feels rather warm. You ask Mrs. Daniels if she knows whether Tiffany has a fever, and she tells you that she didn't take it because she wasn't sure how to take a temperature on such a tiny baby. You are worried that Tiffany may have a serious infection. You place her on the infant scale and find she weighs 4 kg. To complete your vital signs, you take her temperature.

Question

What method would you use to assess Tiffany's body temperature? (Choose one answer.)

1. Oral	3. Axillary
2. Rectal	4. Tympanic membrane

Answer

The correct answer is (2). Rectal thermometers are the most widely available, reliable reflection of core body temperature for infants under 3 months of age. Your selection of methods to measure temperature depends in part on the temperature-measuring device equipment available in your emergency department. The choice of how to measure temperature is a controversial topic.

In older infants and children, where mild elevations of temperature are not as critical in clinical decision making, axillary temperatures may suffice. When properly performed, axillary temperatures are acceptable and tend to be about one degree lower than rectal temperatures.[2]

Oral temperatures, using electronic and glass thermometers, may be obtained in children old enough to cooperate. Glass thermometers present a safety hazard and should not be used for oral temperatures on children who are uncooperative (usually under 6 years of age) because they can easily be bitten and broken inside the child's mouth.[13]

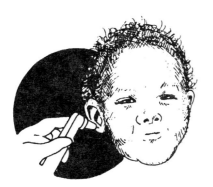

FIGURE 5.2

Electronic infrared tympanic membrane thermometers are increasingly used in emergency departments (see Figure 5.2). They provide a quick, noninvasive alternative for checking core body temperature. Accuracy of these thermometers is dependent, however, on the ability of the user to direct the probe into the outer ear canal toward the tympanic membrane rather than the wall of the ear canal. Current models are not well designed for use on the anatomically variable external ear structures of infants because the probes are rigid and single sized. As a result, significant fevers may be missed. When elevation in temperature is critical to the clinical decision-making process, infrared tympanic thermometer use may not be the best choice.[14–16]

As you check Tiffany's temperature, you show Mrs. Daniels how far to insert the thermometer into the rectum and assure her it will not injure Tiffany. You obtain a rectal temperature of 39.4°C (102.9°F). Your emergency department protocol instructs you to treat any fever of, or above, 38.5°C (101.2°F).

Question

Which of the following interventions would be the most appropriate method(s) of treating Tiffany's fever? (Choose all that apply.)

1. Acetaminophen orally
2. Acetaminophen rectally
3. Aspirin orally

4. Sponge bath (water)
5. Sponge bath (isopropyl alcohol and water)

Answer

The correct answer is (1). Acetaminophen is the antipyretic most widely used for fever therapy in children. It is available in liquid preparations, chewable tablets and rectal suppositories. While rectal acetaminophen administration may be a useful route in the vomiting child, Tiffany should be able to take medication orally (see Table 5.2).

Aspirin is not often used today for fever control in children because its use in the presence of chicken pox or influenza has been associated with development of Reye's syndrome.[5,9]

The use of sponge bathing for fever control is a subject of controversy. Cool or tepid baths induce shivering and often make the child cry, both of which can actually raise core body temperature.[9] Sponging with isopropyl alcohol may result in toxicity because of absorption of the alcohol and is not recommended.[5]

Table 5.2. Antipyretic Dosages[9]

The correct acetaminophen dose for children is 10–15 mg/kg per dose. Acetaminophen doses are usually given every 4–6 hr.	
Acetaminophen products available for use include the following:	
Infant drops	100 mg/mL
Elixir (syrup)	160 mg/5mL
Regular strength chewable tablets	80 mg/tablet
Double-strength chewable tablets	160 mg/tablet
Suppositories	120 mg, 325 mg, 650 mg

You give Tiffany the acetaminophen, and obtain the remainder of your triage history from the mother, using the mnemonic AMPLE.

*A*llergies. Tiffany has no known allergies.

*M*edications. Tiffany takes no medications.

*P*revious history. Despite the fact that Mrs. Daniels obtained no prenatal care, Tiffany was a full-term baby without perinatal complications. She has not yet received any immunizations.

*L*ast meal. Tiffany took only 2 oz of formula at her last feeding and had one wet diaper this morning.

*E*vents preceding the illness. Although she seemed fussy last evening and did not awaken as usual for her 2:00 A.M. feeding, Mrs. Daniels was not alarmed until the baby did not awaken for her midmorning feeding.

Question

Which of the following items would cause you to change your initial triage decision from urgent to emergent? (Choose one answer.)

1. Refused to feed 1 hr ago
2. No stool for 24 hr
3. No wet diaper for 12 hr

Answer

The correct answer is (3). Because decreased urinary output may indicate dehydration, it would change your triage decision to emergent. Infants rapidly become volume depleted in the face of poor intake and extraordinary fluid losses such as vomiting and diarrhea.[8]

Poor feeding is a common response to illness in infants.[8,11] Although refusing *one* feeding does not put Tiffany in danger of dehydration, poor intake is a nonspecific indicator of potentially serious illness.

Some infants normally have only one bowel movement a day. Without signs of intestinal obstruction (e.g., bilious vomiting, abdominal distention, or pain), failure to have a bowel movement would not change your triage decision.

You direct Mrs. Daniels to the first available examination room. Because Tiffany continues to be lethargic and her perfusion appears to be worsening, you put her on a cardiac monitor. After examining Tiffany, Dr. Matthews tells Mrs. Daniels that her baby seems quite ill, and will need to have blood drawn and urine collected to locate the source of the infection that is making her ill. She also tells Mrs. Daniels that Tiffany will need a lumbar puncture to test for meningitis, and will be admitted into the hospital for observation and IV antibiotics. You mentally review the signs and symptoms of meningitis.

Question

If Tiffany has meningitis, you will probably see signs of nuchal rigidity (stiff neck). (Choose True or False.)

_____ True   _____ False

Answer

The correct answer is False. Infants with meningitis seldom develop nuchal rigidity and those under three months of age sometimes remain afebrile.[9] Children older than 2 years of age usually experience nuchal rigidity and headache with meningitis (see Table 5.3).

TABLE 5.3. Clinical Manifestations of Meningitis[1,11]

Infants	Children
Normothermia, fever, hypothermia	Fever and chills
Apnea	Headache
Bulging fontanel	Nuchal rigidity
Vomiting, diarrhea	Vomiting
Poor sucking tone, feeding	Altered mental status
Paradoxical irritability	Seizures
Lethargy	Rash (petechiae, purpura)
Seizures	
Rash (petechiae, purpura)	

> *Note:* Skin lesions such as petechiae or purpura are caused by bacteria invading and damaging blood vessels of the dermal skin layer, and by the effects of toxins circulating in the vascular system.[17]

When Dr. Matthews leaves the room to see another patient, Mrs. Daniels holds Tiffany close to her and with tears in her eyes says, "What is going on here? I don't understand what the doctor is saying. What is meningitis, anyway? It sounds so serious! I don't want Tiffany to have all of those tests." Considering her apparent anxiety, your nursing diagnosis is "anxiety, related to lack of knowledge." Mrs. Daniels will require some time and education to understand and accept the necessity of the tests, and your first intervention is to give her some information about meningitis (see Table 5.4).

TABLE 5.4. Meningitis[1,7,18]

- Meningitis is an inflammation of the membranes lining the brain and spinal cord, usually caused by a bacterial or viral infection. This usually causes severe headache as well as generalized illness.
- Bacterial meningitis is relatively common, and can be very serious, but it usually responds well to treatment if diagnosed early and treated promptly.

You also want to help Mrs. Daniels cope with her anxiety, so you sit down with her for just a moment while you wait for the laboratory technologist and say, "You seem to be worried—is there something...?" She quickly answers, "It's my fault; I should have brought her in last night. I just didn't know that she was this sick!"

Question

What should you say to Mrs. Daniels? (Choose one answer.)

1. "Don't be worried about Tiffany. I'm sure she'll be fine. The tests she's having are just routine, and they often are negative. Even if she has meningitis, most children do very well once they start taking antibiotics."

2. "I can see how worried you are, and that you feel responsible. It's impossible to know whether coming earlier would have made a difference—I wish I could give you more reassurance. Waiting must be so difficult; would it help for you to call someone to be with you?"

3. "It's going to take quite a while for the laboratory to give us the results of Tiffany's tests. After that, Dr. Matthews will look at the results, and will let you know about them. You must feel very concerned, but it's not going to help to be worried all the time you're waiting, and you should try to keep calm for Tiffany."

Answer

The correct answer is (2). It is important to address Mrs. Daniels's needs with support and understanding. Although you can't reassure her that Tiffany is not seriously ill, you can show her that you empathize and that you are on her side. You also can't assuage her guilt, because it might have made a difference if she had come in earlier. You can, however, acknowledge her feelings. Finding someone (family member, friend, or social worker) who can provide emotional support could be helpful. False reassurance should never be given to the parent of a sick child. Encouraging a parent to keep calm for the child can sometimes be helpful, but it is more important to acknowledge Mrs. Daniels's feelings of fear and guilt.

Mrs. Daniels is much calmer now and agrees to let Tiffany have the needed tests. She says she would like to call her husband. You tell her you will stay with Tiffany and show her where the telephone is located. As you watch over Tiffany, you make out the lab slips for the tests ordered by Dr. Matthews and set up for the lumbar puncture.

Question

Which of the following additional tests are usually included in a "routine" sepsis work-up of a febrile infant? (Circle all appropriate answers.)

1. Complete blood count
2. Liver function tests
3. Urinalysis and urine culture
4. Blood culture
5. Blood urea nitrogen and creatinine
6. Chest film

Answer

The correct answers are (1), (3), (4), and (6). A routine sepsis workup is a screen for common serious infections.[2] The blood count is obtained as a nonspecific indicator of infection. Blood, urine, and cerebral spinal fluid (CSF) are cultured, and the CSF is examined for cell count, protein, glucose, and Gram's stain. A chest film is obtained to identify pneumonia, which may be clinically silent in the infant. A blood glucose is drawn to identify hypoglycemia, a common reaction to the stress and septicemia,[7] and to compare with the CSF glucose. Electrolytes may be obtained as a baseline when IV therapy is anticipated.[2,19]

Liver function tests, and blood urea nitrogen and creatinine are obtained only if specifically indicated by the child's history or symptoms.

Question

What other equipment will you need to obtain the specimens for the septic workup? (Circle all appropriate answers.)

1. Sterile urine collection bag and antiseptic wipes
2. "Vacutainer" with attached 19-gauge needle
3. 23-gauge butterfly needle and a 3-cc syringe
4. Heat lamp
5. 5-French feeding tube

Answer

Equipment you will need includes a 23-gauge butterfly needle and a 3-cc syringe, a heat lamp, and a 5-French feeding tube.

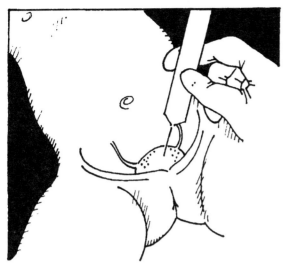

FIGURE 5.3

The 23-gauge butterfly attached to a 3-cc syringe is the preferred device for drawing blood from Tiffany's hand, foot, or antecubital fossa. A 19-gauge needle is too large for use on an infant, and the negative pressure generated by a "Vacutainer" phlebotomy device would collapse a tiny vein.

Infants may quickly become hypothermic in the emergency department setting, and a heat lamp or warming bed will keep Tiffany's body temperature stable while she is undressed for the purpose of examination and diagnostic procedures.

A 5-French sterile feeding tube is appropriate for catheterizing Tiffany. The preferred method of urine collection in infants is suprapubic tap (see Figure 5.3, bladder tap) or urinary bladder catheterization.[20] Urine bag collection is not recommended, especially for infant girls and uncircumcised boys, because of the high rate of specimen contamination by bacteria on the skin folds of the genitalia.

You obtain blood from Tiffany with no difficulty and have no trouble inserting the urinary catheter; 15 mL of clear yellow urine drains into the sterile cup. Because Tiffany will be receiving antibiotics, the emergency department physician orders an IV line, and you gather your equipment for this procedure.

Question

What size and type of catheter would you use to start an IV line on an infant? (Choose one answer.)

1. 23-gauge butterfly
2. 25-gauge butterfly
3. 22-gauge over-the-needle catheter
4. 24-gauge over-the-needle catheter

Answer

You select a 24-gauge IV catheter and decide to attempt it in the dorsum of her right hand, usually the best place in small infants.

Butterfly needles are not recommended because of their tendency to infiltrate, and the 22-gauge over-the-needle catheter would probably be too large. Because your smallest armboard is too big for Tiffany's tiny size, you secure the IV hand on an armboard fashioned from tongue blades taped together and padded with gauze. The IV solution you use is a 250-cc bag of D5 1/4 NS.

Mrs. Daniels returns to the treatment room to be with Tiffany. She asks you why the doctor thinks Tiffany might have meningitis, and you tell her that fever in an infant is unusual. Because meningitis is such a serious illness, it is important not to miss it. You know how difficult it could be if Tiffany had meningitis, and you do your best to reassure Mrs. Daniels realistically. You tell her that it is best to take one step at a time right now, and that you will keep her informed and make sure all of her questions are answered. She asks you more questions including what will happen if Tiffany does not have meningitis. You tell her that it will depend on what is causing Tiffany's infection and that Dr. Matthews will discuss that with her once the source of infection is determined. You check with Dr. Matthews to determine the rate for the intravenous infusion, and she says that Tiffany should be receiving fluids at maintenance rate (see Table 5.5).

Question

Tiffany weighs 4 kg. What will her hourly intravenous infusion rate be if it is run at "maintenance"? (Circle the correct answer.)

1. 10 mL/hr   3. 17 mL/hr
2. 14 mL/hr   4. 21 mL/hr

Answer

The correct answer is 17 mL/hr. The calculation is as follows:

$$100 \text{ mL} \times 4 \text{ kg} = 400 \text{ mL}/24 \text{ hr} = 16.6 \text{ mL/hr, rounded off to } 17 \text{ mL/hr}$$

TABLE 5.5.   Maintenance IV Fluid Requirements

Because many infants are unable to take or retain oral feedings during periods of illness, IV hydration is indicated. IV fluid is selected to provide an appropriate supply of sodium, glucose, and water. D5 1/4 normal saline, run at a "maintenance" rate meets these criteria.
How to figure maintenance IV fluid requirements[22]
Daily maintenance IV fluid requirement calculations are based on the child's body weight in kilograms: 0–10 kg   = 100 mL × kg   11–20 kg   = 1000 mL + (50 mL × weight in kg over 10 kg)   > 20 kg   = 1500 mL + (20 mL × weight in kg over 20 kg)   *The total amount of fluid is delivered on a continuous basis over a 24-hr period.*

Note: A slow IV infusion should ideally be administered with an IV pump. If electronic IV pumps are not available at your hospital, a small bag of IV solution (100–250 mL) and a graduated, volume-controlling administration device will allow you to limit the amount of fluid the infant receives by gravity.

Dr. Matthews comes in to tell you she is ready to do the lumbar puncture. Mrs. Daniels says she doesn't want to stay in the room, and she wants to wait for her husband in front of the hospital. Before she leaves, you tell her that you will be with Tiffany during the procedure.

Question

What size spinal needle is appropriate for use on an infant this size? (Choose one answer.)

1. 18-gauge 3-1/2-inch spinal needle
2. 20-gauge 2-1/2-inch spinal needle
3. 22-gauge 1-1/2-inch spinal needle

Answer

The correct answer is (3). The larger needles would be used on older children and adults.

You prepare Tiffany for the lumbar puncture, taking her clothes off and laying her on her side. Tiffany's irritability may be a sign of increased intracranial pressure, but Dr. Matthews has decided that the spinal tap is essential because she tells you she is fairly certain Tiffany has meningitis.

Question

What concern would there be if a lumbar puncture were performed on an *older child* with increased intracranial pressure? (Fill in the blank.)

_____

Answer

In an older child with increased intracranial pressure, the sudden release of pressure when cerebrospinal fluid is removed may cause herniation of the medulla through the foramen magnum, and death. Infants and children with open cranial sutures are better able to tolerate sudden changes in intracranial pressure.[21]

Holding a child for a lumbar puncture is sometimes difficult. The main purpose of positioning is to maximize the opening between vertebral bodies so that the spinal needle can be inserted. The infant is usually placed on its side, and knees are held as close to the chest as possible, flexing the spine. The child must be held firmly throughout the procedure with continuous observation to ensure that adequate aeration is maintained. Because infectious meningitis can be spread by droplet infection, both persons involved in the lumbar puncture should wear gowns, gloves, and masks.

Dr. Matthews begins the lumbar puncture. As you assist with holding Tiffany, you tell Dr. Matthews that Mrs. Daniels asked you why Tiffany would need admission if it turned out she did not have meningitis. Dr. Matthews talks with you about the risk of Tiffany having a serious infection because of her age. There are other factors that also cause children to be at risk, but Tiffany does not appear to have any of these (see Table 5.6).

TABLE 5.6. Categories of Children at High Risk for Serious Infection[2]

Infants under 3 Months of age
This age group has a higher risk of systemic infection because infants are exposed to organisms for which they have no immunity. Newborns are initially protected by the mother's immune factors transmitted across the placenta. In the first months of life, this passive immunity decreases while the infant's own immune response has not become fully competent. This leaves children a few weeks up to several months of age at increased risk for serious infection.
Immunosuppressed Individuals
Immunosuppression can be congenital (rare) or acquired (AIDS/HIV). It can also be a chemically induced state caused by treatment for a primary disease (chemotherapy, corticosteroids).
Splenic Dysfunction
Children who have had their spleen removed or have developed functional asplenia (e.g., sickle cell anemia) lack the ability to mount an effective response against blood-borne infection.
Presence of chronic disease
Children with chronic diseases (e.g., heart or renal disease) frequently have impaired ability to fight infection.

You and Dr. Matthews notice that Tiffany's CSF is slightly cloudy, which makes you both suspect that she has meningitis. After the lumbar puncture is completed, you recheck Tiffany's vital signs and then go to the waiting room to invite Mrs. Daniels back in. Mr. Daniels has arrived from work so you explain the situation to him and answer his questions. You tell the Daniels that Tiffany will need to be isolated because of her possible meningitis. Mr. and Mrs. Daniels come back into the room with you; you show them how to put on the isolation gowns and masks, and where they will discard their gowns and masks and wash their hands when they want to leave Tiffany's room.

Tiffany's lumbar puncture results show the following:

White blood count	250
Red blood cells	1
Total protein	90
Glucose	25
Gram stain	Moderate polymorphonucleocytes and few gram-positive cocci

Her complete blood count shows a white blood cell count of 29,000 with a left shift (an increase in immature white cells usually indicating infection).

TABLE 5.7. Normal Laboratory Values for a Sepsis Workup[21]

Test	Normal result		
Complete blood count	White blood count 5,000–15,000 per mm^3		
Urinalysis	Less than 5 white blood cells on high-powered field of spun urinalysis		
Cerebrospinal fluid	Appearance	▶	Clear and colorless
	Gram stain	▶	No organisms seen
	Cell count	▶	0–4 white blood cells, 0 red blood cells
	Total Protein	▶	<40 mg/100 mL
	Glucose	▶	40–60 mg/100 mL

Tiffany is admitted to the hospital for IV antibiotics, fluid restriction, strict isolation and close observation with the diagnosis of bacterial meningitis. Dr. Matthews asks you to decrease Tiffany's IV rate to 3/4 maintenance rate and give the first dose of antibiotics before transferring Tiffany to the floor. She explains to Mr. and Mrs. Daniels what they can expect for the next few days. They ask Dr. Matthews what causes meningitis.

TABLE 5.8. Common Causes of Bacterial Meningitis[1,5–7,17,19]

In infants under two months of age:	In children over two months of age:
Group B streptococcus	*Hemophilus influenzae* (H. flu)
Gram-negative enteric organisms (*Escherichia coli*)	*Streptococcus pneumoniae* (pneumococcus)
	Neisseria meningitides (meningococcus)

> **Question**
>
> The doctor orders 200 mg ampicillin IV for Tiffany's first dose of antibiotics. She says that she is basing the dosage on 200 mg/kg/day, to be administered every 4 hr. Tiffany weighs 4 kg. Is this the correct dose for her? (Choose Yes or No.)
>
> _____ Yes   _____ No

Answer

No, the correct amount of ampicillin for Tiffany's first dose is 133 mg. This is how it is calculated:

200 mg × 4 kg (Tiffany's weight) = 800 mg per 24 hr.

Then, 800 mg is divided by 6 (number of doses per 24 hr) = 133.3 mg. This dose is rounded off for ease of administration.

Mr. and Mrs. Daniels leave Tiffany briefly to fill out the paperwork required for admission. You look at her lying quietly on the gurney, and consider her condition. You think about the complications she could have.

> **Question**
>
> What are two serious complications of systemic infections? (Fill in the blanks.)
>
> 1. _____
>
> 2. _____

Answer

Any of the complications listed in Table 5.9 would be appropriate answers.

TABLE 5.9. Serious Complications of Systemic Infections[18,19]

Serious complications can occur with systemic infections such as sepsis and meningitis including the following:
Septic shock
Cerebral edema
Seizures
Disseminated intravascular coagulation
Inappropriate antidiuretic hormone secretion, causing hyponatremia and subsequent cerebral edema

Tiffany remains stable throughout her emergency department stay. She will be admitted to the pediatric unit for continued observation and therapy. As you discuss her admission with the nurses on the floor, you think about what a responsibility they have in watching Tiffany for the early signs of deterioration. The greatest concern for the next few days will be the possibility of Tiffany developing cerebral edema.

Question

What early clinical signs might you expect Tiffany to exhibit if she developed cerebral edema from the meningitis? (Choose all that apply.)

1. Change in heart rate
2. Bulging fontanel
3. Change in blood pressure
4. Cushing's triad

Answer

The correct answer is (2). Because Tiffany's anterior fontanel is still open, swelling of the brain will result in a noticeable fullness of the fontanel to inspection and palpation. Rapid heart rate is a less specific indicator of cerebral edema. Changes in blood pressure and Cushing's triad are late manifestations of cerebral edema, and should not be relied on to diagnose impending herniation. The signs of Cushing's triad are hypertension with a widened pulse pressure, bradycardia, and decrease in respiratory rate and depth.[11,23]

Your hospital is well equipped to take care of Tiffany as long as she remains stable. If her condition deteriorates significantly, she will be transferred to a pediatric center. Intensive care, with personnel specializing in pediatrics, is the appropriate level of care for children who develop complications of systemic infection. Until transport occurs, interim respiratory support, fluid resuscitation, and antibiotic therapy must be provided.

Fortunately, Tiffany does well during her hospitalization. On Day 4 of her hospital stay, you stop by to visit. The floor nurse tells you that Tiffany's blood and CSF have cultured Group B streptococci. Now afebrile and taking oral fluids, she continues to receive antibiotic therapy.

Mrs. Daniels sees you when you come by to visit. She has stayed nearby throughout Tiffany's hospitalization. She thanks you for your care of Tiffany and says she is embarrassed that she was so worried about the testing. You tell her that you have children yourself, and you would be just as worried as she was under the circumstances. Tiffany looks bright and alert, very much improved from when you first saw her.

SICKLE CELL ANEMIA

PREVIEW

Sickle cell anemia is a hereditary blood abnormality (hemoglobinopathy) in which normal hemoglobin is partly or completely replaced by abnormal sickle-shaped hemoglobin.[1] Sickle erythrocytes are inflexible, more fragile, and have a shorter life span than normal erythrocytes (see Figure 5.4, normal and sickled red blood cells).[2]

Sickle cell anemia is diagnosed through a blood-testing process called hemoglobin electrophoresis. Neonatal screening, accomplished by analyzing umbilical cord blood on special plates, identifies infants with sickle cell anemia before complications of the disease develop.[2]

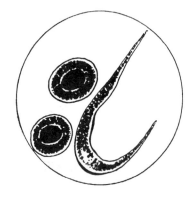

FIGURE 5.4

Approximately 8% of African Americans in the United States, Caribbean, and Latin America carry the sickle cell gene. More than 50,000 individuals in the United States are affected by the actual disease.[2] Sickle cell anemia is also known to affect individuals of Mediterranean descent.[1]

Sickle cell anemia occurs in approximately 1 in 625 births. Before 1900, most individuals with sickle cell anemia died before puberty. In 1970, 20% to 30% of deaths still occurred before 5 years of age, with few individuals surviving through the third decade. Today, it is common for patients with sickle cell anemia to live well into their 40s. This increased longevity is attributed to improved individual health status and better medical management.[2] The most frequent cause of death in individuals with sickle cell disease is infection.[4]

CASE STUDY 2 OBJECTIVES

Once you have completed this case study, you will be able to

- Name the most common cause of death in individuals with sickle cell anemia
- Identify three types of sickle cell crisis
- Identify the most typical type of sickle cell crisis seen in children
- Name three triggers of sickle cell crisis
- Outline two main management components of sickle cell crisis
- Discuss typical medications used to control sickle cell crisis pain in children
- Identify life-threatening complications of sickle cell crisis

CASE STUDY 2

Theodore Has Pain in His Back and Left Leg

Theodore Walters is a 5-year-old African American male child who has been vacationing with his family in your town for the past 3 days. He arrives in your emergency department at 8:00 P.M. on a hot July night complaining of pain in his back and left leg. Mrs. Walters tells you that Theodore has sickle cell anemia.

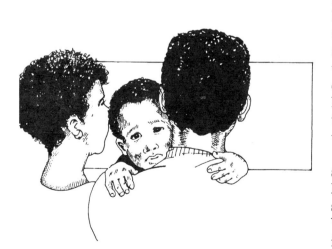

Mrs. Walters says that her son's pain began around noon while the family was picnicking at the state park in the nearby mountains. Although she has been giving him codeine and nonaspirin analgesic every 4 hours, and has encouraged Theodore to drink clear liquids since the pain started, these measures have not provided relief. Mr. Walters mentions that this is a typical crisis for Theodore and that he has required multiple hospitalizations in the past for pain control. He adds that Theodore's most recent crisis occurred about 6 weeks ago.

Theodore is wearing shorts and a green-and-white T-shirt with a big number 4 on it. He is being carried by Mr. Walters and is resting his head on his father's shoulder. You notice that he seems small for his age. While the parents are talking you notice that Theodore is breathing rapidly. When Theodore yawns, you see that the mucous membranes of his mouth are pale (see Figure 5.5).

FIGURE 5.5

TRIAGE DECISION

On the basis of your initial rapid assessment, how would you triage Theodore?

Emergent.   A life-threatening situation in need of immediate intervention.

Urgent.   Patient needs care within 1 hour to prevent further deterioration.

Nonurgent.   Patient is able to wait more than 1 hour without further deterioration.

TRIAGE DECISION ANSWER

Theodore should be triaged as urgent. Your initial impression is that he is breathing rapidly and seems pale; assessment of his *ABCs* show that Theodore is not having any difficulty ventilating, and is awake, alert, and responsive to his environment. You also note that he is in some pain. Because his parents have had much experience with his illness, and they believe he is having a sickle cell crisis, you decide that he will need care quickly to control pain and prevent further deterioration in condition.

Question

What type of crisis do you suspect Theodore is experiencing? (Choose one answer.)

1. Vaso-occlusive crisis   2.   Anemic crisis   3.   Sequestration crisis

---

Answer

The correct answer is (1); pain is a typical presenting symptom of vaso-occlusive crisis. Table 5.10 (facing page) describes the three most common types of sickle cell crisis.

The emergency department and triage area are quiet, so you bring Theodore into a treatment room to continue his assessment. You have seen sickle cell patients before; one patient who had been a frequent visitor to your emergency department died a few months ago from sepsis, so you are very thorough in assessing the seriousness of Theodore's signs and symptoms.

You ask Mr. Walters to sit down with Theodore in his lap. As he does this Theodore grimaces and moans. You prepare to check Theodore's vital signs.

Question

If Theodore were having pain in both arms and both legs, what would you do about taking his blood pressure? (Choose one answer.)

1. Use the limb that hurts least
2. Determine capillary refill
3. Defer taking his blood pressure until later

Answer

The answer is (1) because the nonpainful limb probably has the best circulation. Although it is important to obtain a blood pressure on a child in sickle cell crisis, you should try to avoid using painful limbs because constriction causes stasis of blood and may worsen a vaso-occlusive episode.[3]

You may not be able to obtain an adequate capillary refill time if vessels are occluded, and you should obtain a baseline measure of blood pressure rather than deferring the assessment until later.

TABLE 5.10. Three Types of Sickle Cell Crisis[1,2,5–8]

Vaso-occlusive crisis
Vaso-occlusive crisis presents with severe pain that can mimic a variety of medical/surgical conditions. Stasis of blood flow is caused by entangled sickle-shaped erythrocytes leading to engorgement and enlargement of the affected body part, ischemia, infarction, tissue destruction, and eventual replacement with fibrotic/scar tissue. This can impair function of any tissue or organ. Other symptoms typical of vaso-occlusive crisis include weakness, fever, anorexia, and vomiting. A typical presentation of vaso-occlusive crisis in children between the ages of 6–24 months is dactylitis, a warm, painful swelling of one or both hands and feet caused by infarction of the metatarsals or metacarpals.
Aplastic or anemic crisis
Aplastic or anemic crisis presents with rapid decline in the hemoglobin level and a low or absent reticulocyte count. It is usually caused by viral infections, which results in temporary cessation of red blood cell production in the bone marrow. Because sickled red blood cells are destroyed so quickly (lifespan of 10–20 days as opposed to the normal red blood cell lifespan of 120 days), the child with sickle cell disease already produces new blood cells at 5–8 times the normal rate. Therefore, a decline in bone marrow activity of even 1 day can cause aplastic crisis. Although rare, aplastic crisis can also be caused by folic acid deficiency.
Sequestration crisis
Sequestration crisis is the most life-threatening type of sickle cell crisis. It involves sudden pooling of blood into the spleen resulting in decreased blood volume and shock. Death can occur within hours of onset unless immediate volume expansion and blood replacement is instituted. The potential for sequestration crisis exists until the child's spleen becomes fibrotic and nonfunctional. This usually occurs by the time the child is 5 years of age.

Theodore's mother and father talk reassuringly to their son, promising to stay with him while you make your assessment. Theodore looks at you suspiciously as you check his vital signs.

Heart rate	136 beats/min
Respiratory rate	20 breaths/min
Blood pressure	132/90
Temperature	37.2°C (98.9°F)

Question

How would you describe Theodore's vital signs? (Mark each assessment **1**, **2**, or **3**.)

Heart rate	_____	1.	Normal
Respiratory rate	_____	2.	Abnormally high/fast
Blood pressure	_____	3.	Abnormally low/slow
Temperature	_____		

Answer

The correct answers are *heart rate:* 1; *respiratory rate:* 1; *blood pressure:* 2; and *temperature:* 1. Pain could cause increases in all vital signs. Abnormal vital signs may also be due to preexisting primary cardiovascular, respiratory and renal conditions as well as secondary conditions resulting from damage to major organs from previous vaso-occlusive crises.

To determine what might have precipitated this crisis, you obtain the remainder of the AMPLE history from Theodore's father.

Allergies. None.

Medications. Codeine 15 mg with acetaminophen 160 mg 1 hour ago.

Previous illness. Only problems related to sickle cell disease.

Last meal. Lunch. He has been eating normally and has been drinking only clear liquids since lunch time.

Events preceding illness. Theodore's urine and stools have been normal. He has not been more active than usual and has not had any emotional upsets.

Question

What can trigger a sickle cell crisis? (Choose all that apply)

1. Dehydration	6. Illness or infection
2. Allergy	7. High altitude
3. Emotional upsets	8. Exposure to cold
4. Stress	9. Major burns
5. Immunizations	10. Hypoxia

Answer

All of the items listed *except* (2) and (5) can trigger a sickle cell crisis. It is especially important to keep the immunizations of children with sickle cell disease up to date, because infections may precipitate a crisis. Allergies have not been shown to trigger a sickle cell crisis. Table 5.11 shows some of the precipitants of sickle cell crisis.

TABLE 5.11. Sickle Cell Crisis[6,7,9]

Definition. "Crisis" is the word used to describe the most acute symptoms of sickle cell disease complications. Although the exact cause of sickle cell crisis is unknown, two precipitating factors have been identified.

- *Hypoxia owing to low oxygen tension.* Caused by exposure to high altitudes, strenuous exercise, hyperventilation, or inadequate oxygenation (as with general anesthesia).
- *Increased viscosity of blood.* Caused by insufficient fluid intake, or fluid loss or dehydration.

Sickle cell crises can be triggered by fever, infection, exposure to sudden temperature changes, vigorous exercise, emotional stress, and severe burns.

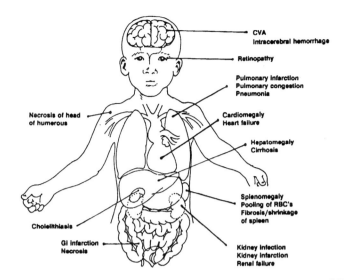

FIGURE 5.6 Body areas affected by sickle cell disease.[1,3,5]

Other serious problems that may result from sickle cell disease include

- Necrosis of the femoral head
- Joint infarction
- Priapism
- Chronic ulcers
- Cellulitis

A classic presentation of vaso-occlusive crisis in infants and young children is hand–foot syndrome. There is localized tenderness and swelling of the dorsal surfaces of hands or feet, which extends to the fingers or toes.

As your assessment continues, Theodore's father and mother watch worriedly. You lift up Theodore's green-and-white T-shirt and listen to his chest carefully in the axillary line on each side to determine whether the two sides are different. His breath sounds are clear and equal bilaterally, and his abdomen is soft and nontender to palpation.

Question

Which of the following items would cause you to change your initial assessment of his condition from *urgent* to *emergent*? (Choose all that apply.)

1. Use of nonaspirin analgesic every 4 hr without relief of pain
2. Father telling you Theodore's stomach seems swollen
3. Recent history of pneumonia requiring hospitalization
4. Parents telling you Theodore is not acting normally

Answer

The correct answers are (2) and (4). Enlargement of the abdomen could be due to sequestration crisis—engorgement of the spleen as it fills with blood, so you would want to treat this as an emergency. If this condition were not recognized and treated immediately with rapid volume expansion and blood transfusion, there would be little hope of survival.[5] Remember that children compensate at first for blood loss, so early recognition is essential. If his parents told you Theodore was not acting normally, you would also consider it an emergent situation, because he could be severely hypoxic, in early hypovolemic shock, or experiencing early signs of a vaso-occlusive crisis.

Taking medication without relief indicates a high level of pain, but considering his other signs, you probably would not change your assessment of the degree of urgency. A recent history of pneumonia would not be a reason to reconsider your evaluation either.

The emergency physician, Dr. Wells, comes in to examine Theodore. Mr. Walters continues to keep Theodore in his lap throughout the examination. After Theodore's examination, he tells you Theodore needs an IV line and tells the Walters that he will be ordering some laboratory tests.

Question

What tests would you expect Dr. Wells to order as part of Theodore's diagnostic workup for vaso-occlusive crisis? (Choose all that apply.)

1. Complete blood count
2. Reticulocyte count
3. Blood culture

4. Urinalysis and urine culture
5. Chest X-ray film

Answer

Dr. Wells will probably order a complete blood count and a reticulocyte count. Although children with sickle cell disease have chronic anemia, a sudden drop in hemoglobin from a previously established "normal" range, typically between 5.5–9.9 g/dL, signals a change indicative of aplastic or sequestration crisis.[2,5]

An abnormally high level of white cells (leukocytosis) of 12,000 to 15,000/μL is normal in sickle cell disease because of granulocytes shifting from the marginated into the circulating compartment. A further increase from previously established "normal" ranges typically occurs with vaso-occlusive crisis and infection.[2]

The reticulocyte count reflects the state of current red blood cell (erythrocyte) production. Reticulocytes are non-nucleated red cells formed in the bone marrow. A high reticulocyte count indicates an accelerated level of erythrocyte production, often as a result of destruction of circulating red blood cells. Baseline reticulocyte counts are normally elevated between 5% to 30% in the child with sickle cell disease. A low or absent reticulocyte count, conversely, indicates that red blood cell production is decreased, as in aplastic crisis.[2,8]

Question

Name three additional tests you would expect the doctor to order if Theodore had a fever. (Fill in the blanks.)

1. _____

2. _____

3. _____

Answer

Any of the following tests might be ordered:

- Blood culture
- Urinalysis
- Urine culture
- Throat culture
- Chest X-ray

The spleen plays an important role in the body's ability to fight infection. Because individuals with sickle cell anemia develop functional asplenia (ineffective spleen) in early childhood because of the sickling phenomenon, they are at high risk for developing overwhelming and potentially fatal infection.[2] Therefore, identifying the infection source is important when a child with sickle cell anemia is febrile. To do this, a blood culture, urinalysis, urine culture, throat culture, and chest X-ray film are usually obtained.[10]

Other diagnostic studies such as electrolytes, kidney and liver function studies, arterial blood gases, lumbar puncture for CSF collection, and stool culture could be ordered if specific pathophysiology is suspected. A type and crossmatch is obtained when the need for a blood transfusion is anticipated.

Dr. Wells inquires about Theodore's current weight. You realize you did not check his weight before placing him in a treatment room. You ask Mr. Walters to carry Theodore to the scales.

Question

What are two reasons why you will need to know Theodore's accurate body weight? (Fill in the blanks.)

1. _____

2. _____

Answer

You will need Theodore's weight to calculate IV fluid requirements and in anticipation of an order for pain medication, because both are calculated on the basis of body weight.

Another reason for weighing him, though less pressing at this time, is to determine his growth percentile. Sickle cell disease is known to cause poor growth and delays in maturation,[5] and you have noticed that he is small for his age. Although it is important to document his size, growth percentile information will not change the treatment plan for Theodore.

Theodore is reluctant to stand on the scale, wanting to stay in his father's arms. Mrs. Walters encourages him, telling him it will just take a minute. You find he weighs 15 kg. You can see from this interaction with Theodore that starting the IV line will not be easy. When Mr. Walters picks Theodore up again, you ask him to return to the treatment room. Because your nursing diagnosis is potential altered tissue perfusion owing to occlusion of vessels by sickled cells (vaso-occlusive crisis), your goal will be improved oxygenation and ventilation, and decrease in pain caused by occlusion of the blood vessels. You wonder whether Theodore should be given oxygen.

Question

Should you administer oxygen to Theodore for comfort? (Choose Yes or No.)

____ Yes   ____ No

Answer

The correct answer is No. Oxygen therapy may not be beneficial to Theodore at this time. In the absence of hypoxemia, tachycardia and tachypnea, oxygen therapy may cause suppression of red blood cell production in the bone marrow.[5]

You make sure Theodore is allowed to maintain any position in which he feels comfortable. You also begin to gather supplies for his IV line.

Question

What are two reasons you would have for starting an intravenous line on Theodore at this point? (Choose two answers.)

1. To treat him for shock
2. To hydrate him thoroughly
3. To give him pain medication
4. To give him packed red blood cells
5. To give him IV antibiotics

Answer

The correct answers are (2) and (3). Because dehydration is known to cause increased sickling, increasing hydration is an important component of vaso-occlusive crisis treatment.[2] The pain of crisis is caused by clogging of the microcirculation with sickled cells, and hydration may act to reduce this phenomenon. Medication is also used to help control pain.[2,5] Because Theodore is in acute pain, this medication should be given intravenously.

Theodore does not appear to be in shock at present, and it has not thus far been determined that he needs either packed cells or antibiotics. Because the possibility that he will need transfusion exists, however, you start as large a line as possible, a 20-gauge over-the-needle catheter.

Mr. and Mrs. Walters are accustomed to the emergency setting, and ask to remain with Theodore when you start his IV line. You encourage them to help keep him calm, and they say they are used to doing that. Because you don't want to start the line on a painful limb, you ask Theodore to show you in which hand he wants to have the IV line started. He reluctantly shows you his left hand. As you start the line, his mother and father get him to sing a silly family song with them. He cries and kicks as you insert the needle, but does not pull his hand away. You give him a sticker that says, "I'm a champ." Dr. Wells tells you that he wants Theodore's intravenous hydration to begin with a fluid bolus.

Question

How much normal saline would you expect to give Theodore over the first hour? (Choose one answer.)

1. 150 mL
2. 300 mL

3. 450 mL
4. 600 mL

Answer

The correct answer is (2). Initial intravenous hydration usually begins with a normal saline bolus of 20 mL/kg, given over the first hour.[11]

Theodore is restless and moans periodically. Mr. and Mrs. Walters are trying to talk to him and comfort him. You make a nursing diagnosis at this point of acute pain. To assess his pain, you use Hester's Poker Chip tool, and Theodore chooses three out of four chips, indicating a high degree of pain. You discuss the need for medication with Dr. Wells.

Question

Match the following medications that are used for sedation or analgesia with the most common routes of administration. (Choose all that apply—there may be more than one route per medication.)

____	Meperidine (Demerol)	(a) Intramuscular injection
____	Morphine	(b) Topical
____	Hydroxyzine (Vistaril)	(c) Intravenous
____	Midazolam (Versed)	(d) po (per oral)
____	Chloral hydrate	(e) pr (per rectal)
____	Nitrous oxide	(f) Intranasal spray
____	Tetracaine/adrenaline/cocaine	(g) Inhalation
____	Lidocaine	(h) Subcutaneous injection
____	Sublimaze (Fentanyl)	
____	Codeine with acetaminophen	

Answer

Meperidine (Demerol)	(a), (c), (d)	Chloral hydrate	(d), (e)
Morphine	(a), (c), (d)	Tetracaine/adrenaline/cocaine	(b)
Hydroxyzine (Vistaril)	(a)	Sublimaze (Fentanyl)	(c)
Lidocaine	(b), (h)	Codeine with acetaminophen	(d)
Midazolam (Versed)	(a), (c), (f)		

Many health care professionals are fearful of overdosing children when ordering and administering pain medication. Analgesic medications can be administered safely when dosages are calculated using the child's body weight. The type of medication most useful for Theodore will probably be meperidine, given intravenously. See Table 5.12 (following page) for medication used in the emergency setting.

Young children are unable to verbalize the need for analgesia. Older children frequently won't ask for pain medication because they fear injections or realize that admitting to continued pain could result in hospitalization. It is therefore imperative that the nurse be able to interpret subtle, nonverbal indicators of pain. Analgesia should never be withheld because the child won't verbalize a need for it.[7]

TABLE 5.12.   Medications Used to Control Pain in the Emergency Setting[5,11,12,15]

Drug	Route	Onset	Duration	Comments
Chloral hydrate	po, pr	30 min–1 hr	4–9 hr	Hypnotic/sedative used to induce sleep for computed tomography or magnetic resonance imaging.
Codeine with acetaminophen	po	30 min–1 hr	3–4 hr	Analgesic. May cause nausea and vomiting.
Sublimaze (Fentanyl)	IV	3–5 min	30–60 min	Analgesic. Causes respiratory depression. Shorter duration than morphine sulfate. Reversible with naloxone. May cause facial pruritus. Potentiates action of midazolam.
Hydroxyzine (Vistaril)	po, IM (never given IV)	po: 30 min to 1 hr; IM: 10 min	7 hr	Decreases anxiety, nausea, and vomiting. Antihistaminic. Enhances effects of opiates. When used with opiates, decrease dosage of opiates. Give by *Z*-track to prevent tissue necrosis. Causes dry mouth.
Lidocaine	sq, topical	5–10 min	90 min–3-1/3 hr	Local anesthetic used for short procedures; 2% jelly used for cleaning scrapes. Not used on burns because of risk of rapid absorption. Addition of epinephrine causes vasoconstriction, delays absorption.
Meperidine (Demerol)	IM, IV, po	IM: 10 min; IV: 3 min; po: 30 min	3–4 hr	Analgesic. Respiratory depression, reversible with naloxone. May cause supraventricular tachycardia.
Midazolam (Versed)	IV	3–5 min	30–60 min	Induces sleepiness/drowsiness. Has amnesic effect, so patients do not remember procedure. Causes respiratory depression, may cause hallucinations, hypotension, nausea. Potentiates action of sublimaze.
Morphine	IM, IV, po	20 min	3–4 hr	Analgesic. Causes respiratory depression, may cause nausea, vomiting.
Tetracaine/ **a**drenaline/ **c**ocaine	Topical	15 min	1 hr	Small laceration repairs; gauze containing solution is pressed onto wound for 10–20 min. Risk of toxicity on large wounds. Not for application on mucus membranes or digits.

po = orally; pr = rectally; IV = intravenously; and IM = intramuscularly.

Dr. Wells orders meperidine 15 mg, to be given intravenously. You check with the Walters to make sure Theodore is not allergic to any medications, and you leave to sign it out of the narcotic drawer.

Question

What two items should you be sure to have on hand before you administer the meperidine? (Fill in the blanks.)

1. _____

2. _____

Answer

When administering any opiate to a child intravenously, you should have both naloxone and a bag-valve-mask device on hand. Severe respiratory depression may occur even if the correct dosage for the child's weight is administered. Because of the acute level of pain, this seldom occurs in patients with vaso-occlusive crisis, however.

When you return to Theodore, you see that the first fluid bolus is complete, and you begin the meperidine infusion over 20 minutes.

Note: After the initial fluid bolus, 5% dextrose in 0.25 to 0.45 saline at two times maintenance rate may be ordered for the child in vaso-occlusive crisis.

Question

If the physician orders twice the maintenance rate of 5% dextrose in 0.45 saline, Theodore's hourly intravenous rate would be: (Choose one answer.)

1. 52 mL/hr
2. 104 mL/hr
3. 26 mL/hr
4. 208 mL/hr

Answer

The correct answer would be 104 mL/hr. Calculation for twice the maintenance rate for Theodore would be

$1000 + (50 \times 5$ kg, the weight in kg over 10 kg$) = 1250$

$1250 \div 24 = 52$ mL/hr (maintenance rate)

52 mL $\times 2 = 104$ mL/hr (2 times maintenance rate)

Fifteen minutes have passed since you began the administration of the pain medication, and you check to determine whether your interventions to relieve Theodore's pain have been successful. Theodore has been given a hand puppet to play with, and he looks less restless. You assess his vital signs.

Heart rate	136 beats/min
Respiratory rate	32 breaths/min
Blood pressure	126/86

You reassess his pain level with the poker chips, and he selects two chips. Mr. and Mrs. Walters are also looking more relaxed. The medication appears to have a good effect on his pain.

Question

What else can you do to help control Theodore's pain? (Mark all the appropriate answers.)

1. Encourage him to rest in bed
2. Assist parents to help him become comfortable
3. Provide diversion for him (toys, books, etc.)

Answer

All of the above answers are helpful. Bedrest is an important component of sickle cell crisis pain control.[3] Parents usually know how to make their child more comfortable, so assisting them in this endeavor is a good option. Diversion and play is another important component. Focusing on a story, television program, music, toy, or game directs attention away from pain. Remember, the "work" of every child is play. Children get bored, restless, and more responsive to pain if they don't have appropriate activities to occupy their attention.

You ask if the Walters would like to have a book to help distract Theodore, and they gratefully say that they would, explaining that because they left for the hospital so quickly they forgot to bring any toys or books with them. They read to him quietly, and Theodore finally falls into a restless sleep 20 minutes later. You observe his respiratory rate every 15 minutes, and it remains stable.

Two hours later Theodore is awake, restless, and moaning constantly.

Question

Based on your nursing diagnoses of altered tissue perfusion and acute pain, what periodic assessments should you perform now, besides vital signs? (Choose all that apply.)

1. The amount of pain Theodore is experiencing
2. Alterations in mental status
3. Temperature
4. Skin color and moisture

Answer

Answers (1), (2), and (4) are correct. Besides monitoring the vital signs and Theodore's mental status, serial assessments of his level of pain will help to determine the effectiveness of treatment or progression of the sickle cell crisis.

You discuss additional medication with Dr. Wells, who orders another dose of intravenous meperidine that you give. This dose keeps Theodore comfortable for less than 2 hours.

Question

What would be the most appropriate plan for Theodore at this point? (Choose all that apply.)

1. Order more pain medication for administration
2. Begin planning for Theodore's discharge with oral pain medication
3. Plan to admit Theodore into the hospital

Answer

Answers (2) and (3) are correct. Failure to control pain with repeated doses of intravenous medication suggests that hospital admission is necessary for continued intravenous hydration and medication.[5,8]

Theodore will probably not be discharged. Discharge might be considered if pain relief had been achieved with one dose of IV medication, but Theodore's pain is not under control.

Theodore has continued to have pain, but it has been limited to his extremities. The type and location of pain experienced by sickle cell patients can be an important indicator of vaso-occlusive events occurring within the body.

Question

If Theodore complained of chest pain and had obvious difficulty breathing, what would you suspect as the cause of his distress? (Choose all appropriate answers.)

1. Myocardial infarction
2. Pulmonary vaso-occlusive crisis

3. Pneumonia
4. Costochondritis

Answer

The correct answers are pulmonary vaso-occlusive crisis or pneumonia (see Table 5.13). Infectious infiltrates and vaso-occlusive infarcts both may present with respiratory distress and localized tissue hypoxia. It may initially be difficult to distinguish one condition from the other. In addition, pneumonia causes localized tissue hypoxia, which increases sickling, vaso-occlusion, and infarction within the lung tissue.[2,5,11]

A sickle cell patient presenting with respiratory symptoms should have chest X-ray films and a blood culture performed. If available at your hospital, an arterial blood gas should be analyzed, and supplemental oxygen should be given on an ongoing basis for saturation of less than 95%.[11] Oxygen should always be given when a child is tachypneic, tachycardic, and hypoxemic.[5]

TABLE 5.13. Pulmonary Vaso-Occlusive Crisis and Pneumonia[2,5,11]

Pulmonary vaso-occlusive crisis and pneumonia can both cause the following manifestations:	
Chest pain	Nasal flaring
Coughing	Tachypnea
Chest retractions	Shortness of breath/labored breathing
Treatment of pulmonary infiltrates include the following:	
Hospital admission	IV antibiotics
Bedrest	Oxygen
IV hydration	

Question

If Theodore had come to the emergency department complaining of sudden onset abdominal pain, what would you suspect as the cause of his problem? (Mark all appropriate answers.)

1. Appendicitis
2. Bowel obstruction
3. Cholecystitis

4. Bowel, liver, spleen vaso-occlusion
5. Gastroenteritis
6. All of the above

Answer

All of the answers are correct. Abdominal pain can be caused by a vaso-occlusive crisis or any number of other medical/surgical problems. Evaluation of abdominal pain should be comprehensive to rule out the possibility of conditions both related and unrelated to sickle cell anemia.[13]

You move Theodore and his parents into the holding room while you await a bed on the pediatric floor. There is a television set, which he is watching. Mrs. Walters suddenly comes rushing down the hall to tell you that Theodore is complaining that his head hurts, and he can't see the picture on the television screen as well as he could before.

Question

What would you suspect as the cause of Theodore's symptoms? (Fill in the blank.)

_____

Answer

Theodore's symptoms may indicate central nervous system vaso-occlusive crisis. This severe complication of sickle cell disease may lead to ischemia, stroke, permanent neurologic deficit, or death (see Table 5.14).

TABLE 5.14.   Neurologic Manifestations of CNS Vaso-Occlusive Crisis[1,5,14]

Vaso-occlusive crisis affecting the CNS presents with any of the following neurologic manifestations:	
Headache	Muscle weakness
Dizziness	Cranial nerve palsies
Visual, auditory, and speech impairment	Parathesias
Intellectual impairment	Paralysis
Ataxia	Seizures
	Coma

The treatment for vaso-occlusive crisis with CNS involvement is blood transfusion to provide a fresh supply of normal erythrocytes.[14] This increases the oxygen-carrying capacity of the blood and decreases the sickling phenomenon and clumping effect of the sickled cells. As a result, microvascular circulation is improved. If instituted rapidly, it is possible to prevent or terminate potentially life-threatening, debilitating consequences of CNS vaso-occlusive crisis.[5,14]

The methods of transfusion commonly used include simple transfusion of packed red blood cells at 15 mL/kg/day and partial exchange transfusion to decrease the concentration of sickled cells in the blood. Because the increased blood viscosity of a high hematocrit increases the incidence of vaso-occlusion, the accompanying hematocrit should be lower than 45%.[5]

You recheck his vital signs.

Heart rate	158 beats/min
Respiratory rate	44 breaths/min
Blood pressure	158/102 mmHg

You quickly tell Dr. Wells, move Theodore back into the treatment room on the gurney and give him oxygen at 10 L/min flow via facemask and turn up his IV fluid rate.

Knowing the treatment for this sort of crisis is a blood exchange transfusion, which is not available at your small community hospital, you realize Theodore will have to be transferred to a facility providing acute care for pediatric patients. This hospital is about 60 miles from your town.

Question

Pending transport, prioritize the following interventions: (Put a **1** by the first priority and so forth.)

_____ Arrange transport to appropriate care facility

_____ Consult with Theodore's primary care physician

_____ Provide large-volume IV hydration

_____ Provide airway management and assisted ventilation

Answer

The answers are, respectively, (3), (4), (2), and (1). Children encountering the life-threatening complications of sickle cell disease need basic supportive measures that provide airway stabilization, adequate ventilation, and oxygen administration. Circulatory support includes IV hydration to dilute circulating blood supply and decrease the clumping effect of the sickled cells until a blood transfusion can be administered. After initial stabilization has occurred, rapid transport to an appropriate care facility that will provide pediatric intensive care and transfusion therapy is imperative for the survival of the patient. Although the child's primary care physician or hematologist should be consulted, timely provision of life-saving measures should never be delayed.

Dr. Wells orders an arterial blood gas, and you increase Theodore's oxygen concentration with the use of a nonrebreathing mask. Dr. Wells orders another 20 mL/kg normal saline bolus. Theodore tells you his head hurts less now. Dr. Wells explains to the Walters that Theodore will be transferred to the receiving facility by helicopter as soon as possible.

You take the Walters into another treatment room and explain the transfer process, and give them the name of the receiving physician. You also give them written directions to the hospital where Theodore is being transferred.

Note: Childhood illness is difficult for any family. Encountering illness while away from home and familiar health care facilities is a stress-producing experience. The nurse can help reduce the stress by making sure that the family receives clear, written directions to the facility where the child is being transferred as well as the name of the physician who will be receiving their child. Providing information about telephone access, rest rooms, and food availability is also helpful.

When you ask the Walters if they have any questions, Mrs. Walters begins to cry, and Mr. Walters struggles not to show his emotions. You sit down with them for a moment, without saying anything. Mrs.

Walters looks at you tearfully and says, "He's so small, and he tries so hard . . . he doesn't deserve this—why him?" Because this is a question you can't really answer, you can only respond empathetically, "I wish I had an answer for you. . . ." She tells you how much they love Theodore, and how difficult this has been. There is not much to say, but you know that just being there for them will be helpful. You offer her some facial tissue, and she dries her eyes saying, "Well, I guess we've been through this before, we'll have to find some way to keep going." She thanks you for helping them and goes to check on Theodore.

You begin to prepare for Theodore's transport. His vital signs are remaining stable, and you obtain copies of his charts and laboratory tests (see Table 5.15).

TABLE 5.15. Interhospital Transport

When transport to the receiving hospital occurs, copies of the following should be sent with the child:
• History and physical findings   • Nurses' notes
• Consultations, progress notes   • Laboratory results
• Medication record   • X-ray films
• Intravenous fluid record
The receiving hospital should be notified by telephone of the *actual* time of departure so they can make final preparations for the child's arrival. An update of the child's condition should also be given at this time.

Once all the paperwork is completed, you go in to talk to the Walters to see if they have any questions. They offer to give back the book they were using, but you tell them that it is for them to keep. Theodore holds on to it tightly.

Theodore is transferred to the regional pediatric center. Two weeks later, you and Dr. Wells receive hand-written notes from Mrs. Walters and Theodore thanking you both for your help during their child's recent illness. She mentions that Theodore recovered from his crisis completely after receiving a series of blood transfusions and was discharged 7 days after admission to the other hospital. She happily reports that Theodore has suffered no permanent damage from the CNS crisis and that he'll be able to start school in September.

NEAR DROWNING AND HYPOTHERMIA

PREVIEW

Each year, drowning claims the lives of nearly 7,000 people in the United States. Drowning is the second most common cause of death related to injury in childhood. Children under 5 years of age encounter the highest incidence of drowning, with a peak occurring in the second year of life. The second highest peak occurs during adolescence, with alcohol consumption related to approximately 50% of these drowning episodes. Adolescents have a high number of surf drownings and incidents involving risk-taking behaviors such as swimming outside marked safety areas.[1]

Childhood submersion episodes typically occur in or near the home. These accidents happen most frequently in bath tubs, hot tubs, and swimming pools.[2] Alcohol consumption by supervising adults may play a role in submersion events of children younger than 5 years of age.[1] Child abuse by submersion also occurs, although the actual extent of this problem is unknown.[3] Ironically, most drowning episodes are preventable.[1]

Submersion episodes can be divided into two distinct categories:

• *Drowning.* Suffocation resulting from submersion in fluid, which leads to death within 24 hours.

- *Near-drowning.* Suffocation resulting from submersion in fluid, which leads to survival for 24 hours or more.

Death from drowning can actually occur by several different mechanisms. Although it is believed that about 90% of all victims die as a result of inhaling water into the alveoli, it is possible to die without getting water into the lungs.[4–6]

CASE STUDY 3 OBJECTIVES

Once you have completed this case study, you will be able to

- Identify the most common location of childhood submersion incidents
- Name the most common methods of assessing core body temperature
- List the components of a submersion history
- Recognize the clinical manifestations of severe hypothermia
- Identify three types of rewarming methods
- Discuss management of the child who has suffered a near-drowning event and is now awake and alert
- Describe three complications that may occur within the first 24 hours after the submersion episode

CASE STUDY 3

I Only Left Lydia Alone for a Minute

It is 7:15 P.M. on a cold February evening. The emergency department where you work is filling up with the usual evening rush of young children with coughs, colds, and sore throats. Suddenly a call comes in from the dispatcher that an ambulance is bringing you an 18-month-old female child whose mother found her floating in the bathtub. Her mother started mouth-to-mouth breathing because the child looked blue and did not seem to be breathing. The child was found awake and alert when the rescue squad arrived at the scene. The prehospital providers tell you that her vital signs were within normal limits for her age at that time. The mother is accompanying the child in the ambulance.

As you wait for the ambulance to arrive, you consider what provisions you should make for the child's arrival, thinking about the major causes of morbidity and mortality in submersion injuries.

Question

You know that Lydia was submerged in bath water. In the emergency setting, the **primary** concern will be the possibility of: (Choose one answer.)

1. Bacterial infection
2. Electrolyte disturbances
3. Hypoxemia
4. Inadequate tissue perfusion
5. Hypervolemia

Answer

The correct answer is (3). Drowning involves sequential events that can ultimately lead to profound hypoxemia and multi-organ failure (see Table 5.16). A significant drop of PaO_2 is seen even when a very small amount of fluid is aspirated.[7] Emergency treatment will focus primarily on assuring adequate ventilation and oxygenation.

TABLE 5.16.   Pathophysiology of Near-Drowning/Drowning[4,9,10]

At first, drowning victims usually struggle to stay afloat and voluntary breath-holding occurs.
Hypoxemia develops and the child gasps, allowing water to enter the airway. Even a small amount of aspirated fluid may cause laryngospasm, and causes significant change in lung mechanics. Lung compliance is markedly decreased, surfactant is inactivated or lost, alveoli collapse, and the PaO_2 drops because of intrapulmonary shunting of blood through nonventilated alveoli.
In younger children, and when the water temperature is below 21°C (70°F), the "diving reflex" may be activated. This mechanism provides transient protection against hypoxia by slowing the heart rate and shunting blood from the peripheral circulation to the heart and brain, thus increasing perfusion of these vital organs.
Water may be swallowed during the submersion. Additional pulmonary morbidity may ensue from involuntary aspiration of stomach contents. This may also occur during resuscitation.
Progressive hypoxemia resulting from laryngospasm or impaired gas exchange leads to CNS ischemia and loss of consciousness within several minutes.
Cardiac rhythm disturbances and myocardial depression result from myocardial ischemia, profound systemic acidosis, and hypothermia.
If adequate ventilation and oxygenation are not quickly restored, hypotension, loss of cerebral or coronary perfusion, cardiac arrest, and brain death follow.

Although inadequate tissue perfusion (shock) may also occur, and must be treated aggressively, it is usually secondary to hypoxemia. Bacterial infection may occur at a later point. There may be electrolyte disturbances but these are usually transient and not life threatening.[8] The child may have aspirated or ingested fluid, but less than 15% of drowning victims aspirate more than 22 mL/kg, which is not enough to cause significant hypervolemia.[9]

You open the pediatric cart, and make sure suction is set up and pediatric-sized oxygen delivery devices are available. The ambulance arrives with a distraught woman holding her child (see Figure 5.7). The emergency medical technician accompanying them tells you that he has brought Lydia Seltzer and her mother, Mrs. Seltzer. Lydia is wrapped in a towel, sucking her thumb and clinging to her

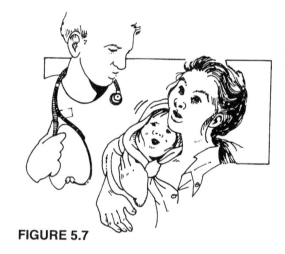

FIGURE 5.7

mother. You move them into the treatment area. When you approach the child to assess her respiratory status better, she bats at you with her hand and screams, "No!" Mrs. Seltzer says "Lydia was only alone in the bathtub for 1 minute when I went to answer the phone, and when I came back, there she was!"

TRIAGE DECISION

On the basis of your initial impression and rapid assessment, you should triage Lydia as

Emergent.   A life-threatening situation in need of immediate intervention.

Urgent.   Patient needs care within 1 hour to prevent further deterioration.

Nonurgent.   Patient is able to wait more than 1 hour without further deterioration.

TRIAGE DECISION ANSWER

Lydia should be triaged as urgent. Although your initial impression is that she is breathing without difficulty or distress, a recent submersion episode requiring mouth-to-mouth resuscitation mandates that she receive care within 1 hour.

Mrs. Seltzer sits down in the treatment room with Lydia on her lap. You notice that although Lydia's face and trunk are pink, her extremities are mottled, and she is shivering. She is wrapped in a damp towel. As you approach Lydia, she turns away crying and presses her face against her mother's chest.

Question

What is your next priority in caring for Lydia? (Choose one answer.)

1. Check vital signs   2. Assess mental status   3. Remove Lydia's damp towel

---

Answer

The correct answer is (3). In any urgent situation, assessment and treatment must go hand in hand. In this case, Lydia is at risk for hypothermia, and you should remove her damp towel and wrap her in a dry bath blanket or towel to prevent heat loss as you continue your assessment.

Formal evaluation of vital signs and mental status will add little to your observations right now. Lydia is alert and responding appropriately to her environment. Stranger anxiety is common for an 18-month-old. A toddler who cries at your approach and finds comfort with her mother is acting in a developmentally appropriate manner.

You give Mrs. Seltzer a gown and diaper for Lydia. You complete your assessment while Mrs. Seltzer dresses her. The *ABC*s are all within normal limits. After Mrs. Seltzer finishes dressing Lydia, you obtain vital signs.

Heart rate	124 beats/min
Respiratory rate	22 breaths/min
Blood pressure	102/68

Lydia's breath sounds are clear and equal bilaterally.

Question

Match Lydia's heart rate, respiratory rate, and blood pressure to the correct description.

_____ Heart rate	1.	Abnormally fast/high
_____ Respiratory rate	2.	Abnormally slow/low
_____ Blood pressure	3.	Within normal range

Answer

All of Lydia's assessments are within normal limits.

Because Lydia's skin is still somewhat mottled, and cool to touch, you obtain a core body temperature. You are especially concerned about hypothermia because children lose heat much more rapidly than adults.

Question

What methods of core temperature measurement are available in your emergency department? (List all available methods.)

1. _____

2. _____

3. _____

Answer

Most emergency departments have only one or two means of assessing core body temperature. The two most common methods are to obtain a rectal temperature by means of

- Glass mercury thermometer
- Electronic probe

Obtaining a rectal temperature is usually considered the most readily accessible and accurate means of assessment. During periods of rapid temperature change, even rectal temperatures may vary considerably from true core body temperature. Because the means of assessment of a true core temperature is rarely available, emergency departments should, as a minimum standard, be equipped with a glass hypothermia thermometer that records very low temperature ranges and allows deep insertion into the rectum.[11] Those readily available at hospital supply houses have a low reading of 23.8°C (74.8°F) and are relatively inexpensive.

More accurate core body temperatures may be obtained via placement of esophageal, nasopharyngeal, pulmonary artery, tympanic membrane (not to be confused with tympanic *infrared* thermometer), or urinary bladder probes. Each of these also has certain limitations.[11]

Mrs. Seltzer places Lydia face down across her lap and helps you by holding the thermometer. You keep Lydia covered with the bath blanket during the procedure. Lydia's temperature is 35°C (95°F). Your nursing diagnosis is alteration in body temperature related to submersion incident. You inform Dr. Miller of Lydia's temperature.

Question

What mechanisms for heat loss could be the cause of Lydia's hypothermia? (Choose all that apply.)

1. Conduction
2. Convection
3. Evaporation
4. Radiation
5. Respiration

Answer

All of the mechanisms listed could be the cause of Lydia's hypothermia. Infants and children are at increased risk for environmentally induced hypothermia owing to their relatively large body surface-to-body volume ratio.[13,14] Even at ambient emergency department temperatures, an undressed child can become significantly hypothermic during routine examination and workup.[11] Pediatric trauma victims resuscitated in the field and babies born in the field or emergency department are particularly prone to hypothermia.[15]

The immersion fluid (bath water) for Lydia may have been warm enough to prevent heat loss during the incident, but you have no means of determining that factor. Submersion in cool or cold water causes rapid heat loss through conductive and convective heat transfer from the body to the water. Lydia certainly was at risk for heat loss through evaporation, radiation, and respiration during resuscitation and evaluation.[16]

Mild hypothermia usually requires little treatment other than to reduce heat loss. A core body temperature of less than 35.0°C (95.0°F) may require more active intervention.[17]

Now that she is in a dry gown and wrapped in a bath blanket, Lydia is no longer shivering, and her extremities look somewhat less mottled. Mrs. Seltzer keeps the bath blanket around her, and you ask her to tuck it around Lydia's head as well, because children have larger heads, proportionately, than adults, and may lose a significant amount of heat via that route. Lydia is still eyeing you suspiciously. You obtain a history, using AMPLE.

Allergies. None.

Medications. None.

Previous medical problems. None.

Last meal. Chicken noodle soup and crackers at 5:00 P.M.

Events preceding injury. Lydia was fine today. She was being given her evening bath when the submersion occurred.

Mrs. Seltzer repeats her account of the submersion episode, telling you that she had just put Lydia into the bathtub when the phone rang. Expecting an important call, she ran to get it and says she was out of the room for only 1 or 2 minutes.

This is not the first time you have heard a parent tell you this. You know all too well how rapidly submersion injuries occur. Lydia does not appear to be seriously ill, and you expect she will do well. However, you know that any submersion injury can be serious.

Question

Which of the following factors significantly affect emergency treatment of a serious submersion injury? (Choose all that apply.)

1. Cold water submersion
2. Submersion time under 5 min
3. Salt water submersion
4. Child under 3 years
5. Fresh water submersion
6. "Dry" drowning vs. "wet" drowning

Answer

The correct answers are (1), (2), and (4).

1. Rapid immersion in cold water may activate a primitive "dive" reflex, shunting blood from the periphery to vital organs and thus improving outcome. For this reason, there are known cases of survival after lengthy submersions. Emergent treatment includes rewarming of severely hypothermic patients even when there are no signs of life.[10]

2. In many cases, submersion time of under 5 minutes is a good sign and means that a child is less likely to need aggressive intervention.[18]

4. Children under 3 years of age are at greatest risk of mortality and morbidity, and are the most difficult to assess, because they are essentially preverbal. Special care should be taken in assessment of respiratory and mental status.

The type of submersion fluid, whether salt water or fresh water, does not appear to be a significant factor in survival, nor is there any difference in the treatment in the emergency setting. There can be significant concern about aspiration when the fluid contains chemicals (such as in bucket submersions) or considerable bacteria in the water, as from sewage.[19,20]

"Dry" drowning results when laryngospasm occurs, effectively closing off the airway until death occurs. The amount of fluid aspirated does not affect outcome, because hypoxemia is the actual cause of death.

Components that should be included in a history of a submersion injury are listed in Table 5.17.

TABLE 5.17. Important Components of a Submersion History[4]

How much time has elapsed since the incident?
How long was the submersion (documented or estimated)?
What was the temperature of the water?
What occurred at the scene and during transport?
What was going on at the time the child became submerged? Is intoxication a factor (especially with adolescent victims)?
Where did the incident occur? (what type of water?)

As you take a detailed history of the incident, Mrs. Seltzer becomes increasingly nervous. She anxiously tells you, "I've never left her alone in the tub before. I've just been so distracted since my husband left. . . ."

Question

Based on this account, what would you do? (Choose one answer.)

1. Reassure Mrs. Seltzer: "This almost happened to me once—it could happen to anyone."
2. Ask Mrs. Seltzer more questions about the incident so you can determine whether neglect or abuse occurred.
3. Ask the emergency department social worker to interview Mrs. Seltzer.
4. Encourage Mrs. Seltzer to say more about why her husband left her so you can determine the degree of family dysfunction.

Answer

The correct answer is (3). If a social worker is not available, however, professionals working in the emergency department must be responsible for careful evaluation of the situation, and for making the decision as to whether to file a report of suspected abuse or neglect.

Although most pediatric submersions are potentially preventable, a subset of cases will reflect violent intent or a pattern of supervisory failure, requiring activation of law enforcement or child protective services. When neglect is suspected, appropriate documentation and referral must be initiated. It is the duty of law enforcement and protective services, not emergency department staff, to determine responsibility and to provide appropriate ongoing counseling for the family.

Note: Health care professionals are not responsible for determining whether abuse or neglect actually occurred but for reporting the suspicion that it **might have occurred**. The legal system is responsible for determining guilt or innocence.

All parents, even those who may be suspected of child abuse, benefit from humane, nonjudgmental care by health care professionals. It is important to remember that many parents feel some frustration with the process of child raising. Those who abuse or neglect their children usually differ from other parents only in having poor impulse control and having been abused themselves as children.

When child maltreatment is suspected, health care personnel must be careful not to make premature judgments about the family situation or about the incident. Superficial reassurances or descriptions of one's own experiences are not advisable.

You take Mrs. Seltzer and her daughter back to an examination room. Dr. Miller pokes her head in on her way to meet an ambulance and asks you to recheck Lydia's temperature, and to obtain a blood gas and a chest film. When you recheck Lydia's rectal temperature, it is still 35°C.

Question

Which of the following rewarming techniques would be appropriate at this time? (Choose one answer.)

1. Wrap her in a blanket
2. Place her under a warming light
3. Administer heated oxygen
4. Warm gastric lavage

Answer

The correct answer is 1. Passive rewarming is considered appropriate for individuals with a stable cardiovascular system and a core temperature above 33°C.[17]

Although controversy exists as to the methods and rates at which patients should be rewarmed,[19] your choice of techniques for rewarming will be based on the resources available for use in your emergency department and the clinical condition of your patient (see Table 5.18). Some experts recommend slow rewarming for the patient with stable cardiopulmonary function, so that tissue temperature remains uniform. Rapid core rewarming is used for the unstable patient.[17]

TABLE 5.18. Rewarming Methods[11,17]

Type	Definition	Technique
Passive Rewarming	No heat application	Remove wet clothing Apply insulation with dry clothes, blankets
Active Rewarming	External heat application	Heated blankets Electric blankets Hot water bottles Heat lamps Warm water submersion
Core Rewarming	Internal heat application	Warm air inhalation Warm IV fluid administration Warm colonic irrigation Warm gastric lavage Warm peritoneal dialysis Hemodialysis

TABLE 5.19.   Effects of Hypothermia on the Human Body[12,15,16]

Temperature Comparisons	Degrees	Effect on body
108° 42° 106° 41° 104° 40° 102° 39° 100° 38° 37° 98° 36° 96° 35° 94° 34° 92° 33° 90° 32° Degrees Degrees Fahrenheit Centigrade	35.0°C (95°F)	Cold skin, poor coordination, shivering, slurred speech*
	33.5°C (92.3°F)	Disorientation, amnesia, shivering, possible bradycardia, atrial fibrillation*
	32.5°C (90.5°F)	Depressed vital signs, severely altered mental status, no shivering
	30.5°C (86.9°F)	Hypoventilation (3–4 breaths/min), dilated pupils
	29.5°C (85.1°F)	Loss of voluntary movement, stiffness, deep tendon reflexes absent
	27.5°C (81.5°F)	Comatose, looks clinically dead, pupils fixed and dilated, risk of ventricular fibrillation
	23.0°C (73.4°F)	Apnea
	21.0°C (69.8°F)	Cardiac standstill

* When hypoxia has resulted in severe brain damage, cardiac and CNS abnormalities will be present at much higher temperatures.

You give Lydia a procedure glove (see Figure 5.8) blown up like a balloon, and you draw a face on it for her. She accepts it but is not willing to meet your eyes, although she seems less apprehensive. Her vital signs remain stable, and her skin feels warmer. The signs of hypothermia have almost entirely disappeared (see Table 5.19).

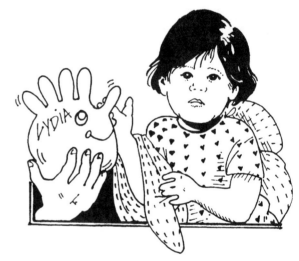

FIGURE 5.8

Question

Specific clinical signs appear as a patient becomes progressively more hypothermic. Number each of the signs listed below from **1** to **6**, indicating the progression of hypothermia (1 = least hypothermic; **6** = most hypothermic).

____ Hypoventilation

____ Poor coordination or shivering

____ Risk of ventricular fibrillation

____ Disorientation

____ Apnea

____ Deep tendon reflexes absent

Answer

The answers are (3), (1), (4), (2), (6), and (5), respectively.

A chest X-ray film and a room air arterial blood gas are obtained. Lydia's arterial blood gas results are

pH	7.31
PCO_2	45 mmHg
PO_2	90 mmHg
HCO_3	22 mEq/L

Question

Lydia's blood gas reflects: (Choose one answer.)

1. Respiratory alkalosis
2. Respiratory acidosis

3. Metabolic acidosis
4. Metabolic alkalosis

Answer

The correct answer is (2). Normal blood gas values are the same in children and adults. Lydia's arterial pH level is slightly below normal, indicating a mild acidosis. Because her PCO_2 level is at the high end of normal, with a fairly high PO_2 level, this is consistent with her history. Her normal bicarbonate level indicates that this is probably acute respiratory acidosis. The hypoxic episode caused the respiratory acidosis, which is now resolving. The next arterial blood gas will probably confirm this assessment.[14,17]

As you discuss the arterial blood gas results with Dr. Miller, you review the drowning sequence leading to respiratory acidosis. Fortunately, her respiratory acidosis is not severe, although it will take some time to be sure she did not suffer significant injury.

Dr. Miller reviews the chest film and arterial blood gases and then examines Lydia. Although no abnormalities are found during the physical examination, she informs Mrs. Seltzer that Lydia will require overnight admission to the hospital for observation. (See Table 5.20, following page.)

When the doctor leaves the room, Mrs. Seltzer starts crying again and asks, "You all seem to be so worried—what's wrong with my baby? Is she going to be all right?" You explain to her that all near-drowning victims are observed in the hospital for 12 to 24 hours because postsubmersion complications can occur without warning.[9]

Note: Children who are awake, alert, and asymptomatic after a near-drowning incident can still develop complications in the later postsubmersion period. Common complications include the following[4,9]:

- Aspiration pneumonia
- Pulmonary edema
- Cerebral edema
- Septicemia

The pediatric unit is ready to receive Lydia. You tell the floor nurse that this will probably be a "short stay" for Lydia, and that she will most likely go home tomorrow.

TABLE 5.20.   Evaluation and Treatment of Near-Drowning Victims[4,6,21]

Group	Management	Nursing interventions
Conscious and alert	Hospitalize 24 hr Arterial blood gas Chest X-ray film Passive rewarming if hypothermic	Assess and monitor for change • Mental status • Respiratory status • Core temperature • Vital signs Maintain passive rewarming
Respiratory distress or altered mental status	All of the above, and may also require • Endotracheal intubation • Ventilatory support with continuous positive airway pressure oxygen • IV infusion • IV antibiotics or steroids as indicated • Intensive care unit admission	All of the above, and may also require • Assistance with intubation • Assessment of tube placement, breath sounds • Monitoring for cardiac rhythm disturbances • Continued ventilatory support • Frequent assessment of — Respiratory rate — Quality and work of breathing
Inadequate ventilation	All of the above, and may also require • Further ventilatory support — Mechanical ventilation — Positive end-expiratory pressure	All of the above, and may also require • Monitoring of ventilatory and perfusion status • Suctioning of endotracheal tube as needed • Monitoring of ventilator
Cardiac rhythm disturbances, asystole	All of the above, and may also require • Cardiac massage • Defibrillation • Cardiac drugs • Core rewarming, if needed	All of the above, and may also require • Assistance with cardiopulmonary resuscitation • Maintenance/monitoring of core rewarming procedures

---

Question

Which of the following are important prognostic indicators for a submersion victim? (Choose all that apply.)

1. Duration of submersion
2. Water temperature
3. Level of consciousness on arrival to emergency department
4. Cardiac rhythm on arrival to emergency department
5. Age of child
6. Field intubation (if needed)

Answer

The correct answers are (1), (3), and (4). The ultimate outcome of a submersion incident depends on the duration of submersion, the degree of CNS damage due to hypoxia, the degree of pulmonary damage resulting from aspiration, and the effectiveness of initial resuscitative measures.

Although many victims appear "dead" on extraction from the water, most are salvageable and have a good neurologic outcome if effective cardiopulmonary resuscitation is started immediately in the field. Conversely, patients who arrive in the emergency department with no spontaneous respiratory effort, coma, and dilated or fixed pupils rarely survive intact, regardless of treatment.[4,9]

Remarkable "saves" have been reported in children who were submerged for long periods in very cold water.[4] For this to happen, the protective effect of hypothermia must *precede* the onset of hypoxemia so that cerebral tissue can maintain a limited metabolism on its store of oxygen.[9] An overwhelming majority of children who present to the emergency department clinically dead with profound hypothermia will not survive.[4]

Lydia was submerged for a short time, according to her mother, and witnesses have been shown to assess submersion times quite accurately.[19] This short submersion time will lessen Lydia's chances for serious sequelae.

Lydia is admitted to the pediatric floor of your hospital where she is observed for 24 hours. She develops no postsubmersion complications. During the hospitalization, Mrs. Seltzer is interviewed by a county protective services social worker. Although no charges of neglect are filed against Mrs. Seltzer, she is referred to a local agency that offers single-parent counseling and support groups.

REFERENCES

Case Study 1

1. Eichelberger, M., Ball, J. W., Pratsch, G. S., & Runion, E. (1990). *Pediatric emergencies: A manual for prehospital providers*. Englewood Cliffs, NJ: Prentice Hall.
2. Jaffe, D., & Torrey, S. (1985). Diagnostic approach to febrile illness. In S. Ludwig (Ed.), *Clinics in emergency medicine: Pediatric emergencies* (pp. 9–28). New York: Churchill Livingstone.
3. Gehlbach, S. (1988). Fever in children younger than three months of age: A pooled analysis. *The Journal of Family Practice, 27*, 305–312.
4. Rosenberg, N., Vranesich, P., & Cohen, S. (1985). Incidence of serious infection in infants under two months with fever. *Pediatric Emergency Care, 1*, 54–56.
5. Foster, R., Hunsberger, M., & Anderson, J. (1989). *Family-centered nursing care of children*. Philadelphia: Saunders.
6. Whaley, L., & Wong, D. (1987). *Nursing care of infants and children* (3rd ed). Washington, DC: Mosby.
7. Fleisher, G. (1988). Infectious disease emergencies. In G. Fleisher & S. Ludwig (Eds.), *Textbook of pediatric emergency medicine*. (2nd ed.). Baltimore: Williams & Wilkins.
8. Kimmel, S. & Gemmill, D. (1988). The young child with fever. *American Family Physician, 37*, 197–206.
9. Kruse, J. (1988). Fever in children. *American Family Physician, 37*, 127–135.
10. Lanros, N. (1988). *Assessment and intervention in emergency nursing* (3rd ed., pp. 131–132). Bowie, MD: Brady Communications.
11. Whaley, L., & Wong, D. (1989). *Essentials of pediatric nursing* (3rd ed.). Baltimore: Mosby.
12. Seidel, J. S., & Henderson, D. P. (1985). *Prehospital care of pediatric emergencies*. Los Angeles: Los Angeles Pediatric Society.
13. O'Brien, E. (1988). Clinical thermometry: In need of nursing research. *Journal of Pediatric Nursing, 3*, 207–208.
14. Rhoads, F., & Grandner, J. (1990). Assessment of an aural infrared sensor for body temperature measurement in children. *Clinical Pediatrics, 29*, 112–115.
15. Ros, S. (1989). Evaluation of a tympanic membrane thermometer in an outpatient clinical setting. *Annals of Emergency Medicine, 18*, 1004–1006.

16. Treloar, D., & Muma, B. (1988). Comparison of axillary, tympanic membrane, and rectal temperatures in young children. *Annals of Emergency Medicine, 17,* 435.

17. Thompson, J., McFarland, G., Hirsch, J., Tucker, S., & Bowers, A. (1989). *Mosby's Manual of Clinical Nursing* (2nd ed.). Baltimore: Mosby.

18. Kaplan, S., & Fishman, M. (1988). Update on bacterial meningitis. *Journal of Child Neurology, 3,* 82–93.

19. Scipien, G., Barnard, M., Chard, A., Howe, J., & Phillips, P. (1986). *Comprehensive pediatric nursing.* New York: McGraw–Hill.

20. Levin, R., Nahlen, B., & Kent, D. (1988). Diagnosis of the child with fever in the emergency department. *Journal of Emergency Nursing, 14,* 359–366.

21. Hazinski, M. F. (1984). *Nursing care of the critically ill child.* St. Louis: Mosby.

22. Einhorn, A. (Ed.). (1989). *House staff manual* (8th ed.). Washington, DC: Children's National Medical Center.

23. Bruce, D., Schut, L., & Sutton, L. (1988). Neurological emergencies. In G. Fleisher & S. Ludwig (Eds.), *Textbook of Pediatric Emergency Medicine.* (2nd ed.). Baltimore: Williams & Wilkins.

Case Study 2

1. Whaley, L., & Wong, D. (1989). *Essentials of pediatric nursing* (3rd ed.). Baltimore: Mosby.

2. Galloway, S., & Harwood-Nuss, A. L. (1988). Sickle-cell anemia—a review. *Emergency Medicine in Review, 6,* 213–226.

3. Rivers, R., & Williamson, N. (1990). Sickle cell anemia: Complex disease, nursing challenge. *RN, 53* 24–29.

4. Nottidge, V. (1983). Pneumococcal meningitis in sickle cell disease in childhood. *American Journal of Disease in Children, 137* 29–31.

5. Charache, S. (Ed.). (1985). *Management and therapy of sickle cell disease.* Bethesda: U.S. Department of Health and Human Services.

6. Scipien, G., Barnard, M., Chard, A., Howe, J., & Phillips, P. (1986). *Comprehensive pediatric nursing.* New York: McGraw-Hill.

7. Foster, R., Hunsberger, M., & Anderson, J. (1989). *Family-centered nursing care of children.* Philadelphia: Saunders.

8. Cohen, A. (1988). Hematologic emergencies. In G. Fleisher & S. Ludwig (Eds.), *Textbook of pediatric emergency medicine.* (2nd ed). Baltimore: Williams & Wilkins.

9. Thompson, J., McFarland, G., Hirsch, J., Tucker, S., & Bowers, A. (1989). *Mosby's manual of clinical nursing* (2nd ed.). Baltimore: Mosby.

10. Kravis, E., Fleisher, G., & Ludwig, S. (1982). Fever in children with sickle cell hemoglobinopathies. *American Journal of Diseases in Children, 136,* 1075–1078.

11. Einhorn, A. (Ed.). (1989). *House staff manual.* (8th ed.). Washington, DC: Children's National Medical Center.

12. Ambulatory Pediatric Association, Emergency Medicine Interest Group. *Sedation and analgesia in the outpatient setting.*

13. Matthews, M. (1981). Cholelithiasis: A differential diagnosis in abdominal "crisis" of sickle cell anemia. *Journal of the National Medical Association, 73,* 271–273.

14. Jayabose, J., Sheikh, F., & Mitra, N. (1983). *Exchange transfusion in the management of CNS crisis in sickle cell disease.* Philadelphia: Lippincott.

15. Hamilton, H. (1992). (Ed.). *Nursing '92 drug handbook.* Springhouse, PA: Springhouse Corp.

Case Study 3

1. Shaw, K., & Briede, C. (1989). Submersion injuries: Drowning and near-drowning. *Emergency Medical Clinics of North America, 7,* 355–370.

2. Fields, A. (1983). *Symposium on Life-threatening episodes in infants and children.* Washington: UpJohn.

3. Griest, K., & Zumwalt, R. (1989). Child abuse by drowning. *Pediatrics, 83,* 41–46.

4. Pearn, J. (1985). Drowning. In J. Dickerman & J. Lucey (Eds.), *Smith's—the critically ill child: diagnosis and medical management.* (3rd ed.). Philadelphia: Saunders.

5. Hoff, B. (1979). Multisystem failure: A review with special reference to drowning. *Critical Care Medicine, 7,* 310–320.

6. Butler, S. (1988). Out of the water, but not out of the woods. *RN, 51,* 26–30.

7. Sarnaik, A. P., & Vohra, M. P. (1986, January). Near-drowning: Fresh, salt and cold water immersion. *Clinics in Sports Medicine. 5,* 35.

8. Modell, J. H., & Davis, J. H. (1968). Electrolyte changes in human drowning victims. *Anesthesiology, 30,* 420.

9. Thompson, A., Mettler, F., & Royal, H. (1988). Environmental emergencies. In G. Fleisher & S. Ludwig (Eds.), *Textbook of pediatric emergency medicine* (2nd ed.). Baltimore: Williams and Wilkins.

10. Bourg, P. (1987). Caring for the near-drowning victim. *Nursing '87, 17,* 24V–24X.

11. Michal, D. (1989). Nursing management of hypothermia in the multiple-trauma patient. *Journal of Emergency Nursing, 15,* 416–421.

12. Zell, S. C., & Kurtz, K. J. (1985). Severe exposure hypothermia: A resuscitation protocol. *Annals of Emergency Medicine, 14,* 49–55.

13. Tron, V., Baldwin, V., & Pirie, G. (1985). Hot tub drownings. *Pediatrics, 75,* 789–790.

14. Whaley, L., & Wong, D. (1989). *Essentials of pediatric nursing* (3rd ed.). Baltimore: Mosby.

15. Eichelberger, M., Ball, J. W., Pratsch, G. S., & Runion, E. (1992). *Pediatric emergencies: A manual for prehospital care providers.* Englewood Cliffs, NJ: Brady.

16. Lanros, N. (1988). *Assessment and intervention in emergency nursing* (3rd ed.). Bowie, MD: Brady Communications.

17. Curley, F., & Irwin, R. (1986). Disorders of temperature control: Hypothermia: III. *Journal of Intensive Care Medicine, 1,* 270–288.

18. Quan, L., Wentz, K. R., Gore, E. J., & Copass, M. K. (1990). Outcome and predictors of outcome in pediatric submersion victims receiving prehospital care in King County, Washington. *Pediatrics, 86,* 586–593.

19. Martin, T. (1984). Near-drowning and cold water immersion. *Annals of Emergency Medicine, 13,* 263–271.

20. Orlowski, J. P. (1979). Prognostic factors in pediatric cases of drowning and near-drowning. *Journal of the American College of Emergency Physicians, 8,* 176–179.

21. Dean, J. M., & Kaufman, N. (1981). Prognostic indicators in pediatric near-drowning: The Glasgow coma scale. *Critical Care Medicine, 9,* 536–539.

22. Pruessner, H., Zenner, G., & Hansel, N. (1988). Management of the near-drowning victim. *American Family Practice, 37,* 251–260.

Chapter Six

Assessment and Intervention of Nontraumatic Surgical Emergencies

Prerequisite Skills

Before studying this chapter, the learner should

- Be able to identify the following anatomic structures:
  - Spleen
  - Umbilicus
  - Small intestines
  - Pancreas
  - Appendix
  - Aorta
  - Common iliac artery
  - Kidney
  - Ureters
  - Liver
  - Stomach
  - Colon
  - Gallbladder
  - Mesentery
  - Inferior vena cava
  - Renal artery
  - Bladder
  - Adrenal glands

- Have knowledge of the normal physiology of the following:
  - Production and destruction of red blood cells
  - Production and destruction of white blood cells
  - Production and excretion of bile
  - Digestion, absorption, and elimination in the gastrointestinal tract
  - Insulin production and utilization in the metabolic chain

- Have a general knowledge of how to evaluate the adult abdomen by means of
  - Auscultation
  - Percussion
  - Palpation

PREVIEW

Acute surgical emergencies in children may be caused by trauma, or may result from abdominal inflammation, obstruction, or perforation. Penetrating trauma is relatively rare in small children, but may result from gunshot or stab wounds, or from motor vehicle accidents. Abdominal pain is always a cause of concern; in adults, obtaining a good history is very helpful. This is not an easy task in small children, especially preverbal children—both the small size of the abdomen and their lack of ability to communicate verbally cause difficulties in obtaining a thorough history.

Despite the problems in obtaining an accurate history from a child, it is always essential to remember the basics of emergency assessment and care. A child with abdominal pain is at risk for shock. The *ABC*s must be assessed and attended to first, and a high degree of suspicion should be maintained for the possibility of hypovolemia and compensated shock. Early and correct diagnosis is important, but nursing diagnosis and care of the patient should be the primary focus.

A few tips on how to examine pediatric patients with abdominal pain may be helpful.

- Approach the patient with abdominal pain as slowly and as nonthreateningly as possible. A few minutes spent in gaining a child's confidence usually will save time at a later point.

- Remove all clothing for the abdominal examination, resisting the temptation simply to pull down the pants and raise the child's shirt. This is even more essential in traumatic injury, because many injuries are not easily seen without removal of all clothing.

- Encourage the performance of the abdominal examination of a small child on the mother's lap; this keeps the patient as calm and relaxed as possible.

- Defer any hands-on abdominal examination until the very last moment, as the patient is not likely to be as cooperative if he or she has experienced pain during an earlier part of the examination.

- Obtain as accurate a chronology as possible from the child, if possible, or from the parents; the sequencing of events may be very important in determining the cause of the child's pain.

This chapter describes three of the most common nontraumatic surgical emergencies in children—appendicitis, intussusception, and pyloric stenosis—and offers some general approaches to categorizing and triaging pediatric patients with abdominal pain.

CASE STUDY 1 OBJECTIVES

On completion of this case study, the learner will be able to

- Make a correct triage decision about a pediatric patient presenting with abdominal discomfort, based on observable evidence

- List the three most common abdominal emergencies by age group for infants, school-age children, and adolescents

- Describe nursing interventions that would address family concerns in a case involving a pediatric surgical emergency

- Identify pediatric disorders associated with abdominal pain

- Describe age-appropriate techniques to facilitate the physical examination of the abdomen

- List historical or physical findings suggestive of a potentially life-threatening abdominal emergency

- List historical and physical findings that might suggest that a child does *not* have a surgical emergency

- Prioritize emergency nursing interventions for the child who may require immediate abdominal surgery

CASE STUDY 1

Joey's Stomach Hurts

Joey DeNato is a 4-year-old white male child brought into your emergency department by his mother and father at 11:30 P.M. (see Figure 6.1). Joey is asleep and is being carried by his father. The DeNatos tell you that Joey has been complaining of a stomachache for 3 days, and has had watery diarrhea and a low-grade fever. They are concerned that he is dehydrated, because he has "taken nothing" for the last 2 days.

You have Mr. DeNato sit down with Joey on his lap. He unwraps Joey's blanket. When he does this, Joey opens his eyes briefly then falls back to sleep. Your initial impression is that Joey is breathing at a slightly faster-than-normal rate, but with good air movement and without difficulty. Joey is in cotton pajamas, and you touch his hands and feet; they are slightly cool to touch, and his skin color seems pale. Because of his parents' complaints about Joey's diarrhea and lack of intake, you assess his capillary refill time to make sure he is perfusing adequately. His capillary refill time is 2 seconds. It is difficult for you to determine Joey's mental status because it is late at night, and his apparent sleepiness may be due to his normal sleeping pattern.

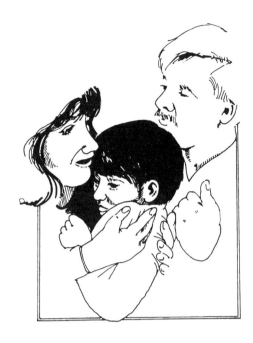

FIGURE 6.1 Joey and his parents.

TRIAGE DECISION

After this initial rapid assessment, would you triage Joey as

Emergent.   A life-threatening situation in need of immediate intervention.

Urgent.   Patient needs care within 1 hour to prevent further deterioration.

Nonurgent.   Patient is able to wait more than 1 hour without further deterioration.

TRIAGE DECISION ANSWER

Joey should be triaged as urgent. He appears to be hemodynamically stable at present but also seems to have signs of possible dehydration. If he is left for a prolonged period of time, dehydration could progress to shock.

Your emergency department is beginning to calm down after the evening rush—the last two hours have been very hectic. You observe this restlessly sleeping child, thinking how uncomfortable he must be, and realize his parents must have some real concerns to bring him in at this hour. You glance at them, and meet their worried eyes. Mr. DeNato says: "We've been trying to get him to drink some water all day, but he just won't take anything, not even a popsicle! Do you think he's dehydrated?"

Question

What are three signs of dehydration you would observe in a 4-year-old child? (Fill in the blanks.)

1. _____

2. _____

3. _____

Answer

In a child this age, the most obvious signs of mild to moderate dehydration would be[1]

- Tachycardia
- Cool hands and feet
- Lack of tears
- Concentrated urine/low urine output

Joey's sleepiness, though potentially a function of dehydration and metabolic imbalance, may be related to the late hour and you have already determined that he can be easily aroused. Although lack of urine output or concentrated urine is a significant sign, it is also more difficult to assess in children this age, because they are able to use the bathroom by themselves, and parents may not know the amount they have urinated.

The other issue that must be addressed is the DeNatos' feelings of responsibility in Joey's illness. You suspect that they are concerned that if they had done something differently, Joey might have fared better.

You reassure them that they were correct in encouraging him to take only clear liquids and that he does not appear to be severely dehydrated. Joey's father holds him carefully, so as not to awaken him, while Joey's mother leaves to complete the necessary paperwork at the admitting desk. Because Joey's *ABCs* are stable and within normal limits, and his mental status seems to be stable at present, you decide to defer taking off his clothes and continue your assessment by taking his vital signs, trying not to awaken him yourself. When you put the blood pressure cuff on his arm, Joey begins to cry and curls up in fetal position. You notice that he does not produce tears as he cries. He goes back to sleep almost immediately. Joey's vital signs are

Heart rate	140 beats/min
Respiratory rate	35 breaths/min
Blood pressure	80/48
Temperature	38.6°C, using an infrared tympanic membrane temperature probe

---

Question

Match Joey's heart rate, respiratory rate, and blood pressure to the correct descriptions. (Answers may be used more than once.)

_____ heart rate   1. Abnormally fast/high

_____ respiratory rate   2. Abnormally slow/low

_____ blood pressure   3. Within normal range

Answer

The answers are (1), (1), and (3), respectively.

Joey's heart rate is somewhat faster than normal for his age, which may be related to his fever, and his respiratory rate is also faster than normal. His blood pressure, however, is within normal limits. (See Table 1.4, Chapter 1).

Since Joey woke up somewhat, you finish your assessment by looking at Joey's body; you remove his pajamas very gently and carefully, because you don't want to upset him any more than necessary. You look at his skin surface, and it appears normal in color, without sign of injury or rashes. His skin turgor seems fair. You put a hospital gown on Joey and put a bath blanket around him. You then ask the DeNatos to wait in the lobby with him until a room is available. Five minutes later Mrs. DeNato approaches you with a worried look asking, "How long will it be?" When you explain to her that there is at least a 15-minute wait, she launches into a detailed account of her concerns, telling you about a neighbor's child who had a perforated appendix the prior month.

Before Mrs. DeNato can complete her story, an examining room becomes available. You take the family back into the examination area, and ask them to sit with Joey until the physician can examine him. As you leave the room, you see Joey moving around in his father's lap and kicking his feet.

There are many concerns when a child has abdominal pain, and a careful history from the parents may help to determine how ill Joey is. When you return, you obtain more details about his illness from the DeNatos.

Question

Of the following historical findings, which would increase your concern that Joey might have acute appendicitis? (Choose all answers that apply.)

1. Lack of appetite
2. Vomiting and diarrhea
3. Intermittent right lower quadrant pain
4. Pain with movement
5. Constant periumbilical pain

Answer

The correct answers are (4) and (5). The first sign of appendicitis in pediatric patients is most commonly periumbilical pain (see Table 6.1, following page).[3] The pain tends to be constant and exacerbated by movement. An indirect way of obtaining a history of peritoneal irritation is to ask if the child complained of pain when there were bumps on the way to the hospital (although with Joey asleep this would be difficult to determine). The fact that Joey appears to move easily weighs against his having peritoneal irritation.

With appendicitis, most children will complain of periumbilical pain in the early stages, with later localization to the right lower quadrant.[3] Intermittent pain or pain that moves from one location to another is less likely to be a sign of appendicitis than gastroenteritis.

Although vomiting is often seen with appendicitis, it generally *follows* the onset of pain. An illness characterized from the onset by nonbilious vomiting and diarrhea is more likely to indicate gastroenteritis.[3,4]

Lack of appetite is not specific to appendicitis, although children with appendicitis almost always complain of lack of appetite.[4] The child who is hungry for pizza, or hot dogs, for instance, probably does *not* have an acute abdominal emergency.

TABLE 6.1.   Signs and Symptoms of Gastroenteritis, Appendicitis, and Urinary Tract Infection[3]

	Gastroenteritis	Appendicitis	Urinary tract infection
Pain	Diffuse, crampy	Periumbilical, right lower quadrant	Flank, dysuria
Vomiting	Coincides with pain	Usually follows pain	Minimal
Diarrhea	Large volumes	Small amounts	Minimal
Fever	Varies	Low-grade early	May be high
Course	Intermittently feels better	Worsens with time	Changes slowly
Physical exam	Soft abdomen, hyperactive bowel sounds	Peritoneal signs, right lower quadrant, rectal localized to right	Costovertebral angle tenderness

Note. From E. H. Hatch, The acute abdomen in children. *Pediatric clinics of North America, 32,* 151–1164. © 1985, Philadelphia: Saunders. Reprinted by permission.

You return to find Joey asleep on the examination table and obtain more information from the DeNatos. Using the mnemonic AMPLE, you ask if he has allergies, and they tell you he has none. He is taking no medications at present, and they tell you that Joey is generally a healthy child who has had only normal childhood illnesses including chicken pox. They say he developed vomiting, diarrhea, and a temperature of 39°C (102.2°F) while at preschool 3 days ago. Although his vomiting stopped after 24 hours, he had persistent watery, nonbloody diarrheal stools, 8 to 10 times a day. They tried to keep him on a liquid diet, with only clear liquids and no solid food over the past 48 hours. Although Joey was well enough to be playing with his building blocks this morning, he started complaining again of abdominal pain this afternoon.

Once she has given you this information, Mrs. DeNato once again begins to tell you about Joey's friend who had appendicitis and asks if her son will need to be operated on tonight.

Question

Based on the detailed history of abdominal complaints and initial evaluation, your best course of action at this time would be to (Choose one answer.)

1. Reassure Mrs. DeNato that it is a good sign that Joey can move around and fall asleep, and that it is very doubtful that he will need surgery.

2. Encourage Mrs. DeNato to tell you more about her neighbor's child so that you will be better able to reassure her about Joey.

3. Tell Mrs. DeNato not to worry, that Joey will need abdominal X-ray films, a complete blood count, urinalysis, and some other tests before a decision about surgery will be made.

4. Discuss Mrs. DeNato's fears about Joey with her, and give her more information about what will happen in the next hour or so.

Answer

The correct answer is (4). When a parent appears to be very concerned, it is best to discuss specific fears related to the child rather than a case that you hear about secondhand. It is also helpful to offer information about what will be happening in the very near future, without making projections any further than that. When parents are anxious, give them concrete information, and encourage them to take one step at a time.

It would not be advisable to offer any predictions, comparisons, or false reassurances, because appendicitis, especially in preschool-age children, is an insidious disease. Perforation rates of up to 60%[5] show how rapidly this disease progresses and how difficult it is to diagnose in very young children.

A general estimate of the speed of progression of appendicitis is

- By 24 hours of onset about 20% of children will have a perforated appendix;
- After 48 hours from onset of symptoms about 80% of children will have a perforated appendix with peritonitis.[3]

Because of the rapid progression of appendicitis, it is very important to consider that pediatric patients may have appendicitis when there is abdominal pain, and it is unwise to exclude the possibility of an acute abdomen until after a thorough physical exam has been completed by the physician. This is true even when the history is highly suggestive of viral gastroenteritis.

You let Dr. Chen know about the DeNato family in room 5, and give her a brief synopsis of Joey's history and presentation. She asks if you have ordered the blood work and urinalysis on the hospital's protocol for patients with suspected appendicitis, and agrees when you explain that you felt that these might not be necessary. Dr. Chen asks you if Joey has had any pain with urination or a sore throat.

Question

What diseases or syndromes other than appendicitis are associated with abdominal pain in children? (Choose all that apply.)

_____ Urinary tract infection

_____ Pneumonia

_____ Ovarian cyst/torsion

_____ Streptococcal pharyngitis (strep throat)

_____ Diabetic ketoacidosis

_____ Pelvic inflammatory disease

Answer

All of the diseases and syndromes listed may be associated with abdominal pain in children. It is often difficult to determine what is causing pain in a child. To complicate matters even further, preverbal children cannot tell you where pain is located, and older children often are not able to distinguish nausea or general malaise from abdominal pain. There are, therefore, many childhood diseases and syndromes that may present with abdominal pain, and several tests may be required to differentiate between these possible causes. Some screening tests for diseases causing abdominal pain are listed in Table 6.2.

TABLE 6.2. Screening Laboratory Tests to Evaluate Pediatric Abdominal Pain

Urinalysis
A positive dipstick for leukocyte esterase, blood, or protein in a clean catch or catheterized specimen is suggestive of urinary tract infection. Several children will have urinary tract infections in the absence of pyuria, so a urine culture should be sent whenever urinary tract infection is seriously suspected.   A dipstick positive for glucose and ketones is suggestive of diabetic ketoacidosis.   Blood in the urine, in the presence of severe colicky pain, is suggestive of a renal calculus (kidney stone).
Complete blood count
The teenager with early appendicitis is unlikely to have a white blood count of >15,000, but an infant may show a white blood count of >20,000 even in the absence of perforation.[4]   Appendiceal perforation is often associated with high white blood count with a shift to the left.[4] Although a normal or low white blood count is more suggestive of a viral process, the complete blood count per se does **not** discriminate between an acute surgical versus medical process.[3,6]
Flat plate and upright abdominal films
Detection of a fecalith (stone in the appendix) is rare in children.[3]   Abdominal films may demonstrate a paralytic ileus, or point to diagnoses other than appendicitis, such as intussusception or volvulus.
Anteroposterior and lateral chest films
Pneumonia, especially in the lower lobes, can cause diaphragmatic irritation and abdominal pain.[3,4]   Because fever and vomiting may also be present, the misdiagnosis of appendicitis may be made.
Urine human chorionic gonadotropin
A pregnancy test should be considered in postmenarcheal females who complain of abdominal pain, regardless of age or history of sexual activity.   Other tests may be necessary on an individualized basis.

You enter the examining room again and find that Joey is still asleep. Mrs. DeNato looks at you hopefully, and you tell her that Dr. Chen is coming to do a physical examination. You assure the DeNatos that they will not have to wake Joey up for a moment, because Dr. Chen will begin her examination by observing him and that most of the examination can be performed with Joey sitting on Mr. DeNato's lap. You suspect that Dr. Chen will be ordering a urinalysis, and you make sure that the equipment is available.

Question

What equipment would you choose if you need to obtain urine from Joey? (Choose one answer.)

1. A pediatric urine bag
2. A sterile urine cup for a clean catch urine
3. A urinary catheter
4. Equipment to perform a suprapubic tap

Answer

The correct answer is either (2) or (3). A urinary catheter would be the preferred method if a urinary tract infection is strongly suspected.

Bagged urine specimens are notoriously unreliable (especially in female infants where the perineum cannot be adequately cleansed). A suprapubic tap would not be recommended in this age child.

Dr. Chen comes into the examining room and introduces herself to the DeNato family. Mrs. DeNato starts to relate the now familiar account of her neighbor's child's appendicitis. Dr. Chen redirects the exchange, and obtains more information about Joey's history and signs and symptoms. After taking a thorough history from the DeNatos, Dr. Chen proceeds to examine Joey on his father's lap. She manages to complete the cardiac and lung examination, as well as auscultating and palpating Joey's abdomen without awakening him. She then asks Mr. DeNato to wake Joey up. After briefly chatting with the sleepy boy, she places him on the examination table and taps the soles of his feet with her fist, asking him if it hurts. He nods, very much awake now, and points to his foot. He irritably pulls himself up so that he is sitting up on the examining table.

Question

What would be an effective method for Dr. Chen to determine how much abdominal pain Joey is having at this point? (Choose one answer.)

1. Ask him how much pain he is having, from 1 to 10
2. Ask him to bend over and touch his toes
3. Ask him to jump down from the examining table
4. Palpate his abdomen and ask him where he has the most pain

---

Answer

The correct answer is (3). Signs of peritoneal irritation can be seen when a child is bumped or jostled. Indirect maneuvers to elicit these peritoneal signs without alerting the child to your objective can be very helpful. The heel strike (tapping the soles of the feet when the child is supine) may elicit complaints of abdominal pain in the child with peritonitis. Likewise, a child with peritoneal irritation will be unwilling to jump (especially more than once!), as this causes abdominal pain.[4]

Young or frightened children may have trouble cooperating with the abdominal examination (see Table 6.3, following page). They may also be unreliable in reporting pain. Having him bend over to touch his toes would not provide useful information.

TABLE 6.3.   Physical Examination of the Abdomen

An ordered approach to the abdominal examination in the child complaining of abdominal pain is critical. The correct order of this examination is
Inspection
Inspection allows the examiner to identify patients with abdominal distention, or, conversely, those with a scaphoid or flat abdomen. It is important that the abdomen be completely uncovered for this portion of the examination, although the examiner must be aware of the potential for hypothermia, particularly in young children.
Auscultation
Auscultation is used to assess the presence and quality of bowel sounds. Bowel sounds are classified as absent, hypoactive, normal, or hyperactive. Absent bowel sounds are commonly associated with peritonitis or other significant intraabdominal pathology. To be classified as absent the examiner must listen for a minimum of 2 min without hearing any bowel sounds. Hyperactive bowel sounds are frequently associated with viral illnesses that produce diarrhea. The presence of tinkles or rushes is consistent with the presence of a bowel obstruction.
Percussion
Percussion is the best method for quickly assessing the patient's abdomen for the presence of air (tympany) or fluid (dullness). It can also be used to assess organ size, particularly the liver, or the size of abnormal intraabdominal masses. In patients with peritonitis, gentle percussion will frequently elicit a painful response, eliminating the need for deep palpation and sudden release to assess for the presence of rebound tenderness.
Palpation
Palpation of all regions in the abdomen allows the examiner to identify abnormal masses, assess organ size, and determine the presence or absence of peritoneal tenderness. In children, abdominal palpation should be performed in a manner that will not preclude later examination or reevaluation. There are several techniques that can be used to identify peritoneal signs in the frightened or uncooperative child including the heel strike or jumping maneuvers described above.

Dr. Chen asks Joey to jump down from the table, and as he reluctantly does so, you notice that Joey does not have pain while doing this. After some further physical examination, Dr. Chen discusses her assessment with the family. She has decided that Joey will not need any laboratory analyses, and that it is a simple case of gastroenteritis. She asks you to check them out with the discharge diagnosis of gastroenteritis with mild dehydration.

Mrs. DeNato seems somewhat reassured about Joey's "appendicitis," and says she has noticed that Joey's diarrhea has slowed down since he came to the emergency department but she has several questions about dehydration and what Joey can eat: "What should I be feeding Joey tonight and tomorrow?"

Question

Which of the following regimens would be recommended for Joey? (Choose any that apply.)

1.   An oral glucose-electrolyte rehydration solution
2.   Clear liquids only for 24 hr
3.   Clear liquids only until the diarrhea stops
4.   High carbohydrate diet as tolerated

Answer

The correct answers are (1) and (4). The American Academy of Pediatrics has recommended "feeding through" in all but severe cases of diarrhea (see Table 6.4).[1,8] Glucose-electrolyte solutions have the best carbohydrate to sodium ratio for repleting fluid losses. They are superior to "clear liquids" such as juices or colas that have inadequate sodium and very high sugar concentration. The high osmolality of juices and colas encourages movement of fluid into the intestinal tract and can make diarrhea worse.

TABLE 6.4. American Academy of Pediatrics Oral Rehydration Recommendations[1]

Glucose-electrolyte solutions (Rehydrite, Pedialyte, Lytren, Resol) are used for rehydration and maintenance therapy
Rehydration fluids can be used in combination with water, breast milk. or low-carbohydrate juice
Feeding should be reintroduced in the first 24 hr of the episode
Initial foods include • *Infants*. Breast milk, diluted formula or milk • *Older infants and children*. Rice cereal, bananas, potatoes, other nonlactose carbohydrate-rich foods

After you explain this protocol to the DeNatos, Mr. DeNato asks you how they can be sure that Joey is getting enough fluid and if he is in danger of getting dehydrated again.

Question

What are three signs of dehydration that you would you tell the DeNatos to watch for with Joey? (Fill in the blanks.)

1. _____

2. _____

3. _____

Answer

The signs you would tell the DeNatos to watch for are[1]

- Decreased urination
- Sunken eyes
- No tears when the child cries
- Extreme thirst
- Unusual drowsiness or fussiness

In addition to these, they should be concerned if Joey's diarrhea gets worse, if he does not take fluid, or if he continues vomiting.

Mrs. DeNato tells you that she is still worried about taking Joey home, because of her neighbor's child's appendicitis. You go over the information about abdominal pain with her.

Question

In giving aftercare instructions for Joey, what signs would you tell the DeNatos are a signal that they should return to the emergency department immediately? (Fill in the blanks.)

1. _____

2. _____

3. _____

Answer

The DeNatos should see their doctor or return to the emergency department immediately if Joey develops any of the following signs or symptoms[1]:

- Persistent or increasing abdominal pain
- Bilious vomiting
- Signs of worsening dehydration (listed earlier)

Any of these would indicate that Joey's condition may require further examination, and possible hospitalization or surgery.

You give the DeNatos your emergency department's written discharge instructions on oral rehydration for diarrhea, as well as those for abdominal pain. Realizing that the DeNatos still seem nervous, you suggest that they call their doctor in the morning to arrange follow-up in the next few days. They thank you for your care, and Joey sleepily waves good-bye.

CASE STUDY 2 OBJECTIVES

On completion of this case study, the learner should be able to

- Make a correct triage decision, based on observable evidence, about the pediatric patient presenting with abdominal distress
- Recognize common diagnoses for abdominal pain in children under 2 years of age
- Identify the specific signs of a surgical emergency in children
- Prioritize interventions for a child with acute abdominal pain
- State a nursing diagnosis for a child with acute abdominal pain
- Identify possible causes for fluid loss in a child with abdominal pain

CASE STUDY 2: INTUSSUSCEPTION

Tabitha Is In Pain

Tabitha Arcenaux is a 16-month-old white female child who is brought to the emergency department by her grandmother, Mrs. Arcenaux, at 4:00 P.M. (see Figure 6.2). Her grandmother seems most worried

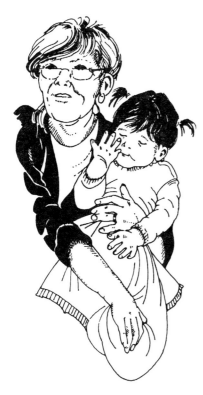

FIGURE 6.2

about the way Tabitha is acting. Mrs. Arcenaux tells you that she has custody of Tabitha and Tabitha's three siblings. She says that Tabitha has been mostly sleeping since breakfast time, intermittently crying inconsolably, and has vomited once. The other children living at home with her have all been well. When you ask about when Tabitha's illness started, Mrs. Arcenaux is very insistent that Tabitha was perfectly fine when she went to bed last night, and that she had a good supper and was acting normally. She said that Tabitha did not eat anything unusual, and went right to bed after supper. Mrs. Arcenaux also tells you that Tabitha has not felt hot or had a fever.

You look at the dark-haired child sleeping in her grandmother's arms. Tabitha appears average in size for her age. Her respiration is unlabored, with good tidal volume. Her color is pale. As you observe her, Tabitha has a large bilious emesis, draws her knees up to her chest, and starts to cry without opening her eyes. Mrs. Arcenaux looks very worried and tries to clean Tabitha with a small towel brought from home. You take them both into the emergency area to help clean Tabitha.

TRIAGE DECISION

On the basis of your initial assessment at this point, you would triage Tabitha as

Emergent. A life-threatening situation in need of immediate intervention.

Urgent. Patient needs care within 1 hour to prevent further deterioration.

Nonurgent. Patient is able to wait more than 1 hour without further deterioration.

TRIAGE DECISION ANSWER

Tabitha's condition is emergent. Your greatest concern at this point is Tabitha's altered mental status, bilious vomiting, and apparently severe intermittent pain as evidenced by Tabitha's crying and the way she draws up her knees. The acute onset of her illness without fever also indicates that this may not be a normal childhood illness, and suggests the need for immediate evaluation and treatment.[1]

You already know that Tabitha's *ABC*s do not require acute intervention at this point, and that you will need to assess her mental status frequently. You bring Tabitha and her grandmother into the examining room, and help Mrs. Arcenaux undress and clean her. Tabitha does not wake up as you change her and take her vital signs—even when you use the blood pressure cuff. Her vital signs are

Heart rate	140 beats/min
Respiratory rate	30 breaths/min
Blood pressure	90/58

Temperature   37.4°C, (99.4°F), rectal

Capillary refill time   <2 s

Question

Mark Tabitha's heart rate, respiratory rate, and blood pressure as either normal or abnormal for her age. (Use **N** for normal and **A** for abnormal.)

_____   Heart rate

_____   Respiratory rate

_____   Blood pressure

Answer

The answers are (A), (N), and (N), respectively.

Although Tabitha's vital signs would not be normal for an adult, her respiratory rate and blood pressure are within normal limits for a 16-month-old child. Her heart rate is higher than normal, which needs further assessment. A rectal temperature of 99.4°F is also normal for a child, because rectal temperatures are higher than oral temperatures.

Tabitha's hands and feet feel comfortably warm to touch. Tabitha is quiet right now, so you weigh her on the small scale in the examining room and find that her weight is 11 kg. When she is placed on the scale, Tabitha wakes up somewhat and begins to cry, and you quickly give her back to Mrs. Arcenaux, who rocks her back and forth, and talks to her quietly, trying to soothe her. Tabitha does not stop crying, despite her grandmother's efforts to console her. After about 5 minutes, Tabitha suddenly stops crying and is once again responsive only to painful stimuli.

You notify the emergency physician of Tabitha's urgent need for attention, and you take a brief AMPLE history from Mrs. Arcenaux.

Allergies. None.

Medications. None currently. Up to date on immunizations.

Previous medical history. Tabitha has no history of other medical problems.

Last meal. Tabitha ate well last night and has not eaten today.

Events preceeding injury/illness. Tabitha seemed fine when put to bed, and was found listless in her crib this morning.

Mrs. Arcenaux tells you that as far as she knows there has been no recent history of significant trauma, although Tabitha is becoming more adventurous about walking without holding on and falls frequently. Mrs. Arcenaux says Tabitha has not hit her head recently, as far as she knows. When you ask about a possible ingestion, Mrs. Arcenaux doesn't think that Tabitha could have "gotten into anything." She says she is with Tabitha most of the day, they keep all medications and cleaning solutions on the top shelves and lock the cupboards, and she seldom lets Tabitha out of her sight.

Mrs. Arcenaux tells you that Tabitha has always been a healthy child and has been followed for regular checkups by a family physician at the Health Department. She assures you she raised four children herself so she knows how children act when they are sick. She also tells you she can't remember ever seeing anything like this with any one of them. You are becoming more concerned about Tabitha, and you give Mrs. Arcenaux an emesis basin and a washcloth for Tabitha, and tell her that you are leaving her to find one of the emergency physicians to examine Tabitha right away.

Question

Which of the following would you consider as possible illnesses/injuries at this point? (Check all that apply.)

1. Acute abdomen
2. Central nervous system injury/illness
3. Nonaccidental trauma (child abuse)
4. Toxic ingestion
5. All of the above

Answer

The correct answer is that all of the illnesses and injuries listed are possibilities. This is a confusing picture. The combination of altered mental status and vomiting could be consistent with an ingestion or CNS trauma or disease (e.g., meningitis, increased intracranial pressure). Head injury or intraabdominal injury owing to nonaccidental trauma could also explain some of the signs and symptoms in this afebrile child, although there are no obvious indicators for abuse in this history. Tabitha's apparent intermittent pain and vomiting should alert you to the possibility of a serious abdominal emergency. Paroxysmal pain occurring at frequent intervals, accompanied by straining and vigorous crying is typical of intussusception (see Table 6.5).[2]

TABLE 6.5.   Causes of Abdominal Pain in Children[3]

	Under age 2 years	**Age 2–5 years**	**Age 5–16 years**
Common causes	Gastroenteritis Viral syndrome Bowel obstruction	Gastroenteritis Appendicitis Urinary tract infection Pneumonia Asthma Viral syndrome Otitis	Gastroenteritis Appendicitis Urinary tract infection Constipation Viral syndrome Otitis Pelvic inflammatory disease
Less common causes	Sickle cell crisis Strangulated hernia Trauma/abuse Lead poisoning	Strangulated hernia Intussusception Pyelonephritis Meckel's diverticulum Hepatitis Diabetic ketoacidosis Bowel obstruction Lead poisoning	Pneumonia Asthma Ectopic pregnancy Ovarian cyst Cholecystitis Diabetic ketoacidosis Gastritis
Least common causes	Appendicitis Volvulus Ovarian torsion	Strangulated hernia Rheumatic fever Myocarditis Pericarditis	Rheumatic fever Ovarian or testicular torsion

You find one of the emergency physicians in another examining room and tell him about Tabitha; he says he will be right in to see her, but right now he is involved in stabilizing an elderly patient with a cardiac rhythm disturbance. When you return to the Arcenaux family, you see that Tabitha is quiet now, but you are becoming more concerned about the possibility that this may be a surgical emergency. You call the operating room to ask about the schedule there.

Question

What specific sign is most indicative of a possible surgical emergency? (Choose one answer.)

1. Paradoxical irritability
2. Bilious vomiting
3. Intermittent abdominal pain
4. Lack of fever

Answer

Bilious vomiting, in particular, should always alert you to the possibility that there may be a surgical emergency. Vomiting of gastric contents alone should be *nonbilious*.[4] Bilious emesis implies obstruction distal to the site where the bile duct empties into the duodenum and is often a sign of bowel obstruction (see Figure 6.3).

Paradoxical irritability and intermittent abdominal pain are signs that may indicate serious illness in children, and should be carefully explored, but these are not specific to surgical emergencies and may have many causes.[5] Lack of fever, when combined with signs and symptoms of abdominal pain, can be suggestive of a surgical emergency but is not as clear an indication as bilious vomiting.

The emergency department physician has not yet seen Tabitha, and although he can't come in right now, you describe Tabitha's condition to him, and suggest that it may be wise to initiate some interventions according to your protocols. Dr. Wallace concurs.

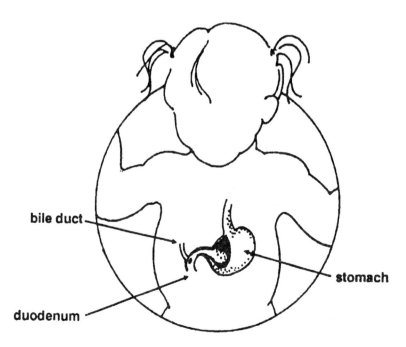

FIGURE 6.3   Location of bile duct emptying into duodenum.

Question

What would your first three priorities be at this time? (Place a **1** by your first priority, **2** next to your next priority, etc.)

_____ Obtain an order for an analgesic for Tabitha

_____ Reassess the arterial blood gases

_____ Administer supplemental oxygen

_____ Start an IV line

_____ Order laboratory analyses

Answer

The answers are: (1), reassess Tabitha's *ABC*s; (2), administer supplemental oxygen; and (3), start an IV line.

The priorities in any emergently ill patient are always the same: to assess and reassess the *ABC*s for potentially life-threatening problems, and then to intervene to correct those problems. Although Tabitha has shown no evidence of respiratory compromise, it is better to err on the side of safety and administer supplemental oxygen while you sort out this case. An IV line is a safety net in the event that her condition worsens. When there is any risk of cardiovascular compromise, it is wisest to start an IV line. It is easier to obtain venous access *before* Tabitha's condition deteriorates.

Analgesics are not generally given to children before the cause of their pain is identified. The administration of an analgesic to a child with abdominal pathology may mask her symptoms and delay diagnosis and definitive treatment.[6] If Tabitha's extreme lethargy persists, a head CT may be in order. However, cardiopulmonary stabilization is the priority at this time.

When you return to the room, Mrs. Arcenaux shows you an emesis basin containing bright green fluid, and tells you that Tabitha has vomited twice since you left. You are becoming increasingly worried about Tabitha. Tabitha's radial pulse seems a bit less strong, her hands and feet are cool, and her heart rate is up to 155 beats/min. You start giving her oxygen by blow-by with Mrs. Arcenaux holding the tubing.

Question

What is your nursing diagnosis at this time? (Fill in the blank.)

_____

Answer

The most appropriate nursing diagnosis at this time is alteration in perfusion related to possible volume loss and pain. Your immediate interventions at this time need to be directed to improving perfusion, which includes assuring adequate oxygenation and administration of fluid.

You explain to Mrs. Arcenaux that you are going to start an IV line as a precautionary measure, because you may want to give Tabitha some fluid. You use a 22-gauge intravenous catheter and place it in the back of Tabitha's hand. You also draw blood through the cannula for laboratory analyses: glucose, amylase, electrolytes and complete blood count. You use a dextrostick to determine her blood sugar, which is approximately 120. The emergency physician is still occupied in the other room, and you start her on the IV fluid indicated by your hospital's protocols.

Question

Which of the following IV fluids is usually recommended for a child with signs and symptoms of dehydration? (Choose all that apply.)

1. Ringer's lactate
2. Normal saline
3. Dextrose 5%, 0.9 normal saline
4. Dextrose 5%, 0.45 normal saline

Answer

Either Ringer's lactate or normal saline would be appropriate. Tabitha is showing signs of progressive volume loss and circulatory compromise (progressive tachycardia, weaker pulses, cool extremities), and needs immediate fluid administration.[7] Isotonic fluids (crystalloid) should always be chosen.

Dextrose 5%, 0.9 normal saline and dextrose 5%, 0.45 normal saline are hypertonic solutions. Neither of these should be used in this case.

Once you have established Tabitha's IV line, you stabilize it carefully with tape. Mrs. Arcenaux has stayed with Tabitha during the procedure, talking to her and comforting her when she cries. The emergency physician tells you to go ahead and give Tabitha a fluid bolus.

Question

How much fluid would you give Tabitha as a fluid bolus?

1. 500 mL
2. 220 mL
3. 110 mL
4. 250 mL

Answer

An appropriate approach to volume resuscitation in a child is to give a bolus of 20 mL/kg of Ringer's lactate or normal saline over less than 20 min, and then reassess clinical signs of perfusion and repeat the bolus if needed.[8] Because Tabitha's weight is 11 kg, 220 mL over 20 min represents a 20 mL/kg bolus. A "keep open" rate for a child is 10 mL/hr.

Question

Tabitha's volume depletion could be accounted for by the following losses. (Choose True or False for each question.)

1. External blood loss   T   F
2. Occult blood loss in the abdomen   T   F
3. Vomiting   T   F
4. "Third spacing" in the gut   T   F

Answer

The correct answers are

1. *False.* Tabitha has not had any obvious blood loss by history or physical examination.
2. *True.* Occult bleeding in the abdomen can occur into the bowel lumen, the peritoneal space, or the retroperitoneum, and may be difficult to detect on physical examination.[4] Vomiting and poor oral intake can rapidly lead to dehydration in this age group.
3. *True.* However, if the history is reliable, the short duration of complaints and the occurrence of only four episodes of emesis make it unlikely that this is the only source of fluid loss for Tabitha.
4. *True.* "Third spacing" involves leakage of fluids from the inside of the intestinal tract into the peritoneal space, and occurs when there is inflammation or vascular compromise of the bowel.

While you are taping Tabitha's IV, she has a large bloody stool. As you rapidly clean this up, you realize how serious this is. You estimate that she has lost about 80 mL of bright red blood in the stool.

Question

How much crystalloid would generally be recommended to replace a 80-mL blood loss in a child? (Choose one answer.)

1. 80 mL   2. 160 mL   3. 240 mL

Answer

The correct answer is (3). As in an adult, about three times the amount of fluid lost is a reasonable guideline as fluid replacement for blood loss.[8] All fluid replacement requires continuous assessment of the patient, however. If the patient did not improve after 240 mL of fluid, the need for another bolus, and the need for colloids or blood should be assessed.

As you continue to give Tabitha fluid, you retake her blood pressure; it is unchanged, at 90/58. Mrs. Arcenaux looks at you very anxiously. "She's losing blood! Why aren't you doing something about it?" You explain that the fluids you are giving will help, and that if Tabitha continues to bleed you may also have to give her some blood. She asks you what could possibly cause this type of bleeding in a child, and tells you that she has always heard that bleeding from the rectum is a sure sign of cancer.

You tell her that this type of bleeding in a young child is rarely caused by cancer, and that there are many other possibilities, some more serious than others. You tell her that Dr. Wallace will be in right away, and he may be able to give her a better idea of what may be wrong once he has examined Tabitha.

Question

What are three likely causes of bloody stool in a child Tabitha's age? (Fill in the blanks.)

1. _____

2. _____

3. _____

Answer

The likely causes of gastrointestinal bleeding are shown in Table 6.6.

TABLE 6.6. Causes of Lower Gastrointestinal Bleeding in Pediatric Patients[5]

Newborn	Toddler	Any age
Hemorrhagic disease Hemorrhagic gastritis Necrotizing enterocolitis Milk allergy colitis Midgut volvulus Milk allergy Swallowed blood Anal fissure Esophagitis	Intussusception Meckel's diverticulum Duplication Nodular lymphoid hyperplasia	Gastroenteritis Infectious diarrhea Vascular malformation Mallory-Weiss syndrome
Preschool	**School Age**	
Juvenile polyps Schonlein-Henoch purpura Hemolytic-uremic syndrome Esophageal varices Foreign body	Peptic ulcer Crohn's disease Ulcerative colitis Hemorrhoids	

In Tabitha's case, her stool shows fresh blood. Because the blood has not been digested in any way, it is most likely to be a lower gastrointestinal problem, and at her age, the most likely cause is intussusception.[9]

At this point, Dr. Wallace hurries into the room. You update him on Tabitha's course and your interventions. Tabitha has now received 20 mL/kg of Ringer's lactate and has a heart rate of 140 beats/min. Dr. Wallace thanks you for your help and quickly examines the child. He says there is something interesting you might want to see and tells you to feel her right upper quadrant. He shows you where to palpate, and you feel a sausage-shaped mass. He explains to Mrs. Arcenaux that this is the typical presentation for an intussusception, the most common form of bowel obstruction in this age group.[3] He tells Mrs. Arcenaux that he needs to make arrangements for a special X-ray film for Tabitha. He asks you to give Tabitha another 20 mL/kg fluid bolus, a dose of a broad-spectrum IV antibiotic, and to place a nasogastric tube. He leaves to call the surgery consultant and the radiologist on call.

Mrs. Arcenaux seems mystified. She asks you what the doctor meant, how her granddaughter could have gotten a "blocked bowel," and what they're going to do to Tabitha. She says that Tabitha didn't eat anything that would have stopped up her intestine. As you attempt to complete the multiple tasks requested by Dr. Wallace, you try to explain how an intussusception occurs and what steps will be taken to correct it.

Question

Which of the following statements about intussusception are true? (Select all that apply.)

1. A barium enema is generally used to diagnose the presence of an intussusception.
2. Most children with intussusception require bowel resection.
3. If bilious vomiting and bloody diarrhea are not present, the diagnosis of intussusception is unlikely.
4. Intussusception involves a malrotation (twisting) of the small bowel.

Answer

The correct answer is (1). A barium enema performed under fluoroscopy will demonstrate the obstruction, with failure of the contrast medium to pass through the involved segment of bowel. In approximately 75% of cases,[2] the barium enema will also be therapeutic, causing sufficient hydrostatic pressure to reduce the obstruction by unfolding the involved bowel. This is usually most successful within the first 24 hours.[3] Because of the risk of perforation of the bowel with this procedure, antibiotics are often given prophylactically to decrease the risk of peritonitis.

When a barium enema is not successful in relieving the obstruction, a laparotomy under general anesthesia is performed to permit manual reduction of the intussusception. Rarely, the bowel will have become sufficiently ischemic that a surgical resection is necessary.

Intussusception involves the telescoping of a segment of the bowel into the segment just caudad to it (see Figure 6.4). This occurs most commonly at the level of the ileocecal valve.[2] Intussusception is a "great pretender." Although the textbook description includes crampy abdominal pain, bilious vomiting, and "currant jelly" stools, many children will present with only one of these signs or symptoms. Lethargy may be the most striking feature of the child with intussusception, although the cause of this alteration in mental status is not clearly understood.[5]

Volvulus refers to twisting of the intestine onto itself, which may result from malrotation of the gut because of a problem in embryologic development. Midgut volvulus may occur when there is a lack of mesenteric attachment and the loops of intestine twist onto themselves—producing obstruction. The rotation of the bowel may include the superior mesenteric artery (see Figure 6.5) and may progress to bowel necrosis from inadequate perfusion. Volvulus is a surgical emergency and usually occurs at birth or in the first year of life.[2]

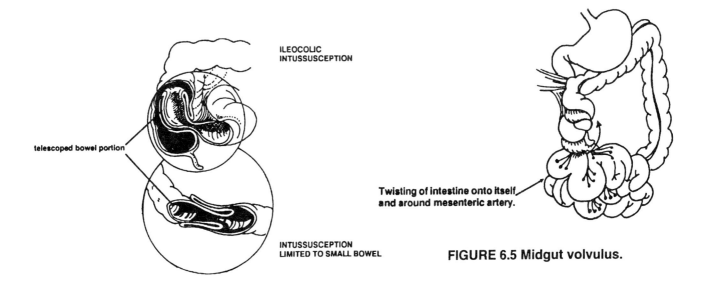

ILEOCOLIC
INTUSSUSCEPTION

telescoped bowel portion

INTUSSUSCEPTION
LIMITED TO SMALL BOWEL

FIGURE 6.4 Intussusception.

Twisting of intestine onto itself
and around mesenteric artery.

FIGURE 6.5 Midgut volvulus.

After the second bolus of fluid, Tabitha's perfusion is much improved; her skin appears less mottled, and her heart rate drops to 120 beats/min between bouts of pain. The nasogastric tube is draining bilious fluid. The surgeons arrive, and after a brief examination they obtain consent from Mrs. Arcenaux for laparotomy in the event that the barium enema does not reduce the intussusception. Tabitha is wheeled off to the fluoroscopy suite by the surgical intern. Forty-five minutes later, Dr. Wallace lets you know that the barium enema was successful and that Tabitha has been admitted to the floor for overnight observation.

Mrs. Arcenaux is greatly relieved and asks when she can see Tabitha. You walk with her over to the fluoroscopy suite and find that Tabitha will be moved upstairs shortly. Mrs. Arcenaux asks you why Tabitha will have to spend the night, and you spend some time telling Mrs. Arcenaux about your hospital's procedures for overnight observation. Mrs. Arcenaux decides to let her other grandchildren stay with a friend so that she can spend the night with Tabitha. The X-ray technician brings Tabitha out, and her grandmother holds her hand. She tells you she is embarrassed that she was so worried and thanks you for all your help.

CASE STUDY 3 OBJECTIVES

At the end of this chapter, the learner should be able to

- Recognize common signs and symptoms of pyloric stenosis
- List two abnormal laboratory test results that might suggest the diagnosis of pyloric stenosis
- Recognize the significance of bilious versus nonbilious emesis
- Select appropriate responses to parents' questions about pyloric stenosis

CASE 3

Why Won't Roberto Stop Vomiting?

It is early in the morning on a Sunday in October. You are triage nurse for the day, but because there are no patients yet, you are helping to check the equipment in the emergency department, preparing for what you expect to be a busy day ahead. The nurse working with you has gone to have a cup of coffee in the lounge. Suddenly, you hear a noise at the front desk, and look out to the triage area to see a frantic young Latino woman holding a small baby (see Figure 6.6). She begins ringing the bell at the triage desk repeatedly, and you hurry out to see what is wrong. You look at the mother inquisitively, and she starts talking in rapid Spanish. Although you speak a little Spanish, you cannot keep up with her, and she begins to point frantically at her baby and shows you the child's blanket, which appears to have a small quantity of regurgitated milk on it. She keeps pointing to her baby, Roberto, and saying that maybe he has "empacho." This is something with which you are unfamiliar, and you make a note that when you find someone who speaks Spanish you will ask about it.

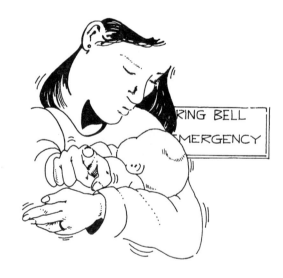

FIGURE 6.6

As you take a quick look at the baby, you see no signs of respiratory distress and feel somewhat relieved. The baby also seems to have normal skin color, and is awake and crying. You use your limited Spanish to try to obtain more information, and you ask the emergency department clerk, who is just returning from breakfast, to see if he can find a Spanish interpreter. You do manage to find out, using a combination of sign language and your broken Spanish, that Roberto is only 3 weeks old, that he is vomiting "everything he eats," and that this has been going on since yesterday.

TRIAGE DECISION

On the basis of this quick look and brief history would you triage this baby as

Emergent.   A life-threatening situation in need of immediate intervention.

Urgent.   Patient needs care within 1 hour to prevent further deterioration.

Nonurgent.   Patient is able to wait more than 1 hour without further deterioration.

TRIAGE DECISION ANSWER

You should triage him as urgent. Roberto seems to have no respiratory distress, his circulatory status seems adequate, and he is awake and alert. In addition, the mother does not seem to be indicating that Roberto has had any sort of acute injury as far as you can tell.

Because the other nurse on duty is still taking her coffee break, you decide to take the family into the emergency department treatment area. The emergency physician is checking up on a trauma patient admitted last night to the intensive care unit.

As you continue to assess Roberto, you find out that his mother's name is Blanca Garcia. She seems calmer now that she is in the emergency department, and you ask her to hold Roberto while you take his vital signs. You have managed to establish a good relationship with her, using mostly nonverbal communication.

Respiratory rate	30 breaths/min
Heart rate	140 beats/min
Capillary refill	<2 s
Temperature	99.6°F

You do not take Roberto's blood pressure because he is still crying, and his capillary refill is brisk. You begin to feel a little annoyed at Mrs. Garcia, because you suspect this will turn out to be the case of a new mother worrying needlessly about her child spitting up a little after feedings.

A Spanish-speaking nurse arrives from the labor and delivery area to help you talk with Mrs. Garcia.

Question

What would be three appropriate question(s) to ask Mrs. Garcia? (Select three questions.)

1. Is your baby vomiting at every feeding?
2. Is your baby losing weight?
3. Is this your first baby?
4. How many times a day does your baby have a wet diaper?
5. Have you ever heard of this happening to anyone in your family before?

Answer

The correct answers are (1), (4), and (5). It is important to determine whether Roberto is becoming dehydrated, which would be a serious consequence of his vomiting, and can happen very rapidly in a small child. Both questions (1) and (4) may be helpful in determining hydration. Question (5) is appropriate because some diseases tend to run in families, and family members are often aware of the diagnoses.

Whether it is Mrs. Garcia's first baby is pertinent information and is appropriately asked as part of history taking. When asked at the very beginning of an interview, however, it is often taken as an insult by patients in emergency settings, because it may be perceived as an implication that the parent is simply inexperienced. It is very rare for parents to know the weight of their child, so this question is not usually worth asking. If the patient is a frequent visitor to the hospital, such as a child with a chronic illness, this may be useful.

Mrs. Garcia tells you that Roberto is vomiting after every feeding, although he always seems hungry and has been taking several ounces of milk before he starts vomiting. The last wet diaper he had was last night. He cried most of the night, and his diaper was dry this morning when she dressed him to bring him in. You continue to take a more complete history from Mrs. Garcia with the help of Celia, the nurse from labor and delivery.

Allergies. None known.

Medications. None.

Previous history of illness. None–normal, uncomplicated delivery.

Last meal. Mrs. Garcia tells you she gave Roberto about 3 ounces of milk just before she brought him to the emergency department.

Events preceding injury/illness. None.

It is difficult for you to communicate with Mrs. Garcia and the labor and delivery nurse over Roberto's vigorous crying, but she tells you (mostly showing you with hand gestures) that she is so worried because Roberto is vomiting his entire feedings—not just a little bit of them. You ask Celia what "empacho" means, and she tells you that this is commonly believed among Hispanics that this childhood malady is due to a "ball of food" sticking to the stomach wall, usually caused by being forced to eat against one's will.[1]

Roberto spits up a little milk, and as you help Mrs. Garcia clean up Roberto, Celia quickly describes several other problems you may encounter with Hispanic patients. Some Hispanic cultural health care beliefs, along with their traditional treatments are listed in Table 6.7.

TABLE 6.7. Some Childhood Maladies and Traditional Treatments Common in the Hispanic Culture[1]

Type of ailment	Description/translation	Cause	Treatment
Caida de mollera	Sunken fontanel	Fall, rapid removal of child from breast or bottle	Prayers, pressure on the hard palate, suction over the fontanel
Empacho	"Ball of food"; indigestion	Being forced to eat against one's will	Massages along spinal cord, castor oil with citrus juice
Malaire or *pasmo*	"Bad air"; symptoms include pain, muscle spasms, paralysis	Exposure to cold air	Prevention; keeping child warm
Malojo	"Evil eye"; symptoms include crying, fever, fretfulness	Caused by gaze of a person with "strong eyes"	Prayers, charms, rubbing raw egg over body, person causing evil eye touching child
Susto	"Fright"; causes loss of appetite, restless sleep, pallor	Frightening event that causes soul to leave body; can also be caused by cold, sun, hunger	Ritual cleansing with herbs, prayers, invocations
Ataque	"Attack"; causes seizures, hyperventilation, altered mental status	Stress, anxiety	Spiritualist can assist in cure
Bujeria/ embrujo	"Witchcraft/sorcery"; causes exhaustion, restlessness, lack of sleep	Witchcraft/sorcery	Folk healers

You check Roberto's diaper and see that it is still dry. Knowing this is a sign of dehydration, especially in this age child, you begin to list the laboratory analyses that will probably be needed.

Question

What laboratory analyses would be likely to be ordered for Roberto? (Select all that apply.)

1. Electrolytes
2. Complete blood count
3. Type and crossmatch
4. Blood cultures
5. Urinalysis

Answer

The correct answers are (1), (2), and (5). Any child who is vomiting or who may not be taking adequate fluids is likely to have an electrolyte imbalance, which can become rapidly fatal in small children, so electrolytes are usually measured.[2] A complete blood count should be done to consider the possibility of infection or other illness in an infant. Urinalysis should also be performed, although it may be difficult to obtain a sample right now. Type and crossmatch will not be necessary right now because Roberto has no history of trauma, and he does not appear to be severely volume depleted. Obtaining blood cultures is not a priority; although it is possible for a baby to have infection without fever, it seems highly unlikely that Roberto's signs and symptoms are related to systemic infection, so blood cultures would probably not be ordered routinely.

You have taken all of Roberto's clothes off, and as you observe his abdominal area, you see waves of muscle contractions passing from right to left across his upper abdominal area. You have never noticed this before in a patient. Roberto suddenly vomits about 20 mL of white fluid mixed with curds. There is no evidence of blood in his vomitus. You are surprised at how vigorously he vomits. As he continues to vomit, you hold his head to the side toward you to keep him from aspirating. Although you are holding an emesis basin close to his head, his emesis reaches beyond it to the pant leg of your scrubs, about 2 feet away.

You begin to feel a little sheepish about this, because you have really had it in the back of your mind that the problem was Mrs. Garcia's inexperience rather than that Roberto might have a serious illness. Now that you have seen Roberto vomit, you realize that he may be very ill—the force with which he was vomiting was unusual.

Question

Place the letter *I* (for intussusception) or *P* (for pyloric stenosis) or both (*I* and *P*) next to each sign. (Signs may be used more than once.)

Signs

_____ Bilious vomiting

_____ Nonbilious vomiting

_____ Projectile vomiting

_____ Jaundice

_____ Rectal bleeding

_____ Dehydration

_____ Altered mental status

_____ Alkalosis

_____ Hypochloremia and hypokalemia

Answer

The answers are: (*I*), bilious vomiting; (*P*), non-bilious vomiting; (*P*), projectile vomiting; (*P*), jaundice; (*I*), rectal bleeding; (*I,P*), dehydration; (*I,P*), altered mental status; (*P*), alkalosis; and (*P*), hypochloremia and hypokalemia.

Although both surgical emergencies involve intestinal obstruction, the location of the obstruction is quite different, and affects the signs and symptoms (see Figure 6.7).[3] In intussusception, the obstruction is distal to the outlet of the bile duct; in pyloric stenosis, the obstruction involves hypertrophy, or thickening, of the pyloric sphincter muscle above the outlet of the bile duct.[4] In pyloric stenosis, therefore, the infant vomits stomach contents, and develops hypochloremic alkalosis through loss of hydrochloric acid in the emesis.[4] Note that both illnesses could cause dehydration and altered mental status, however, resulting from fluid loss.[4]

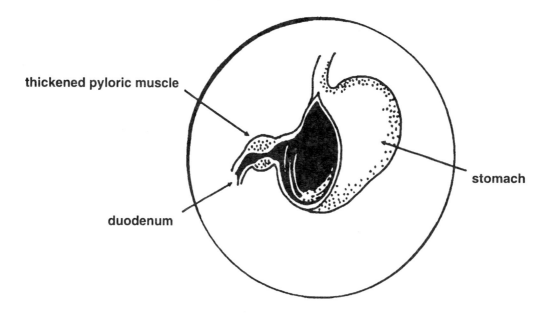

FIGURE 6.7 Thickening of the pyloric muscle blocks the stomach contents.

You clean up Roberto's emesis, and give him to Mrs. Garcia to hold, along with a damp washcloth and an emesis basin. Dr. Morris arrives in the emergency department. Before he enters the room, you describe Roberto's case, and tell him about the abdominal contractions you noticed and about the projectile vomiting. He asks you about the emesis, specifically if there was any blood. There was none, you tell him, although you did not test the emesis for occult blood. He assures you that won't be necessary, and you ask him what diagnoses he is considering. While he examines Roberto, he tells you that right now he is considering pyloric stenosis as the most likely possibility.

Question

What are two likely causes of bloody emesis in children?

1. _____

2. _____

Answer

Bloody emesis at this age would be highly unusual. The most likely reasons for bloody emesis in a child Roberto's age would probably be acute gastritis or gastroenteritis, but any disease in which some blood might be swallowed should also be considered a possibility (see Table 6.8).

TABLE 6.8. Possible Causes of Upper Gastrointestinal Bleeding in Children[4]

Acute gastritis, gastroenteritis	Mallory-Weiss syndrome
Pharyngitis	Esophageal varices
Candidiasis	Esophagitis
Epistaxis	Peptic ulcer
Postsurgical complication	Ingestion (aspirin, alcohol, etc.)
Postdental procedures	Bleeding disorders
Swallowed foreign bodies	

Dr. Morris speaks some Spanish and talks with Mrs. Garcia as he examines Roberto. Once he has completed his exam, he orders laboratory analyses and an abdominal ultrasound. You remind him that the X-ray technician who does the ultrasound exams is on call because it is Sunday, so it will be at least an hour before this examination can be performed.

When Dr. Morris leaves, Mrs. Garcia looks very worried again. She asks several questions you don't understand, and the interpreter tells you Mrs. Garcia wants to know what is wrong with her baby. You tell her that you don't know for certain yet, but the doctor will be able to give her a better idea after the lab tests and sonogram. She then asks you what medicine is given for this, and how soon she will be able to take her baby home.

Question

On the basis of what you know at this point, your best answer would be:

1. There is a very good probability that she will be able to take her baby home once the tests are done.
2. You can't give her any idea at present about whether she can take her baby home or not.
3. Her baby will probably have to stay in the hospital for several days at least.
4. The doctor will talk to her about whether Roberto needs to be hospitalized when the test results are back.

Answer

The correct answer is (3). It seems there is a very high likelihood from Roberto's clinical presentation that he has an obstruction that will require hospitalization at the least and probably will require surgery. The surgery of choice for pyloric stenosis is a pyloromyotomy—incision into the muscle fibers leaving the mucous layer intact.[5] In any case, Roberto will have to be hospitalized because he is becoming dehydrated—he has had no urine output for several hours.

It would be very unusual for a child with Roberto's clinical presentation to be sent home. Although the exact diagnosis is not yet certain, you can safely inform Mrs. Garcia that Roberto will probably require hospitalization. Parents need information about what is ahead, because they must make plans for meals, family members, and their other activities.

Once he has written his notes on Roberto's examination, Dr. Morris returns to examine Roberto once again, palpating Roberto's abdomen slowly and carefully. After he vomited, Roberto relaxed somewhat and is lying quietly in his mother's arms during the examination. As Dr. Morris palpates the right upper quadrant, Dr. Morris tells you he can feel a small density and that he is fairly certain Roberto has pyloric stenosis. He asks you to find the interpreter and help him explain to Mrs. Garcia that Roberto will probably require surgery.

Question

Because Dr. Morris is considering pyloric stenosis as the most likely diagnosis, which of the following questions might yield very valuable information at this point?

1. Have you noticed blood in Roberto's stool?
2. Was Roberto born prematurely?
3. Have any other family members had this type of problem?
4. What type of formula is he being given?

Answer

Although (1), (2), and (4) are important questions that Dr. Morris will ask as a part of the history, the most pertinent question is whether this type of illness has occurred in the family previously (3). His main reason for asking this question would be that pyloric stenosis is much more likely with a positive family history.[4]

TABLE 6.9   **Some Facts About Pyloric Stenosis**[4,5]

Occurs in 4 to 5 per 1,000 live births
Is more likely to occur when there is positive family history
Is more common in boys than in girls (4 or 5 to 1 ratio)
Frequently occurs in firstborn children
Is usually managed surgically in the U.S., but is often managed medically in Europe

Luckily, it is quiet in labor and delivery, and you ask the Spanish-speaking nurse, Celia, to come back to interpret for Dr. Morris. She translates Dr. Morris's explanation, and Mrs. Garcia begins to cry. She tells you that she cannot consent to surgery without her husband there. Dr. Morris tries to explain the seriousness of the problem to Mrs. Garcia, and Mrs. Garcia says she understands, but she wants to leave and come back tomorrow, after she has discussed this with her family, especially her husband.

You are beginning to have some concerns about the legal issues involved in this discussion including patient's rights, the urgent need for care of the child, and the risks of Mrs. Garcia leaving the hospital. Celia offers to call Roberto's father, who is at work managing a coffee shop, so Mrs. Garcia can talk to him.

As Mr. and Mrs. Garcia converse on the telephone, Mrs. Garcia calms down visibly, and when she finishes talking to him, she says that her husband will be in to sign the admitting papers and to discuss the surgery with Dr. Morris. You give Mrs. Garcia directions to Radiology, where Roberto will be having his sonogram. Celia tells you she will help take Mrs. Garcia over there, and puts her arm around Mrs. Garcia, walking slowly over to Radiology with her.

REFERENCES

Case Study 1

1. American Academy of Pediatrics, Committee on Nutrition. (1985). Use of oral fluid therapy and posttreatment feeding following enteritis in children in a developed country. *Pediatrics*, *75*, 358–361.
2. Seidel, J. S., & Henderson, D. P. (1985). *Prehospital Care of Pediatric Emergencies*. Los Angeles: Los Angeles Pediatric Society.
3. Hatch, E. H. (1985). The acute abdomen in children. *Pediatric Clinics of North America*, *32*, 1151–1164.
4. Behrman, R. E., & Vaughan, V. C. (1987). *Nelson textbook of pediatrics* (13th ed.). Philadelphia: Saunders. 781–788.
5. Janik, J. S., & Firor, H. V. (1979). Pediatric appendicitis: A 20-year study of 1,640 children at Cook County (Illinois) Hospital. *Archives of Surgery*, *114*, 717–719.
6. Reynolds, S. L., & Jaffee, D. M. (1990). Children with abdominal pain: Evaluation in the pediatric emergency department. *Pediatric Emergency Care, 6*, 8–12.
7. Snyder, J. D. (1991). Use and misuse of oral therapy for diarrhea: Comparison of U.S. practices with American Academy of Pediatrics recommendations. *Pediatrics, 87*, 28–33.
8. Schnaufer, L., & Mahboubi, S. (1988). Abdominal emergencies. In G. Fleisher & S. Ludwig (Eds.), *Textbook of pediatric emergency medicine*. Baltimore: Williams & Wilkins.
9. Spitz, L. (1987). Acute abdominal emergencies. In J. A. Black (Ed.), *Paediatric emergencies*. Boston: Butterworths.

Case Study 2

1. Spitz, L. (1987). Acute abdominal emergencies. In J. A. Black (Ed.), *Paediatric emergencies*. Boston: Butterworths.
2. Behrman, R. E., & Vaughan, V. C. (1987). *Nelson textbook of pediatrics* (13th ed., pp. 781–782, 787–788). Philadelphia: Saunders.
3. Reynolds, S., & Jaffe, D. (1990, August 15). Quick triage of abdominal pain. *Emergency Medicine*, 39–42.
4. Hazinski, M. F. (Ed.). (1984). *Nursing care of the critically ill child*. St. Louis: Mosby.
5. Felter, R. A. (1991). Nontraumatic surgical emergencies in children. *Emergency Medicine Clinics of North America, 9*, 589–610.
6. Fleisher, G., & Ludwig, S. (1988). *Textbook of pediatric emergency medicine* (2nd ed.). Baltimore: Williams & Wilkins.
7. Chameides, L. (Ed.). (1988). *Textbook of pediatric advanced life support*. Dallas, TX: American Heart Association.
8. Emergency Nurses Association. (1986). *Trauma nursing core course (provider) manual* (2nd ed.). Chicago: Award Printing Corporation.
9. Foster, R. L., Hunsberger, M. M., & Anderson, J. J. (1989). *Family-centered nursing care of children*. Philadelphia: Saunders.

Case Study 3

1. Silva, G. C. (1984). Awareness of Hispanic cultural issues in the health care setting. *Children's Health Care, 13*, 4–9.
2. American Academy of Pediatrics, Committee on Nutrition. (1985). Use of oral fluid therapy and posttreatment feeding following enteritis in children in a developed country. *Pediatrics, 75*, 358–361.
3. Hazinski, M. F., (Ed.). (1984). *Nursing care of the critically ill child*. St. Louis: Mosby.
4. Felter, R. A., (1991). Nontraumatic surgical emergencies in children. *Emergency Medicine Clinics of North America, 9*, 589–610.
5. Schnaufer, L., & Mahboubi, S. (1988). Abdominal emergencies. In G. Fleisher & S. Ludwig (Eds.), *Textbook of pediatric emergency medicine*. Baltimore: Williams & Wilkins.

Chapter Seven

Trauma Assessment and Intervention

Prerequisite Skills

- Knowledge of the basic anatomy and physiology of pediatric patients
- Ability to perform primary and secondary trauma survey
- Knowledge of trauma resuscitation for adult patients
- Understanding of crisis intervention theories

PEDIATRIC TRAUMA ASSESSMENT AND INTERVENTION

PREVIEW

Trauma assessment and intervention has become a very standard procedure in communities where there has been trauma center designation. Central to this type of well-coordinated effort is the commitment of the community and each designated hospital. Pediatric trauma is especially difficult for most health care providers, because pediatric trauma patients are rare. There is much to be gained, therefore, from development of clear protocols and guidelines for care. All emergency departments that care for critically injured pediatric patients should be well prepared in advance to minimize the inevitable chaos that accompanies pediatric trauma. Preparations should include

- Clearly identified areas for pediatric resuscitation equipment
- Equipment and supplies appropriate for pediatric patients
- Medication charts showing dosages on a per kilogram basis
- Scales and measuring tapes to determine the length and weight of pediatric patients accurately
- Pediatricians or general practitioners available for consultation
- Training and education of emergency department staff in pediatric trauma and resuscitation

Although there are many similarities between adult and pediatric trauma resuscitation, particular attention should be given to the differences between the anatomy of the pediatric and adult airway, and the recognition of compensated shock in the pediatric patient. This chapter should help to clarify some of these very important issues.

CASE STUDY 1 OBJECTIVES

On completing this case study, the learner will be able to

- List three special considerations in caring for the pediatric trauma patient
- Prioritize nursing actions during a trauma resuscitation
- Describe the assessment parameters to be used in the evaluation of a child with head trauma
- List the priorities of management of the head-injured child
- Identify pediatric considerations in the assessment and stabilization of thoracic injuries
- Describe principles of assessment and management in a child with abdominal trauma
- Develop two nursing diagnoses for the pediatric trauma patient
- Identify appropriate interventions to help the child and the family deal with the emotional factors involved in pediatric trauma

CASE STUDY 1

Yoshiko Has Been Hit by a Car

You are working evening shift in the emergency department when the paramedics bring in Yoshiko, a 3-year-old Asian female, who is unconscious with multiple bruises and lacerations (see Figure 7.1). They report to you that they were called to respond to the scene of an accident where a child had been hit by a car traveling at approximately 20 miles/hr. Witnesses at the scene say that Yoshiko was thrown about 20 feet. The paramedics tell you that when they arrived Yoshiko was unconscious lying in the street. Her vital signs at the scene were

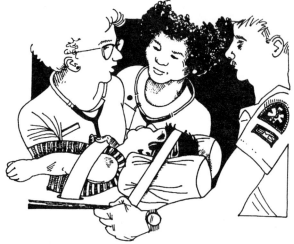

Blood pressure	60/palpation
Heart rate	165/min
Respiratory rate	20/min
Pupils	Equal but slow to react

FIGURE 7.1

Yoshiko is on a backboard, with her head immobilized with sandbags and tape. The paramedics have inserted an oral airway, and she is breathing on her own. You touch Yoshiko's arm and call her name loudly with no response. She has some bruising on her forehead and a gauze wrapped around her head shows a small amount of blood. Your emergency department estimates weight by length of the child. Yoshiko is about 39 inches, and you estimate her weight at about 15 kg.

TRIAGE DECISION

Based on your initial rapid assessment, you would triage this patient as

Emergent.   A life-threatening situation in need of immediate intervention.

Urgent.   Patient needs care within 1 hour to prevent further deterioration.

Nonurgent.   Patient is able to wait more than 1 hour without further deterioration.

TRIAGE DECISION ANSWER

Yoshiko's condition is emergent; she needs immediate intervention. Any unconscious patient has a potentially life-threatening condition because of the risk of airway compromise.

Although your hospital is not a trauma center, trauma patients are brought in several times a month, and you have done your best to prepare for them. You have pediatric equipment in a designated area, and a pediatric crash cart with a list of medication dosages calculated for the kilogram weights of children. Yoshiko is brought into the trauma resuscitation room and moved with the backboard onto a gurney. You call for the emergency physician, but he is caring for a patient with a myocardial infarction in the other treatment area. You ask the paramedics to stay and help for a few minutes, and begin your primary trauma survey, beginning with the *ABCDE*s.

Question

What are the *ABCDE*s for a pediatric patient? (Fill in the blanks.)

A _____

B _____

C _____

D _____

E _____

Answer

The primary trauma survey for a child is much the same as for an adult (see Table 7.1). A major difference is to remember that children often suffer from hypothermia, either from exposure in the field or from being uncovered in the emergency department.

TABLE 7.1.   Primary Survey for Trauma

Airway. Is the child's airway positioned well, open and clear of debris? (Remember that the tongue is the most common cause of airway obstruction in the child.)

Breathing. Is the child's chest rising equally and is there adequate tidal volume?

Circulation. Is the child's perfusion status adequate? Is there any external hemorrhage to be controlled?

Disability. What is the child's neurologic status? Have any drugs been used?

Exposure. Are there any other injuries? Remove all clothing and check. *E* also stands for **environment**—consider possible hypothermia resulting from exposure to cold temperatures. Children are much more susceptible than adults to hypothermia. Make sure to keep the child warm enough in the emergency department—rewrap immediately after assessment.

Your first step is to assess Yoshiko's airway and breathing. She now has a respiratory rate of 14, with pronounced intercostal retractions and audible inspiratory stridor.

Question

How would you describe Yoshiko's respiratory status? (Choose one.)

1. Normal respiratory rate, with increased work of breathing.
2. Abnormally slow respiratory rate, with increased work of breathing.
3. Slightly rapid respiratory rate, with increased work of breathing.

Answer

Yoshiko has a slow respiratory rate for her age, and she is showing increased work of breathing with the intercostal retractions. She also has abnormal breath sounds (stridor), which may indicate some type of upper airway obstruction (see Table 7.2).

TABLE 7.2. Rapid Assessment of Airway and Breathing[1, 2]

Airway
Is the airway patent—is air moving freely through the large airways?
Is the airway maintainable with head positioning, suctioning, or adjuncts such as an oral airway or bag-valve-mask ventilation?
Is the airway unmaintainable so that advanced airway interventions such as foreign body removal, intubation, or cricothyroidotomy are required?
Breathing
Is the respiratory rate normal for age? (See Pediatric Vital Signs Chart, Table 1.4, Chapter 1)
Is there increased work of breathing?   • Presence of retractions?   • Use of accessory muscles in neck and chest?   • Nasal flaring?   • Seesaw abdominal and chest movement?

It is clear that Yoshiko needs immediate airway intervention. Unfortunately, the other emergency department nurse is assisting the physician in the other room. You call the nursing supervisor for help and begin your interventions using your trauma protocol. The nursing supervisor arrives and tells you she is not very experienced in emergency nursing, but she will help you until she can send you a nurse from the intensive care unit. You ask one paramedic to help you in maintaining immobilization of Yoshiko's spine, and you ask the nursing supervisor to assist in ordering lab work and X-ray films according to your standard trauma protocols.

Question

What method would you use to improve patency of Yoshiko's airway? (Choose one answer.)

1. Reposition her airway using head-tilt chin-lift maneuver and place a folded towel under her shoulders.
2. Use in-line cervical immobilization and reopen her airway using the jaw-thrust maneuver.
3. Place her head in the "sniffing position," and prepare for needle cricothyroidotomy.
4. Remove her oral airway and insert a nasopharyngeal airway using in-line cervical spine immobilization.

Answer

The first step in assuring a patent airway is to stabilize the cervical spine and open the airway, because the most common cause of airway obstruction in a pediatric patient is the tongue. The jaw-thrust maneuver is used so that spinal immobilization can be maintained (see Figure 7.2). Use of the "sniffing position," with the head flexed on the neck and the neck slightly extended, optimizes opening of the pediatric airway, but extreme caution must be taken to maintain stability of the cervical spine until spinal cord injury is ruled out.

The head-tilt chin-lift maneuver is not used because of possible damage to the cervical spine when the neck is extended. A needle cricothyroidotomy would be the choice after attempting other methods including endotracheal intubation without success. Insertion of a nasopharyngeal airway is not recommended for the unconscious patient, and insertion can be traumatic to a child.

One of the paramedics helps you to place a cervical collar on Yoshiko and remove the sandbags (see Table 7.3, following page). They tell you, apologetically, that they do not carry cervical collars in pediatric sizes. As you place the collar on Yoshiko, you explain to them why sandbags are not recommended for stabilizing the cervical spine of a child, and show them how to use towels instead, if the correct size of cervical collar is not available (see Figure 7.3). You leave the muslin wrap immobilizing her body in place. She will have to remain immobilized until the cervical spine is definitely cleared both radiologically and clinically. You will continue to maintain immobilization until a full assessment of Yoshiko's neurologic status can be made. There is a slight risk of cervical spine injuries in children with negative X-ray films, a syndrome called spinal cord injury without radiologic abnormality[3] This is because most pediatric cervical spine injuries are ligamentous, not bony. You use the jaw-thrust maneuver to make sure her airway is open.

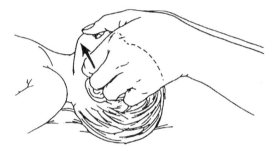

FIGURE 7.2

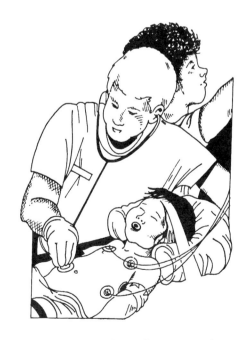

FIGURE 7.3 Towels and tape may be used if the appropriately sized cervical collar is not available.

TABLE 7.3.   Pediatric Spinal Immobilization

The cervical spine is stabilized by manual in-line immobilization and the application of an appropriately sized cervical collar.
The bottom edge of the collar should rest on the shoulder while the chin is held in alignment. A collar that is too short will not offer adequate support. A collar that is too long will hyperextend the neck and may compromise the airway.
The cervical spine of a pediatric patient can be stabilized by taping the head of the child to a backboard, with a roll of towels or blankets around the head to eliminate the dead space between the tape and the patient.
Sandbags should not be used to maintain correct head position for in-line cervical immobilization.
Spinal immobilization means that the patient must be kept on the backboard, and *both* the head and body must be maintained in a neutral position.

You notice that after your last efforts to improve her airway, the respiratory distress does not improve significantly. Her respiratory rate is now 12 breaths/min, her stridor is worse, and her retractions remain about the same.

Question

What will be your next interventions to stabilize Yoshiko's airway? (Choose one answer.)

1. Intubate, ventilate with a bag-valve-mask device, suction and place on a ventilator.
2. Suction, ventilate with a bag-valve-mask device, and intubate.
3. Perform a needle cricothyroidotomy and ventilate.
4. Intubate, suction, and place on a ventilator.

Answer

The correct sequence would be to suction, ventilate with a bag-valve-mask device, and intubate. In the pediatric patient, mucus can easily plug the airway because of the small diameter of the airway (see Figure 7.4). More invasive procedures should not be considered until you have cleared the airway, made sure the airway is positioned optimally, and provided 100% oxygen by bag-valve-mask and reassessed. It may also be helpful to assure that the oral airway is the correct size (see Figure 7.5).

FIGURE 7.4   Because the diameter of the pediatric airway is smaller than the adult's, the airway is more easily blocked by mucus. Obstruction is even more likely when the airway is narrowed by edema. (Reproduced with permission. *Textbook of Pediatric Advanced Life Support.* 1988, 1990. © American Heart association.)

A needle cricothyroidotomy would only be done as a last resort when an airway cannot be obtained by any other method; the procedure is rarely used for children. Endotracheal intubation will be necessary for the unconscious patient, but adequate ventilation can be obtained with a bag-valve-mask device until preparations are made for this procedure (see Table 7.4).

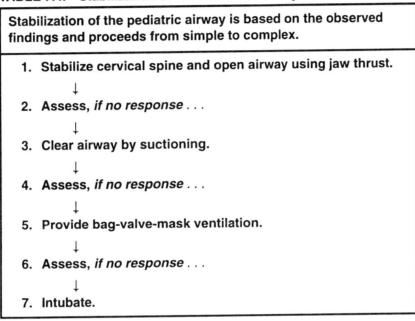

TABLE 7.4.   Stabilization of the Pediatric Airway

Stabilization of the pediatric airway is based on the observed findings and proceeds from simple to complex.
1. Stabilize cervical spine and open airway using jaw thrust. ↓ 2. Assess, *if no response* . . . ↓ 3. Clear airway by suctioning. ↓ 4. Assess, *if no response* . . . ↓ 5. Provide bag-valve-mask ventilation. ↓ 6. Assess, *if no response* . . . ↓ 7. Intubate.

Yoshiko is not responding well enough to the initial noninvasive airway interventions, so one of the paramedics is giving her bag-valve-mask ventilation, and she will require endotracheal intubation. You have the intensive care unit nurse help you, and you begin to assemble the equipment necessary for this procedure as she monitors Yoshiko and attempts to start an IV line. The emergency physician tells you he will come in right away to intubate.

Question

1. What is the appropriate size endotracheal tube for Yoshiko?
2. Should this be a cuffed or uncuffed tube?

Answer

A 4.5-mm uncuffed endotracheal tube would be approximately the right size. You may determine the correct size using a chart, or by obtaining a tube roughly the size of the child's little finger or nostril.

Uncuffed tubes are generally used for patients under 15 kg. Although cuffed tubes are available in all sizes, they are usually not recommended for infants and small children because of the potential for damage to tissue in the airway from pressure resulting from overinflation of the cuff. Some intensive care units use the cuffed tubes, however, making sure the cuff is slightly underinflated, indicated by an audible air leak (see Figure 7.6).

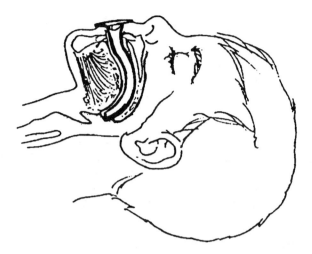

FIGURE 7.5 Oral airway effects of the tongue. (Reproduced with permission. *Textbook of Pediatric Advanced Life Support.* 1988, 1990. © American Heart association.)

The emergency physician rapidly intubates Yoshiko without difficulty. Once intubated, Yoshiko is ventilated manually with a bag-valve-mask device while cervical spine immobilization is maintained by the paramedic. You ask for a ventilator, but find out it will be 15 minutes before one is available. As you listen to Yoshiko's chest, you notice that the breath sounds on the right are more audible than on the left.

Note: Because the chest wall of a child is thin, you may hear breath sounds from one area transmitted throughout the chest. Listening to breath sounds in the axillary line on each side helps to determine differences between the two sides of the lungs.

Because this is a trauma case, you consider the possibility of hemothorax or pneumothorax.

Question

Other causes for Yoshiko's unequal breath sounds could be (Fill in the blanks.)

1. _____

2. _____

Answer

Two other causes for unequal breath sounds could be intubation of the right mainstem bronchus or obstruction of the left bronchus by mucus or blood. Pediatric airways are more easily obstructed by mucus, blood, or edema because of the small diameter.

After hyperventilating Yoshiko for a few moments, you suction her endotracheal tube carefully and recheck its position. The tube seems to have descended somewhat further than the original placement, and you hear diminished breath sounds on the left side. The emergency physician backs the tube out by about 1/2 inch. After this, you reassess and find that Yoshiko's breath sounds are equal bilaterally. You assess her further for signs and symptoms consistent with a hemothorax or pneumothorax.

- Continued signs of respiratory distress
- Unstable vital signs
- Recurrence of unequal breath sounds

If a hemothorax or pneumothorax were suspected, Yoshiko should have needle decompression of the chest performed immediately, without waiting for a chest X-ray films, and then a chest tube would be inserted. You check the trauma cart to make sure that you have a chest tray and pediatric sizes of thoracostomy tubes ready in case she continues to have problems.

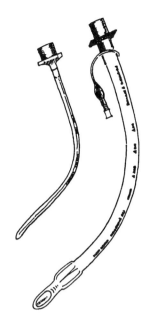

FIGURE 7.6 Cuffed and uncuffed endotracheal tubes.

Question

About what size of thoracostomy tube would be correct for Yoshiko? (Fill in the blank.)

_____ French

Answer

Any size from 20 to 28 French would be approximately the right size for Yoshiko, although it is useful to have several sizes ready (see Table 7.5).

TABLE 7.5.   Average Thoracostomy Tube Sizes[4]

Age	Tube Sizes (French)
Up to 1 year	10–12
1 to 3 years	16–20
3 to 8 years	20–28
8 to 12 years	28–32
12 to 14 years	32–42

Ten minutes have passed. The intensive care unit nurse has not been able to start an IV line. Listening to Yoshiko's breath sounds, you hear equal breath sounds bilaterally, with no indication of hemothorax or pneumothorax at the moment. While Yoshiko's airway and breathing are being stabilized you are also assessing her circulatory status. You note the following:

Heart rate	170 beats/min
Capillary refill	>3 s
Peripheral pulses	Weak
Skin color	Pale
Blood pressure	90/palpated

Question

Which of the above assessments does **not** indicate possible hypovolemic shock? (Fill in the blank.)

_____

Answer

Blood pressure 90/palpated; this blood pressure is within normal limits for a 3-year-old child. The fact that her capillary refill is prolonged, her skin is pale, and her heart rate is increased indicate that she is probably in compensated shock.[1]

Yoshiko now has a stable airway, and your focus is on cardiovascular stability. Your next priority is to obtain venous access (see Figure 7.7, facing page) so that you will have a route for administration of IV fluid and medication.

Question

Does Yoshiko's condition indicate the need for fluid resuscitation at this time? (Choose Yes or No.)

_____ Yes   _____ No

Answer

Yes. Yoshiko will probably need fluid resuscitation. *Any child who has a normal blood pressure, but is demonstrating signs of impaired perfusion should be considered to be in compensated shock and should receive fluid resuscitation.*

Because children can compensate well for volume loss, up to 25% of total blood volume may be lost before a change in blood pressure. A child's estimated blood volume is 80 mL/kg. Because total normal blood volume is determined by weight, it is obvious that children have a small total amount of blood when compared with adults. What might be a relatively small amount of blood loss for an adult can therefore actually represent a large percentage of the child's total volume.

Note: **Blood pressure is often the last parameter to change when there is volume loss in a pediatric patient.**

You have determined that Yoshiko is in compensated shock and will need fluid resuscitation, so you mentally review your venous access and fluid resuscitation protocols. You are relieved to see that Yoshiko is now being effectively ventilated, and her color is improving slightly.

> **Question**
>
> List four methods for obtaining venous access in a pediatric patient. (Fill in the blanks.)
>
> 1. _____
>
> 2. _____
>
> 3. _____
>
> 4. _____

Answer

Four methods that can be used to obtain venous access in a child are:

1. Percutaneous peripheral IV line placement
2. Cutdown
3. Central line insertion
4. Intraosseous line placement

As you set up Yoshiko's IV lines, you talk to her as you would to an alert patient, reassuring her and telling her you are trying to help. You do not know how much she can hear or understand.

> **Question**
>
> What size catheter is appropriate for Yoshiko? (Choose one answer.)
>
>   1. 22–24 gauge
>   2. 20–22 gauge
>   3. 18–20 gauge

Answer

The correct size of intravenous catheter would be 18 to 20 gauge. Small children have quite sturdy veins, and often a larger size catheter can be used than one might expect. Table 7.6 shows appropriate sizes of intravenous catheters for children.

TABLE 7.6. Equipment for Venous Cannulation

Age (years)	Weight (kg)	Over-the-needle catheters (gauge)
<1	<10	20, 22, 24
1–12	10–40	16, 18, 20
>12	>40	14, 16, 18

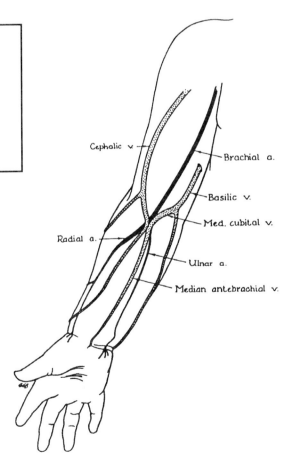

FIGURE 7.7 Obtaining venous access.

Because you want to use the largest size catheter possible, you place a peripheral line in Yoshiko's right antecubital fossa, withdrawing enough blood for diagnostic tests.

The tests include complete blood cell count, electrolytes, coagulation studies, blood urea nitrogen, creatinine, glucose, bilirubin, and serum amylase. Because there is the possibility of hemorrhage in any trauma, type and crossmatch is included in your trauma protocol.

Yoshiko is still being ventilated manually, and you call once again for a ventilator. You have succeeded in starting a second IV line in her left hand. The emergency physician orders a fluid bolus, which you give her, and then assess her response.

Question

Yoshiko's estimated weight is 15 kg. How much fluid would you give her? (Choose one answer.)

1. 150 mL
2. 300 mL
3. 400 mL
4. 500 mL

Answer

The dose for fluid resuscitation is 20 mL/kg of Ringer's lactate, or 300 mL. This would be an appropriate amount even if you are concerned that Yoshiko may be have increased intracranial pressure related to a closed head injury. When a patient is in shock, you must restore the circulating blood volume to assure adequate perfusion to the brain as well as to other organs.

Question

Which of the following parameters would you use to assess Yoshiko's response to fluid resuscitation? (Mark the correct parameters.)

1. Capillary refill
2. Heart rate
3. Anterior fontanel
4. Peripheral pulses
5. Pupillary reaction
6. Temperature of extremities

(Choose one of the following answers.)

a. 1, 2, 3, 4
b. 1, 2, 4, 5
c. 2, 3, 4, 6
d. 1, 2, 4, 6

Answer

Assessment of capillary refill, heart rate, peripheral pulses, and temperature of extremities all may be used to assess cardiovascular status (d). Yoshiko is too old to have an open anterior fontanel—that usually closes by 18 months of age. Pupillary reaction is not a valid parameter for assessment of perfusion but is a parameter used in neurologic assessment.

The X-ray technician arrives to take the portable X-ray films of Yoshiko's cervical spine. Your assessment findings following the fluid bolus are

Heart rate	160 beats/min
Capillary refill	3 s

Peripheral pulses	Weak
Color	Pale
Blood pressure	80/palpation

The unit coordinator comes into the treatment room to tell you that Yoshiko's mother and father will be arriving at the hospital shortly.

Question

What would be the next procedure? (Choose one answer.)

1. Start a Dopamine drip.
2. Give a second fluid bolus of 40 mL/kg.
3. Give a second fluid bolus of 20 mL/kg.
4. Give packed red blood cells at 10 mL/kg.

Answer

A second fluid bolus at 20 mL/kg should be given. If Yoshiko does not respond to the second bolus, a likely order would be to give packed cells at 10 mL/kg. Dopamine should not be given at this time because a vasopressor should not be started while she is still hypovolemic (see Table 7.7).

TABLE 7.7. Fluid Resuscitation in the Pediatric Trauma Patient

1. **Establish vascular access.**
   ↓
2. **Give 20 mL/kg of Ringer's lactate.**
   ↓
3. **Reassess, *if no response*. . .**
   ↓
4. **Give 20 mL/kg of Ringer's lactate.**
   ↓
5. **Reassess, *if no response*. . .**
   ↓
6. **Give 10 mL/kg of packed cells.**

If Yoshiko does not respond to the administration of fluid and blood, then you will consider the possibility of a newly formed or previously undetected pneumothorax. Another possibility is undetected bleeding into the abdomen, chest, or pelvis. Your assessment of Yoshiko at this point shows the following:

Heart rate	120 beats/min
Respiratory rate	Manually assisted, 16 breaths/min
Capillary refill	Less than 2 s
Peripheral pulses	Palpable
Skin color	Pink
Blood pressure	100/palpated

Now that fluid resuscitation is well underway and cardiovascular status is improving, you reassess *D*—disability or neurologic status. The *D* also may be a reminder that the possibility of drug abuse should be considered, especially in older children.

Question

What are two methods you could use to assess the neurologic status of a 3-year-old child? (Fill in the blanks.)

1. _____

2. _____

Answer

Any of the following answers would be correct:

- Assessment of mental status
- Observation of pupillary size and reactivity
- Observation of abnormal body movements

A useful tool to use for nursing assessment of mental status is the mnemonic AVPU (see Table 7.8).

TABLE 7.8. Rapid Assessment of Mental Status

A	*A*lert
V	Responds to *V*erbal stimuli
P	Responds to *P*ainful stimuli
U	*U*nresponsive

At this point, Yoshiko's pupils are equal but react sluggishly. She opens her eyes, withdraws and moans with words you cannot understand in response to pain. Because of the mechanism of injury, you are fairly certain that she has a closed head injury.

Question

Because Yoshiko is intubated, an intervention that you can initiate immediately is hyperventilation at a rate 10 above her normal respiratory rate. (Choose True or False.)

_____ True   _____ False

Answer

True. It would probably be helpful to hyperventilate Yoshiko. Hyperventilation causes lowering of the $PaCO_2$ and constriction of the cerebral blood vessels, lessening the volume inside the closed and unyielding cranial vault, thereby lowering the intracranial pressure.[5] Some interventions for the head-injured child are listed in Table 7.9.

TABLE 7.9. Stabilization of the Pediatric Head Truma Patient

Any alteration in mental status may indicate severe head injury, so early consultation with a neurosurgeon is a priority.
Hyperventilate to a $PaCO_2$ of 25 to 30 mm Hg. This will reduce cerebral blood flow enough to decrease intracranial pressure without completely cutting off blood supply to the brain.[5]
Monitor the child's $PaCO_2$ level to ensure that the $PaCO_2$ does not drop to a level that would impair blood flow to the brain.
Elevate the head of a head-injured patient. Although this may not be advisable when there is suspicion of spinal injury or shock, elevating the head may help to lower intracranial pressure.
Any traumatized child who is not oxygenating or ventilating adequately, has no gag reflex, is unconscious, or is unable to manage his or her secretions adequately will require endotracheal intubation.

> *Note:* When endotracheal intubation is needed for a child with a suspected head injury, rapid sequence intubation should be used to prevent further increase in intracranial pressure (see Rapid Sequence Intubation at the back of this chapter).

Question

If Yoshiko experiences seizures at this time, she should probably be started on antiseizure medications. (Choose True or False.)

_____ True   _____ False

Answer

False. Seizures are relatively common in the first 24 hr after head injury; this type of seizure activity usually does not require medication unless it is prolonged or recurrent. If the child does progress to frequent seizures, then IV medication will probably be given.

Your last assessment of Yoshiko showed that her circulatory status was close to normal. Now that her blood pressure has been stabilized, you want to change her fluid and decrease the rate of her intravenous infusion.

Question

Which of the following fluid and rate would be appropriate for Yoshiko? (Choose one answer.)

1. Dextrose 5% in water with 1/2 normal saline at 1/2 maintenance rate
2. Dextrose 5% in water at maintenance rate
3. Dextrose 5% in water with 1/2 normal saline at maintenance rate
4. Dextrose 5% in water at 1/2 maintenance rate

Answer

As long as the child's cardiovascular status remains stable, the best choice for maintenance is dextrose 5% in water with 1/2 normal saline at maintenance rate.[6] Because she has been given a large amount of fluid, you want to be careful not to overload her cardiovascular system at this point.

Note: Dextrose 5% in water is not recommended as an IV solution at any point in the treatment of the child with head injury.

At present, Yoshiko's lungs are clear, and you will continue to assess her respiratory cardiovascular status at frequent intervals. In the meantime, your full assessment of Yoshiko continues with *E*—exposure. You undress her completely to look for further injuries, keeping in mind the importance of preventing hypothermia. You take Yoshiko's temperature; it is 35.4 °C. (See Temperature Conversion Table at the end of Chapter 1.)

Question

Which of the following interventions is most appropriate to improve Yoshiko's hypothermia? (Choose one answer.)

1. Do nothing at this point because there are other priorities.
2. Cover Yoshiko with a bath blanket and keep the ambient temperature warm.
3. Use a radiant warmer, warm IV fluids, and warm humidified oxygen.
4. Prepare for peritoneal lavage with warm saline.

Answer

Because Yoshiko is mildly hypothermic, it would be helpful to keep her from losing any heat and to make sure the room temperature is warm. The correct answer is cover Yoshiko with a bath blanket, and keep the ambient temperature warm (see Table 7.10). In a case such as this, however, where she may have to remain largely uncovered for procedures, a radiant warmer may be helpful in maintaining normothermia. Yoshiko's lowered temperature must not be ignored, nor does it need to be treated aggressively or invasively at this point.

TABLE 7.10. Treatment of Hypothermia

Degree of hypothermia	Temperature °C (°F)	Rewarming method	Procedures
Mild	33–35 °C (91.4–95 °F)	Passive external (surface)	Prevent active movement to help conserve body heat Use coverings—blankets and towels to conserve heat Maintain warm environment
Moderate	30–32 °C (86.0–89.6 °F)	Active external (surface)	**In addition to passive external methods use** Heat lamp Warm bath to trunk Use stockenet hat to keep head warm
Severe	<30 °C (<86 °F)	Active internal (core)	**May use any of the passive procedures initially,** *plus* Heated, humidified air Warm IV fluids Gastric, bladder, colonic lavage Severest cases may require extracorporeal rewarming with cardiac bypass

Note. From Henderson, D. P. Submersion Injuries. In C. Joy (Ed.), *Pediatric trauma nursing.* © 1989, Rockville, MD: Aspen. Adapted by permission.

Small children are at very high risk for hypothermia because of their high ratio of body surface area to body weight. This allows for rapid heat loss because of conductive and convective losses during a trauma resuscitation. The resulting hypothermia can cause metabolic acidosis, hypoxia, cardiac rhythm disturbances, and poor response to resuscitation.

When you recheck Yoshiko's temperature a few minutes later, it is 36°C. At this point Yoshiko is stable; your assessment is

Heart rate	110 beats/min
Blood pressure	110/60
Capillary refill	< 2 s
Peripheral pulses	Palpable
Skin color	Pink

Her pupils are equal and reacting more quickly to light. You have now completed the primary survey, and Yoshiko has been stabilized for the time being.

Question

Based on the results of your primary survey, you decide on at least two nursing diagnoses appropriate for Yoshiko. What are they? (Fill in the blanks.)

1. _____

2. _____

Answer

Any of the following would be correct:
- Ineffective breathing pattern
- Impaired gas exchange
- Alteration in cardiac output: decreased
- Alteration in tissue perfusion: cardiopulmonary, peripheral, cerebral
- Fluid volume deficit: actual
- Altered body temperature

Question

What are the expected outcomes for the nursing interventions related to the nursing diagnoses listed above? (Fill in the blanks.)

1. Ineffective breathing pattern
   Desired outcome _____

2. Impaired gas exchange
   Desired outcome _____

3. Alteration in cardiac output decreased
   Desired outcome _____

4. Alteration in tissue perfusion
   Desired outcome _____

5. Fluid volume deficit actual
   Desired outcome _____

6. Altered body temperature
   Desired outcome _____

Answer

1. The child will have an effective breathing pattern or assistance of breathing will occur.
2. The child will have normal gas exchange as evidenced by pulse oximeter and arterial blood gas results.
3, 4, and 5. The child's perfusion status will be normal as evidenced by normal color of skin and mucous membranes, skin temperature, peripheral pulses, capillary refill, level of consciousness, urine output, and blood pressure.
6. The child's body temperature will be maintained within normal limits.

Although it seems longer, only 15 minutes have passed since Yoshiko came in, and now that Yoshiko is more stable, you are ready to move onto the secondary survey. This will allow you to perform a head-to-toe assessment to identify previously undetected injuries and to reassess your primary survey findings. The X-ray technician returns to take X-ray films of Yoshiko's chest and abdomen.

Question

What is the first step of your secondary survey? (Choose one answer.)

1. Look for fractured extremities.
2. Examine the chest and abdomen for injuries.
3. Begin diagnostic tests.
4. Try to obtain a more thorough history.

Answer

A history will give you further information concerning the mechanism of injury that will be helpful in considering potential injuries during your secondary survey. Examination of the chest and extremities will follow examination of the head and neck. Diagnostic tests should occur in conjunction with or following the secondary survey.

Note: Mechanism and type of injury is important!

- Remember that most pediatric trauma is blunt; as a result, multiple organ injuries are common.[7]
- During the secondary survey, it is important to consider the likelihood of additional occult injuries.

Along with determining the mechanism of injury, you will need a brief history to determine if there are other problems that may affect Yoshiko's care. (Remember, one easy way to recall some of the essentials in obtaining a history is the mnemonic AMPLE.)

You talk with the paramedics about the accident. They reiterate that Yoshiko was struck by a car and was thrown a distance of at least 20 feet, although they really couldn't determine the exact distance. They say apparently she lay there unconscious until they arrived. They mention also that she seemed to have been hit on the left side, and that the front bumper of the car was dented slightly. Police officers have arrived at the hospital, and a paramedic leaves to ask them whether they have any more details. At this point, you have not been able to speak to the parents regarding allergies, medications, previous illnesses, or last meal. You continue with the secondary survey. The secondary survey begins with examination of the head and neck.

Question

What signs specific to a basilar skull fracture would you expect to see in a head-injured patient? (Circle all that apply.)

1. Battle's sign
2. Raccoon eyes

3. Rapid respiratory rate
4. Dilated and fixed pupils

Answer

You might see Battle's sign (ecchymosis in the mastoid area behind the ear) (Figure 7.8) or raccoon eyes (ecchymosis in the orbital area) (see Figure 7.9) if the patient had a basilar skull fracture. Sometimes these do not appear until later in the course of treatment, however. Rapid respiratory rate and dilated pupils may be signs of increased intracranial pressure, but would not necessarily indicate a basilar skull fracture (see Table 7.11).

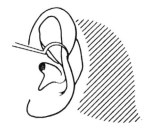

FIGURE 7.8 Battle's sign.

FIGURE 7.9 Raccoon eyes.

TABLE 7.11.   Secondary Survey: Head and Neck

Head and face	Inspect for	Palpate for
	Swelling	Tenderness
	Abrasions	Depressions
	Bruising	Bulging or depressed fontanel
	Lacerations	(<2 years old)
Eyes	**Inspect for**	**Check pupils for**
	Periorbital ecchymosis	Symmetry
	Subconjunctival hemorrhage	Size
		Shape
		Reaction to light
Ears	**Inspect for**	
	Ecchymosis behind the ears	
	Blood or clear fluid draining from the ear	
Nose	**Inspect for**	
	Bleeding or drainage of clear fluid	
Neck	**Inspect for**	**Palpate for**
	Bruising	Tracheal deviation
	Edema	Subcutaneous emphysema
	Tracheal deviation	Tenderness
	Distended neck veins	

> *Note:* Spinal immobilization must be maintained until X-ray results and clinical assessment have ruled out a spinal cord injury.

Without disturbing spinal immobilization, you complete the head and neck assessment for Yoshiko. All findings are normal except for the slight scrape on Yoshiko's left forehead. You move on to examination of her chest, and note a large bruise on her left chest. You also note that as she is being ventilated there is decreased movement on the left side again, with breath sounds slightly diminished. Her vital signs are remaining stable.

Question

You are certain that the endotracheal tube is correctly placed—what would you suspect the problem might be at this time? (Choose one answer.)

1. Flail chest
2. Pulmonary contusion
3. Open pneumothorax
4. Tension pneumothorax

Answer

You would suspect pulmonary contusion. Children have a compliant thorax because of their very flexible, elastic ribs and sternum. The elasticity of the chest wall makes actual fractures less common but increases the potential for internal injuries to the thoracic organs. A pulmonary contusion should be suspected with any chest injury, particularly when bruising is noted. A direct blunt injury as seen with an automobile–pedestrian accident is the most common cause.[8]

Yoshiko's cervical spine X-ray films have been read by the radiologist as negative. The emergency physician agrees that her cervical collar can be removed. You are still concerned about her chest and consider what other causes there might be for the diminished breath sounds.

Question

In addition to pulmonary contusion, what is another common chest injury to suspect in children? (Choose one answer.)

1. Flail chest
2. Rib fractures
3. Pneumothorax
4. Traumatic asphyxia

Answer

Pneumothorax is also a common chest injury seen in children. The most frequent cause of pneumothorax is blunt trauma. Again, because of the flexibility, actual rib fractures and flail chest are not commonly seen. Traumatic asphyxia usually occurs as the result of a compression injury, such as being run over by a vehicle (see Table 7.12).

TABLE 7.12.   Secondary Survey of the Chest

Inspect for	Observe breathing for	Auscultate for	Palpate for
Bruising	Rate	Breath sounds	Tenderness
Swelling	Rhythm		Subcutaneous
Deformities	Effort		Emphysema
Lacerations	Symmetry of chest wall movement		Deformities
Abrasions			

Clinical signs and symptoms of respiratory distress may be the result of chest wall, pulmonary, or pleural injuries. Indicators of chest wall injury include:

- Hypotension
- Tachycardia
- Bruising
- Crepitus
- Paradoxical chest wall movement
- Tachypnea
- Chest wall tenderness

To your great relief, Yoshiko's vital signs are remaining stable. Her chest X-ray film shows that her lungs are clear, and that there is no pneumothorax. The patient in the next room has been transferred upstairs so the emergency department physician and nurse are back to assist you.

Question

The finding of a clear chest on X-ray film suggests that Yoshiko does not have a pulmonary contusion. (Choose True or False.)

_____ True   _____ False

Answer

False. Initial symptoms in a child with pulmonary contusion are few, if any. Within a few hours, the child will begin to develop wheezing, rales, decreased breath sounds, and an increased temperature. Hemoptysis may also be seen. Within 2 to 6 hours, the PaO_2 will decrease, and the $PaCO_2$ will increase. The child will exhibit further clinical signs of respiratory distress. The chest X-ray film will reveal a clear lung in the first few hours, with subsequent development of consolidation.

You know now that Yoshiko may have a pulmonary contusion. The goal of initial treatment of a pulmonary contusion is to prevent worsening interstitial pulmonary edema. Now that Yoshiko has been stabilized, further fluid administration must proceed carefully. Albumin may be used for osmotic purposes and diuretics would be appropriate to further restrict the amount of pulmonary interstitial fluid.

You are continuing your secondary survey to determine the extent of other injuries. The next step is examination of the abdomen.

Question

Your first priority is to prepare for a peritoneal lavage. (Choose True or False.)

_____ True   _____ False

Answer

False. A peritoneal lavage is not indicated at present. As long as the child is hemodynamically stable, then a clinical physical assessment including radiologic evaluation by means of an abdominal CT scan is required. A peritoneal lavage is indicated for an unconscious patient when

- Emergent neurosurgic intervention is required
- There is no time for an abdominal CT
- There are signs of abdominal bleeding (see Table 7.13) requiring immediate laparotomy[9]

TABLE 7.13. Secondary Survey of the Abdomen

Inspect for	Auscultate for	Palpate for
Distention Lacerations Abrasions Bruising Protruding tissue	Bowel sounds (absent bowel sounds are more indicative of underlying injury than increased bowel sounds)	Tenderness Rigidity

You are continuing to monitor Yoshiko's vital signs, which are stable. She continues to mumble incoherent words when stimulated by pain or movement. A CT scan has been ordered along with skull X-rays, and an abdominal CT is being considered for Yoshiko. CT scans are noninvasive, clinically reliable, and injury-specific, and they allow for the classification of the nature and the extent of the injury with a high degree of accuracy. You know that the CT of the abdomen is being considered because head and abdominal injuries occur together frequently in children.

Because Yoshiko's condition is remaining stable, the CT of her abdomen is not ordered. After assessment of Yoshiko's abdomen, her genitourinary tract is assessed. Genitourinary injuries occur frequently in children, and although they are rarely life-threatening, they can be the cause of significant morbidity.

Question

If Yoshiko had required an abdominal CT scan that revealed a liver or spleen injury, would she have been considered a candidate for immediate surgery? (Choose Yes or No.)

_____ Yes   _____ No

Answer

The correct answer is No. Yoshiko would not necessarily have been considered a candidate for immediate surgery. When a child is hemodynamically stable, nonoperative management is preferred for both liver and spleen injuries. The child should be hospitalized and then closely observed. Serial hematocrits and physical examinations of the abdomen are performed (see Table 7.14).

TABLE 7.14. Genitourinary Assessment

Indications of genitourinary injury	Examine abdomen and flanks for	Examine the external genitalia for
Abdominal or flank pain	Tenderness	Swelling
Pelvic fracture	Masses	Ecchymosis
Lower rib fracture	Abrasions	Blood at the meatus (suggests a urethral injury)
Perineal bruising or swelling	Contusions	
	Flank ecchymoses (these indicate retroperitoneal bleeding.)	

Examination of Yoshiko's genitourinary tract indicates that she does not have an injury in this area. You prepare for urinary catheterization to send urine for analysis and to monitor her urine output.

Question

What is the main contraindication to urinary catheter insertion? (Fill in the blank.)

_____

Answer

The main contraindication for urinary catheterization is the suspicion of a urethral injury, indicated by bleeding from the genital area (or the meatus in a male child), or bruising of the perineum. When a urethral injury is suspected, consultation with a urologist is usually required. You also might need a specialist in attendance if there is a history of surgery on the urethra.

You and the other nurse prepare Yoshiko for urinary catheterization. You use her name when talking to her and telling her that her parents will soon be with her and that you are all there to help her. You also tell her that the procedure may be uncomfortable, but it will let you know how she is doing so you can help her better. You notice that some of her dark hair is sticking to her face, and you move it away and gently clean her face with a damp washcloth.

Your urinary catheterization kit comes with an adult-size catheter, so you look for the pediatric catheters.

Question

What size urinary catheter would be appropriate for Yoshiko? (Choose one answer.)

1. 14 French   2. 10 French   3. 8 French

Answer

The correct answer is (2), 10 French. Table 7.15 shows the correct sizes of urinary catheters.

TABLE 7.15. Pediatric Foley Catheter Sizes

Age	Catheter size
Newborn	5
6 months	5
1 year	8
18 months	8
3 years	10
6 years	10
8 years	10
10 years	10
12 years	12
14 years	12

You talk reassuringly to Yoshiko as you insert the catheter. The initial output of urine is 50 mL of clear yellow urine. You test a small amount with a dipstick and send the rest for analysis. The dipstick reading is negative. You now begin to examine Yoshiko's extremities for signs of injury to the extremities.

Question

Which of the following fractures carries special risk for pediatric patients? (Choose one answer.)

1. Femur   3. Epiphyseal plate
2. Humerus   4. Skull

Answer

Epiphyseal fractures are found in children and not in adults. The cartilaginous epiphyseal plate (see Figure 7.10), or growth plate, is present in the long bones of growing children (girls < 14 years, boys < 16 years). Fractures through the epiphyseal plate carry a special risk as they may result in lifelong deformity. A specialist should be consulted when such a fracture is suspected.

Your assessment of Yoshiko's extremities shows that her left leg is slightly shorter than the right, and it is slightly swollen. She grimaces and becomes agitated when you touch her upper leg. You suspect she has a fractured femur. This type of fracture is relatively common in children, partially because of the slender diameter of the bone. Diagnosis is usually made through the classic symptoms of angulation, external rotation, and shortening of the affected leg. You immobilize her femur with a pediatric splint to prevent injury to the femoral artery and obtain a portable X-ray film, which shows a small fracture.

At this point, you have completed a full assessment of Yoshiko and have stabilized her to the point where you are ready to consider preparing her for transport to a pediatric trauma center. Although trauma scores are sometimes used in determining which children should be transported to another center, policies vary from institution to institution, and your hospital does not have a specific protocol. Because this is a recurring problem you make a mental note to talk about this with the emergency department supervisor to see if such a protocol could be developed collaboratively with the physicians.

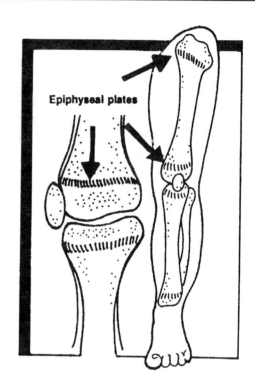

FIGURE 7.10 Epiphyseal plate.

Meanwhile, you receive word that Yoshiko's parents are in the waiting room. Because Yoshiko's condition is now stable, you ask the other nurse to watch Yoshiko so you can speak with her parents. You find Mr. and Mrs. Watanabe sitting next to one another—they both look very worried. When you introduce yourself, Mrs. Watanabe says "I went into the house for just a moment, I thought that the front gate was closed and the next thing I knew the car had hit her. It's all my fault! Is she going to die?"

Question

What would be the most appropriate response to Mrs. Watanabe's statement? (Choose one answer.)

1. "Oh, don't say that, it's not your fault."
2. "Well, let's put that behind us for now. We need to worry about Yoshiko."
3. "I know you're very upset. Yoshiko has been seriously injured, but she is stable now. We are cleaning her up, and you will be able to see her in a few moments."
4. "Can you tell me what happened? She is very sick, but it would help her treatment if we knew exactly how she was injured."

Answer

It is important not to discount a parent's feelings of guilt and anger, which responses (1) and (2) tend to do. The correct answer is (3). Parents of injured children need information concerning their child. They need to realize that their child is receiving care that is appropriate, and they need as much information as possible.[10] Mr. and Mrs. Watanabe need to see their injured child as soon as possible.

Family-centered care should be initiated from the first contact with the parents. Help parents realize their unique role in the care of their child. They need to be reassured that they are irreplaceable in meeting their child's needs. Your role is to support the parents in the care of their child. Incorporating parents into the care of the child can reduce their anxiety and diminish the psychological trauma that the child may experience.

You return to the resuscitation area with Mr. and Mrs. Watanabe, explaining the equipment to them. They are very upset, but calm down quickly. Although you know that Yoshiko is still unconscious, she seems somehow calmer now that her parents are with her. They visit with Yoshiko for awhile, holding her hand and comforting her. Once you have answered their questions, you explain to them that Yoshiko is stable enough to be transferred to a pediatric trauma center where she will receive the best care possible. You make the arrangements for transfer, giving Mr. and Mrs. Watanabe directions and a map to the trauma center, and reassuring them that you will be sending all of her tests and X-rays, and that you will follow up to find out how Yoshiko is doing.

CASE STUDY 2 OBJECTIVES

On completing this case study, the learner will be able to

- Prioritize nursing interventions to be used in caring for the pediatric burn patient
- Classify burns according to current burn assessment methods
- Describe three different methods for estimating the body surface area of burns
- Use a formula to determine the amount of fluid maintenance required for a burn victim

TRAUMA CASE STUDY 2: BURN

Jerome Spilled Boiling Water on Himself

Jerome, a 2½-year-old African-American male child (see Figure 7.11), is brought into the emergency room by his father, Mr. Johnson. Jerome is wearing only the lower half of a pair of pajamas, and has a towel over his shoulders. It is 6:45 P.M., and Mr. Johnson explains to you that he was preparing dinner and had a pot of boiling water on the stove. While Mr. Johnson's back was turned, Jerome reached up and grabbed the handle of the pot, pouring the boiling water onto himself.

Jerome is crying vigorously, and has obvious areas of burn injury on his right upper arm, chest, and legs. The burns are a combination of pink, dry areas and areas where the skin is red and moist with blisters developing. Observing his breathing carefully, you see that he is not showing any signs of respiratory distress.

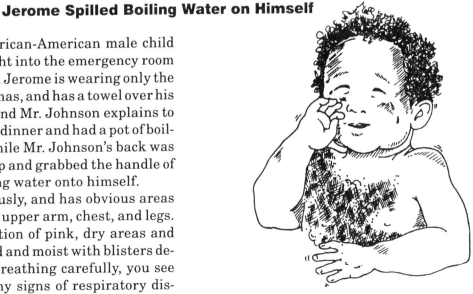

FIGURE 7.11 Jerome.

TRIAGE DECISION

Based on your initial rapid assessment, you would triage this patient as

Emergent.   A life-threatening situation in need of immediate intervention.

Urgent.   Patient needs care within 1 hour to prevent further deterioration.

Nonurgent.   Patient is able to wait more than 1 hour without further deterioration.

TRIAGE DECISION ANSWER

The patient should be triaged as emergent. Although his condition may not appear to be life-threatening at this moment, Jerome should be triaged as emergent because of his pain, to assess the depth and extent of his burns more accurately, and to assure that his burns are kept as clean as possible. Jerome definitely could not wait longer than 1 hour for care.

A flash burn in an enclosed space and any type of burn when there is the possibility of smoke inhalation would require immediate intervention, because respiratory problems are common. The appearance of Jerome's burn is consistent with the father's story, and there are no signs of soot in his nose or singed nasal hairs, so you rule out this possibility.

Because of Jerome's pain, and to continue your assessment, you bring him to the treatment area immediately. You quickly pick up two bottles of sterile saline solution and some sterile towels as you take him in. As you lie Jerome down on towels on the gurney, you begin your assessment of his airway, breathing, and circulatory status. You carefully remove his pajamas and wet down the affected areas with saline solution to help relieve the pain. Jerome's father stays with him, standing at the head of the bed.

Continuing your assessment of the *ABC*s, you find that Jerome's airway is clear, he is breathing well, and he has warm extremities with a capillary refill less than 2 seconds. His vital signs are

Respiratory rate	44, with no retractions or stridor
Heart rate	130/min, regular
Blood pressure (by palpation)	90/palpated

Question

Does this assessment indicate that Jerome is in the early stages of compensated shock? (Choose Yes or No.)

____ Yes   ____ No

Answer

No. These may not be indicators for shock. Even though Jerome's heart rate and respiratory rate are higher than normal for his age group, the increase in these parameters is probably caused by pain and anxiety. Other clinical signs, including no respiratory distress and good systemic perfusion, indicate a hemodynamically stable child.

You cover Jerome's burns lightly with soft, dry dressings to prevent loss of body heat, and keep him warm with a clean bath blanket. An important nursing diagnosis to consider for Jerome during this phase of his treatment is alteration in body temperature related to his burn. Children are at risk for hypothermia because of their relatively larger body surface area and smaller body mass. In burn patients, a heat loss also occurs through the burned area. Although it is a warm day, and the ambient temperature in your emergency department is warm, you cover Jerome lightly with a bath blanket so there is less risk of his becoming hypothermic.

Jerome is somewhat calmer now that the burned area is covered. Because he continues to cry and move around restlessly, however, you suggest to the emergency department physician that he may need medication for pain.

Question

A pediatric burn patient may become agitated for several reasons, which may include: (Choose all that apply.)

1. Pain
2. Head injury
3. Hypoxia
4. Ingestion

Answer

All of the choices are correct. When assessing a patient with any type of traumatic injury, all of these possibilities should be considered. The first concern is always the adequacy of oxygenation and ventilation. Head injury may also cause alteration in mental status, and ingestion should be considered—this could be by accidental ingestion in a toddler, or from experimentation by older pediatric patients. Because giving some types of pain medication may cause some respiratory depression and alteration in mental status, it is important to establish baselines for comparison, and assure adequacy of oxygenation and ventilation before administration.

You continue your assessment to determine whether there are any additional injuries, and you continue to assess the depth, extent, location, and severity of his burns. You note that on Jerome's right upper arm, his chest, and his right thigh, he has large patches of red, moist, erythematous areas. You also notice that blisters are starting to develop in several areas. There are also some areas of redness that look like sunburn surrounding the moist areas.

Question

How would you classify the type of burns you see on Jerome? (Circle all that apply.)

1. Superficial
2. Partial thickness
3. Full thickness

Answer

Based on current classifications of burn wounds, most of Jerome's burns are "partial-thickness" burns involving the epidermis and the dermal layer. He may also have some superficial burns. Until recently, burns were classified as first, second, third, and fourth degree. More current usage is to classify first-degree burns as "superficial," second-degree burns as "partial thickness," and to group third- and fourth-degree burns together as "full-thickness" burns. Burn wound classification is provided in Table 7.16.

It can be difficult to assess the burn correctly, however, in the emergency setting. "Full-thickness" burns extend all the way through the skin and dermal elements. One way to determine whether a burn is partial or full thickness is to press on the burned area with your finger in a sterile glove. If the capillaries refill after pressure is released, it is a partial-thickness burn. A full-thickness burn will not blanch and become pink again.

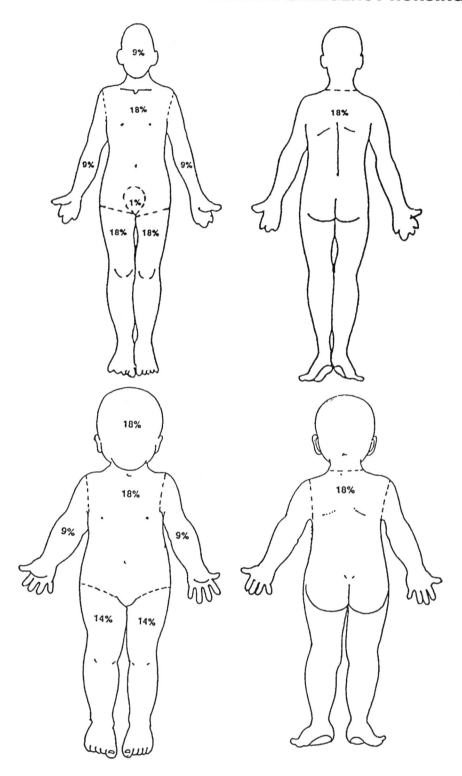

FIGURE 7.12   Rule of Nines.

TABLE 7.16. Classification of Burn Injuries[1]

Degree	Structures involved	Depth (inches)	Clinical appearance	Cause	Sensation
Superficial (first degree)	Epidermis	0.002	Red, dry, erythematous	Sunburn, scald	Normal, or sensitive to pain and temperature
Partial thickness (second degree)	Superficial dermis, deep dermis	0.02	Red, blisters, moist, erythematous; blanches with pressure	Scald, immersion, contact, grease, flash fire	Sensitive to pain and temperature
Full thickness (third degree)	Subcutaneous tissue and muscle	0.035–0.040	Dry, white, brown, black, or dark waxy yellow; skin surface cracked; avascular; if red, does not blanch with pressure	Prolonged immersion, flame, contact, grease, oil	Anesthetic to pain and temperature

You continue to assess Jerome's burns, documenting his burned areas with a line drawing in your notes. To document Jerome's condition correctly and to assist in decisions about admission, you will need to determine the approximate body surface area (BSA) of Jerome's burns. There are several methods you may use for this.

> *Note:* It is especially important to examine Jerome's scalp carefully. Scalp burns may be overlooked when a child's hair is very dense and tightly curled.

METHODS TO DETERMINE THE EXTENT OF BURN INJURY

Method 1: Rule of Nines

In the adult, the relative percentages of the distinct body surface areas are all divisible by nine (see Figure 7.12, previous page). In the child, the head accounts for a larger percentage of total BSA, and the legs account for a smaller percentage, so the Rule of Nines is not as precisely applicable. It is helpful to post a chart such as this one on the wall to aid in estimating the BSA of burns.

Method 2: Rule of the Palm

The Rule of the Palm (see Figure 7.13) is probably the easiest method to use when determining the size of a child's burn. As a general rule, the surface of the child's palm is approximately 1% of the total body surface area. By approximating the number of times the child's palm would fit into the burn area, you can estimate the percentage of BSA burned.

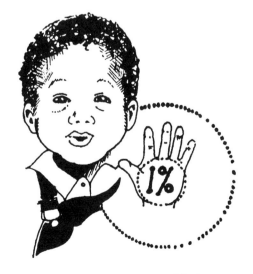

Figure 7.13 The Rule of Palm

> *Note:* When calculating the size of a burn, the areas of superficial partial-thickness (first-degree) burns are *not* included in the total.

Method 3: Lund and Browder Chart for Assessment of Burn Area

The Lund and Browder Chart (see Table 7.17) is also an accurate method for burn assessment and may be made into a fill-in sheet for use in the emergency department. The main disadvantage of this method is that although it tends to be more accurate, it may also be more time-consuming than the use of other assessment tools.

TABLE 7.17.   Lund and Browder Chart

AREA	0–1 year	1–4 years	5–9 years	10–15 years	Adult	Second degree (%)	Third degree (%)	Total (%)
Head	19	17	13	10	7			
Neck	2	2	2	2	2			
Anterior trunk	13	13	13	13	13			
Posterior trunk	13	13	13	13	13			
Right buttock	2.5	2.5	2.5	2.5	2.5			
Left buttock	2.5	2.5	2.5	2.5	2.5			
Genitalia	1	1	1	1	1			
Right upper arm	4	4	4	4	4			
Left upper arm	4	4	4	4	4			
Right lower arm	3	3	3	3	3			
Left lower arm	3	3	3	3	3			
Right hand	2.5	2.5	2.5	2.5	2.5			
Left hand	2.5	2.5	2.5	2.5	2.5			
Right thigh	5.5	6.5	8	8.5	9.5			
Left thigh	5.5	6.5	8	8.5	9.5			
Right leg	5	5	5.5	6	7			
Left leg	5	5	5.5	6	7			
Right foot	3.5	3.5	3.5	3.5	3.5			
Left foot	3.5	3.5	3.5	3.5	3.5			
Total								

Question

Using the Lund and Browder chart, determine the extent of Jerome's burn. What percent of body surface would you estimate is burned? (Fill in the blank.)

_____ %

Answer

About 20% of Jerome's BSA is burned. In a 2½-year-old, the right upper arm accounts for 4%, the chest (anterior trunk) 13%, the right thigh 6.5%, for a total percentage of 23.5%.[2] Note the decreasing percentage of the head and increasing percentage of the thigh as the child gets older—compare with the Rule of Nines diagrams.

You continue to try to keep Jerome calm and as comfortable as possible. The emergency physician orders morphine sulfate to help relieve Jerome's pain. Mr. Johnson stays at the head of the bed talking to him and stroking his head. You explain the importance to him of not touching his burn, because of his lack of protection from infection in the burned areas.

Mr. Johnson asks you what will happen next, and you explain that, depending on the assessment of the extent and severity of Jerome's burns (see Table 7.18), he will either be transferred or admitted to your hospital. He says he hopes Jerome will stay here because it is close to his home.

TABLE 7.18. Classification of Burn Severity

Minor	Moderate	Major
<10% BSA covered with superficial burns	10–20% BSA covered with partial-thickness burns <10% BSA covered with full-thickness	>20% BSA covered with partial-thickness burns >10% BSA covered with full-thickness burns Burns to hands, feet, face, or perineum[*] Electrical burns Inhalation injuries Burns complicated by other injury

* Sometimes burns to major joints and circumferential burns of the extremities are included in this category.

Question

Based on the depth and extent of Jerome's burns, you would determine that his burn is: (Choose one answer.)

1. Minor   2. Moderate   3. Severe

Answer

From your determination of the depth and the extent of the burn, you classify Jerome's burn as moderate.

An essential nursing diagnosis for Jerome at this point is alteration in skin integrity, related to his burn. There is always serious concern about infection with a burn, and your nursing interventions should include covering and protecting the exposed areas. Another nursing diagnosis for Jerome during this phase might be alteration in body fluid level. If Jerome showed signs of shock, fluid resuscitation would be necessary. There are several formulas available for fluid resuscitation for burn patients (see Table 7.19).

TABLE 7.19.   **Formulas for Fluid Resuscitation for Burn Patients**

Parkland formula
4 mL of Ringer's lactate per kilogram of body weight per percent of BSA burned given in the first 24 hr (4 mL × kg × %BSA).
<ul><li>½ the amount given in the first 8 hr;</li><li>¼ in the second 8 hr</li><li>¼ in the third 8 hr</li></ul>
Duke formula
3 mL of Ringer's lactate per kilogram of body weight per percent of BSA burned, *plus* one-half ampule of sodium bicarbonate per liter of replacement fluid given in the first 24 hr
<ul><li>½ the amount given in the first 8 hr</li><li>¼ in the second 8 hr</li><li>¼ in the third 8 hr</li></ul>

Note: When calculating the rate of administration over 24 hours, **the time of the burn injury** is the starting point, not the time of admission to the hospital. The child must receive one half the fluid requirement in the first 8 hours after the burn. If there is a delay in starting fluid resuscitation, the child must receive one half the fluid replacement *in the remaining time of the 8-hour period.*

Question

Jerome's weight is estimated to be 15 kg. Using the Parkland formula, what would be the appropriate amount of fluid for him to receive in his first 8 hours? (Choose one answer.)

1. 7,050 mL
2. 705 mL
3. 1,410 mL
4. 2,820 mL

Answer

The answer is (2). The calculation for the amount in 24 hours is 4 mL/kg/BSA burned, one half given in the first 8 hours.

4 mL × 15 (patient's weight in kg) × 23.5 (% BSA burned) = 1,410 mL

1410 × 1/2 = 705 mL

If Jerome required this type of fluid resuscitation, you would need to monitor his response to therapy closely. Your continuing assessment would include these parameters.

- Skin signs and capillary refill

- Level of consciousness
- Urine output (a urinary catheter should be inserted for any burn over 20% BSA)
- Blood pressure

You want to assess Jerome's urine output. The emergency physician has decided Jerome does not need a urinary catheter, so you carefully place a urine bag to determine Jerome's urinary output.

Question

What amount of urine output would indicate that you are keeping up with fluid loss in a pediatric burn patient? (Choose one answer.)

1. Urine output > 1 mL/kg/hr
2. Urine output > 5 mL/kg/hr
3. Urine output > 10 mL/kg/hr
4. Urine output > 30 mL/kg/hr

Answer

You would want to see at least 1 mL/kg/hr in a pediatric patient. Urine output can give you a good idea of whether you are keeping up with fluid loss from burns.[3] The trends in urine output are watched over several hours to make decisions about fluid infusion rates.

Jerome is stable at this point with a normal respiratory status and no signs of shock. You have just been informed that he will be transferred to the regional burn center because of the extent of his burn.

Question

Which of the following medications might be ordered before Jerome leaves your Emergency Department? (Choose all that apply.)

1. Application of topical lidocaine
2. Application of silver sulfadiazine
3. Intravenous antibiotic
4. Tetanus toxoid

Answer

The child should receive tetanus toxoid if there is no record of his immunization status. A child who is being transferred to a burn center should not have a topical agent applied to the burn, because it will only have to be removed on arrival at the burn center. Some emergency department physicians use a Xeroform dressing to protect the wound during transport,[3] but most burn centers prefer the wound to be cleaned to remove any debris and covered with sterile gauze or slightly moist sterile dressings. This will allow for immediate visualization of the wound on arrival at the burn unit.[4]

Silver sulfadiazine (Silvadene) should not be applied in this case, because it would have to be removed on arrival at the burn unit. It is the most commonly used topical antibacterial agent when a patient will be cared for at home. Application of this medication may be painful, especially with partial-thickness burns; keeping Silvadene refrigerated and spreading it on gauze before application may help to eliminate some of the pain.

The application of topical lidocaine is *not* recommended because it carries a significant risk of seizure— a toxic level may be rapidly reached by absorption through damaged skin. Antibiotics are not usually recommended prophylactically but may be used at the burn center if an infection develops.

Question

You notice several blisters on Jerome's burns. Should you break the blisters? (Choose Yes or No.)

_____ Yes   _____ No

Answer

It is best not to break blisters. When blisters are broken, the layer of dead skin promotes the growth of bacteria, leading to further tissue destruction.[1] All open blisters should be completely debrided.

As mentioned earlier, Jerome is to be transferred to a regional burn center for further care. Table 7.20 provides the American Burn Association criteria for admission to the hospital and admission to a burn center.[3]

TABLE 7.20.   Criteria for Admission to Hospital or Burn Center[3]

Criteria for admission	Consider admission to the hospital	Consider transfer to a burn center
Age	<5 or >60	<5 or >60
Airway	Present	Severe
Electrical injury	Present	Present
Significant associated injury or preexisting disease	Present	Present
Burns of face, hands, feet, or perineum	Present	Present
Suspected child abuse	Present	Present
Burned area (second and third degree)	> 15%	> 20%
Burned area (third degree only)	> 2%	> 10%

Question

From the history that you received, you know that Jerome has experienced a scald burn. In toddlers, a hot water scald is the most common type of burn. (Choose True or False.)

_____ True   _____ False

Answer

True. The most common type of burn among toddlers is the scald burn. Toddlers are naturally curious and can easily pull a pot of hot liquid onto themselves. A scald wound is often scalloped in shape, and has blisters and an uneven depth of injury. It looks as if the water has splashed and cascaded downward—as water runs downhill. The depth may vary from a superficial (first-degree) burn to a deep dermal full-thickness (second- or even third-degree) injury.

Note: If the pattern of the burn is inconsistent with the history given by the caretaker, the possibility of child maltreatment should be considered.

Mr. Johnson continues to stay with Jerome, comforting him. You assess his response to the pain medication; it has been effective—Jerome is less agitated, although he remains awake and is still breathing well. Mr. Johnson takes you aside and asks you quietly what will happen with Jerome's burns. "Will he have a lot of scarring? Will his skin grow back?"

Question

The answer you should give Mr. Johnson is: (Choose one answer.)

1. Usually the skin grows back normally from this type of burn.
2. It is difficult to tell, because you don't know the exact depth of the burn, and children respond differently to this type of injury.
3. Jerome will probably need extensive skin grafting, probably with skin from other parts of his body (autologous grafts), and may need a series of surgeries.

Answer

Each individual responds differently, so prediction is not advisable. Unfortunately, it is almost impossible to give Mr. Johnson, at this point, any idea of how well the burned area will heal. Some children develop keloids (more common in black patients), some pigmentation may be lost, and the depth of the burn cannot be precisely determined in the emergency setting. You can reassure Mr. Johnson that partial-thickness burns usually do not require skin grafting, and children tend to heal rapidly. You also mention that the burn fortunately is not on Jerome's face and will be covered most of the time by clothing even if there is some scarring.

You tell Mr. Johnson that Jerome will be transferred to a burn center to provide him with the best care available. He is very upset and says over and over again, "How could I let this happen? What could I have done to prevent this?"

You tell Mr. Johnson that you can see how painful it is for him to feel so responsible and that you are sure he did not intend to hurt Jerome. This seems a good moment to give him some information about scald burn prevention.

Question

List at least two ways to prevent scald burns in children. (Fill in the blanks.)

1. _____

2. _____

Answer

There are several measures that can be taken to prevent scald injuries. Kitchen scalds are very common in children. Recommendations to prevent these injuries include:

1. Keep the handles of pots on the stove turned so that children cannot reach them.
2. Keep cups of hot liquids away from children.
3. Do not warm baby's formula in the microwave. The liquid can become dangerously hot even though the container remains cool.[5]

Another consideration is the prevention of tap water scalds. It is recommended that antiscald devices be installed on hot water faucets and that hot water heaters be preset for 120°F.[6]

Jerome is transferred to the regional burn center by ambulance along with copies of all his emergency department records and laboratory tests. Mr. Johnson follows behind the ambulance in his car.

The burn center sends you a follow-up letter describing his recovery. Jerome apparently had no complications, did not require any skin grafts, and returned to his home 3 weeks later.

REFERENCES

Case Study 1

1. American Heart Association. (1988). *Pediatric advanced life support provider manual.* Dallas, TX. American Heart Association.
2. Seidel, J., & Henderson, D. (1987). *Prehospital care of pediatric emergencies.* Los Angeles: Los Angeles Pediatric Society.
3. Pang, D., & Wilberger, T. (1982). Spinal cord injury without radiographic abnormalities in children. *Journal of Neurosurgery, 57,* 114.
4. Moloney-Harmon, P. (1990). The pediatric trauma patient. In R. Welton & K. Shane (Eds.), *Case studies in trauma nursing.* Baltimore: Williams & Wilkins.
5. Foster, R. L. R., Hunsberger, M. M., & Anderson, J. J. T. (1989). *Family-centered nursing care of children.* Philadelphia: Saunders.
6. Hazinski, M. F. (1987). *Nursing care of the critically ill child.* St. Louis: Mosby.
7. King, D. (1985). Trauma in infancy and childhood. *Pediatric Clinic of North America, 32,* 1299.
8. Mancuso, L. (1989). Chest trauma. In C. Joy (Ed.), *Pediatric trauma nursing.* Rockville, MD: Aspen.
9. Peckham, L. & Kitchen, L. (1989). Abdominal and genitourinary trauma. In C. Joy (Ed.), *Pediatric trauma nursing.* Rockville, MD: Aspen.
10. Philichi, L. (1988). Supporting the parents when the child requires intensive care. *Focus on Critical Care, 15,* 34.

Case Study 2

1. Coren, C. V. (1987). Burn injuries in children. *Pediatric Annals, 16,* 328–339.
2. Emergency Nurses Association. (1986). *Trauma nursing core course (provider) manual,* (2nd ed.). Chicago: Award Printing Corporation.
3. D'Italia, J. G. (1989). Burns. In C. Joy (Ed.), *Pediatric trauma nursing* (pp. 154–172). Rockville, MD: Aspen.
4. Woolley, S., & Drueck, C. (1990). Burn injuries. In S. Kitt & J. Kaiser (Eds.), *Emergency nursing: A physiologic and clinical perspective* (pp. 755–781). Philadelphia: Saunders.
5. McLoughlin, E., & Crawford, J. D. (1985). Burns. *Pediatric Clinics of North America, 32,* 61–75.
6. McLoughlin, E., & McQuire, A. (1990). The causes, cost, and prevention of childhood burn injuries. *American Journal of Childhood Diseases, 144,* 677–683.

RAPID SEQUENCE INTUBATION

Rapid controlled anesthesia induction is used to relax muscles and render the child unconscious rapidly, increasing ease of intubation and lessening the child's stress.[6]	
Medications that may be used before intubation include	
To prevent fasciculation	*Pancuronium*, *vecuronium*, or *atracurium*: are nondepolarizing agents. Given in low dosages, they prevent fasciculation.
Adjunctive agents: to block vagal stimulation	*Atropine* is commonly used to prevent bradycardia and decrease secretions. *Lidocaine* lowers intracranial pressure and suppresses the cough reflex.
To paralyze muscles: to facilitate intubation	*Succinylcholine* is given for paralysis. It has many side effects that need to be considered.[6]
For sedation	*Fentanyl*, *lorazepam*, or other short-acting barbiturates or narcotics are usually given to treat pain and anxiety associated with intubation and paralyzation.
Performing rapid sequence intubation	
A team approach and proper equipment is necessary. There should be protocols for IV access, preoxygenation, cardiac monitoring, and use of pulse oximetry.[6] Nurses and physicians should be familiar with the drugs used, their contraindications, and side effects.	
Ventilation after intubation	
One of the common errors that occurs after intubation of a child is aggressive ventilation at a rapid rate in an effort to decrease the $PaCO_2$ rapidly. This may result in a tension pneumothorax because of increased lung and airway pressures.[7] The goal is to lower the CO_2 level and increase the PaO_2, but this must be done without overexpansion of the lungs. The best rule to follow is to ventilate with each breath only until the chest begins to rise. Careful attention should also be given to providing time for exhalation to occur. Oxygen powered ventilators ("elder valves") are not used on small children, because they are more difficult to control.	

Chapter Eight

Growth and Development: Psychosocial Aspects of Pediatric Emergency Nursing

Prerequisite Skills

- Knowledge of the basic stages of child development and their significance in the care of pediatric patients in the emergency setting
- Knowledge of the major developmental tasks of childhood and adolescence
- Ability to recognize the signs and symptoms of physical pain in adults
- Understanding of the effects of psychosocial intervention for pain in adults
- Understanding of basic family dynamics and processes
- Ability to appreciate and facilitate the grieving process in families who have suffered the sudden death of a family member

PREVIEW

Approximately one third of all patients cared for in emergency departments are under 18 years of age. The treatment these children receive ranges from primary health care to the treatment of life-threatening illnesses and injuries. Coming to the emergency department can be a frightening experience for these children and their families who are unaccustomed to this busy and (to them) scary place. The initial response of a child to a strange or painful situation is usually fear. In the emergency department these fears often include

1. Fear of pain
2. Fear of separation from parents
3. Fear of unknown people
4. Fear of the unfamiliar environment and equipment

Children frequently respond to their fears by trying to avoid, escape, or resist examination and treatment. If fear can be overcome, however, the next response will generally be curiosity. In a safe situation, children love to see new things, learn how equipment works, and explore the immediate surroundings.

Children coming to the emergency department are often accompanied by concerned, anxious family members. Because each family member reacts in his or her own way in coping with the crisis, nursing assessment should consider the needs of the family system as well as those of the child. Advance preparation may also be helpful; suggestions to prepare children and parents in advance of the emergency department visit are included at the end of this chapter.

When interacting with children of all ages, some guiding principles are:

- *Talk in a calm, low voice.* A soft voice repeating comforting or supporting phrases has a quieting effect. Avoid threatening children or talking to them harshly. When you model calm, controlled behavior, you help to minimize uncontrolled fear in the child and gain the trust of the parents.

- *Try to avoid surprises.* It helps children when you identify sensations they will feel during treatments: how the alcohol swab feels (cold), how medication smells (sweet), tastes (sour), or how equipment sounds (buzzing noise); and when you let them know what will happen next ("Now I'm going to listen to your heartbeat").

- *Never tell children that they are not experiencing pain.* Pain is an individual, subjective experience that can be totally unrelated to the amount of tissue damage. If a procedure is likely to hurt, say so. Unexpected pain will cause increased fear, loss of trust, and make further treatment more difficult.

- *Assume that children can understand*, even the very young ones. Be honest and open, and answer questions in an age-appropriate manner. Encourage children to ask questions and allow them to participate in the decision-making process when possible.

- *Provide reassurance, encouragement, and praise* ("You're really helping us by being so still," "Let's take some deep breaths together," or "This will be done when we finish counting to ten"). Children of all ages need to be helped through painful or frightening procedures and reassured afterward.

As an emergency nurse, you have an opportunity to make a difference in the child's and parent's perception of the emergency department experience. Through appropriate intervention, emergency department nurses have an opportunity to ensure the most positive physical and psychosocial outcomes possible.

This chapter will help to integrate developmental/behavioral theories with nursing care to provide you with the skills necessary to create a positive emergency department experience for the child, the family, and the staff. On completion of this chapter, the learner should be able to

- List the major developmental tasks of infants, toddlers, preschoolers, school-age children, and adolescents

- Recognize the way in which infants, children, and adolescents experience and manifest the following:

  - Pain

  - Body image and major fears

  - Relationships with significant others

- Determine nursing diagnoses based on a psychosocial assessment of the child and family

- Identify nursing interventions to assist infants, children, and adolescents in coping during the emergency department visit

- Identify interventions to assist the family in beginning their grieving process following the death of their child

THE INFANT IN THE EMERGENCY DEPARTMENT

Infancy is a time of rapid growth and psychosocial development. In the span of 12 months, infants triple their birthweight, increase in height by 50%, begin to walk, start using monosyllabic words, and become increasingly independent. Babies have different temperaments, activity levels, and feeding patterns. They must rely on their often very anxious parents to provide the nurse and physician with the history of their illness or injury.

CASE STUDY 1 OBJECTIVES

The purpose of this case study is to review the psychosocial aspects of care surrounding an infant who is brought to the emergency department by her concerned parents. Ways to help the infant cope and to assist the family are highlighted. At the end of this case study, the learner will be able to

- Identify one developmental task of infancy
- Recognize how infants experience body image, major fears, pain, and relationships with significant others
- Specify nursing interventions that will promote coping during emergency procedures
- Name one intervention to assist the family in parenting their infant in the emergency department

CASE STUDY 1

Amanda and Her Mother

Amanda Smith, a 9-month-old infant, has been seen by the emergency department physician and has been diagnosed as having possible bacteremia/sepsis. Amanda is feverish and fussy, but Mrs. Smith is able to comfort her with rocking and cuddling. Amanda will require further evaluation including a lumbar puncture, blood tests, and a bladder tap. As you are preparing the room for the sepsis workup, you observe Amanda and her parents. With tearful eyes, Mrs. Smith is holding Amanda.

Mrs. Smith is asked to wait outside the treatment room during the sepsis workup. She agrees somewhat reluctantly. As you reach for Amanda, she clings to her mother, hides her head in her mother's shoulder, and screams.

Question

Is Amanda's reaction (Choose one answer.)

1. Normal for her age?
2. Indicative of underlying psychological problems?

Answer

This reaction would be normal for her age. Amanda's reaction is typical of a 9-month-old infant. In the first 2 years of life, the infant relies on parents for comforting "explanations" for anything that is unexpected, confusing, or painful. Because Amanda is not critically ill, she forcibly clings to her mother and protests the separation. The infant who did not protest separation from the mother would be of more concern because this lack of protest might be an indication of serious illness or lack of appropriate attachment to caretakers (see Table 8.1, following page).

TABLE 8.1. Developmental Assessment of the Infant

The infant is learning to feel safe and to trust the environment.[1] This trust develops from the mother's appropriate and reliable response to the infant's needs.
The infant's body image is at a feeling level only (comfort/discomfort, hunger/satiation, etc.).[2] Somatosensory stimulation, such as touch, cuddling, and play, helps the infant develop a healthy body image.
The infant's immediate needs are for relief of hunger, relief of discomfort, sleep, and the need to suck. The infant has little tolerance when these needs are not met.
The infant is developing his or her senses, integrating environmental stimuli, and performing purposeful movement.[3]
The older infant shows signs of separation anxiety (clinging and protesting separation from the mother) as well as stranger anxiety (crying or being wary of strangers).

Question

Which behaviors would be normal or abnormal in infancy? (Choose either **N** for normal behavior or **A** for abnormal behavior.)

1. _____ Crying with painful stimuli

2. _____ Clinging to the mother

3. _____ Avoidance of eye contact

4. _____ Going willingly to a stranger

Answers

1. **N** It is normal for infants to respond rapidly and vigorously to painful stimuli by crying. Older children learn to control their responses to some degree.

2. **N** Stranger anxiety is common in late infancy, and parents represent safety, so the child will cling to the mother.

3. **A** Infants will usually meet your eyes, often even when they are afraid.

4. **A** As infants learn to separate from their parents, they become fearful of unfamiliar faces. After about 8 or 9 months of age children develop stranger anxiety and are rarely friendly to strangers until late toddlerhood.

Because of Amanda's behavior, you believe she is experiencing separation and stranger anxiety. You consider how to help Amanda cope in this situation.

Question

What interventions might help Amanda cope with the separation from her mother? (Fill in the blanks.)

1. _____

2. _____

3. _____

TABLE 8.2. Interventions to Promote Infant Coping

Intervention	Rationale
Keep parents in sight, if possible (parents must not be required to stay)	Decreases separation anxiety
Use warm hands, warm stethoscope, and keep room warm	Decreases stress and provides sensory comfort[4]
Provide sensory stimulation (rock/hold/cuddle) if possible[2]	Helps to promote comfort and decreases time of being restrained
Speak in a lighter tone of voice	Infants respond favorably to lighter, higher pitched voices[5]
Provide distractions if infant shows an interest in the environment	Maintaining interest in the environment may help to lessen noxious stimuli

Answer

Several measures can be initiated to help Amanda cope with her separation. Some of the possibilities are listed in Table 8.2 (see Figure 8.1).

You lay Amanda on the stretcher to begin the workup. Amanda cries and tries to cling to you as she is positioned for the lumbar puncture. The physician, as he is preparing for the procedure, asks, "Could you keep her more still?" You are concerned that her vigorous movements might cause injury during the lumbar puncture.

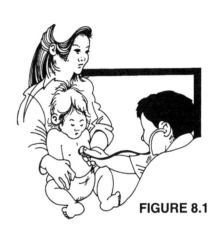

FIGURE 8.1

Question

Would sedation generally be recommended for a lumbar puncture? (Choose Yes or No.)

_____ Yes   _____ No

Answer

The correct answer is No. Sedation is not recommended in infants being evaluated for meningitis because there is concern that sedation might mask signs of neurologic deterioration. Amanda will probably cry and struggle throughout the sepsis workup; this is her way of coping with separation and pain. If you are unable to secure her adequately for the workup, ask for assistance from another nurse. Restrain her in a firm but unhurried manner while speaking quietly to her.

Question

What are two age-appropriate interventions that would help Amanda to cope and to minimize pain with this procedure? (Fill in the blanks.)

1. _____

2. _____

Answer

There are many interventions that may help. Infants respond mainly to sensory comfort, and older children develop many strategies themselves. Table 8.3 shows some interventions to help infants cope with painful procedures.

TABLE 8.3.   Interventions to Help Infants Cope With Pain[7]

Intervention	Rationale
• Hold infant securely	• Promotes body image/body boundaries
• Offer opportunities for self-comfort; for example, sucking provides comfort through oral stimulation	• The infant can "tune out" some noxious stimuli through sucking
• Allow infant to move as soon as possible after being restrained for a procedure	• Infants diffuse stress and frustration through motor activity[6]
• Touch, rock or cuddle infant	• Provides cutaneous stimulation; helps infant organize self
• Play a musical toy in the infant's field of vision	• Serves as a distraction technique

Note: Despite early assumptions that infants did not experience pain because of immaturity of the neurologic system, it is now generally accepted that they do experience pain to the same degree as adults, although localized pain may be experienced as "whole body" pain, and there is less modulation of the pain response.

Table 8.4 lists the behavioral responses of newborns and infants to pain.

TABLE 8.4.   Behavioral Responses of Newborns and Infants to Pain[7]:

Age	Nonverbal behavior	Verbal behavior	Child's description of pain
Newborn	Generalized body movements; withdrawal of extremity; irritability	Crying	None
Infant	Withdrawal of extremity; anticipatory fear (eyes widen, body tenses); irritability; regression (not making eye contact, etc.)	Crying	None

Note: Pain is also manifested by physiologic changes: increased heart and respiratory rates, pallor, diaphoresis, and dilated pupils.

The sepsis workup has been completed. When you enter, Mrs. Smith immediately takes Amanda from your arms, talking to her softly and cuddling her. You explain that it will take awhile for the results of the tests, and Mrs. Smith says to you, "Whatever happens, from now on, I'm going to be much more careful and keep a much closer watch on Amanda; at the first sniffle, I'll call the doctor."

Question

How would you respond to Mrs. Smith? (Choose one answer.)

1. "Watching Amanda more carefully may not really help—all children get sick quite often at this age."
2. "Sometimes parents feel responsible for their children's illnesses—are you feeling that you might have been responsible in some way for Amanda's?"
3. "That's a good idea—it's hard to tell when a child is really sick, and there is often a risk of something serious."

Answer

The correct answer is (2). The message Mrs. Smith seems to be giving is that she might have changed the course of Amanda's illness by earlier intervention. Allowing Mrs. Smith the opportunity to discuss her concerns may help in allaying guilt, and gives you an opportunity to provide appropriate education in recognition of serious illness and appropriate emergency department use. Answer (1) may promote a sense of helplessness, and answer (3) may set Amanda up for vulnerable child syndrome, where the child is overprotected by parents who believe something "bad" will happen to the child—it could make her overly cautious and overprotective of Amanda.

You can reassure Mrs. Smith by telling her that she was timely in seeking care. Providing anticipatory guidance (through pamphlets, demonstrations on how to use and read a thermometer, and fever reduction, injury prevention, etc.) will also help Mrs. Smith feel comfortable as a new parent.

Amanda and her mother wait in the holding area for the results of the sepsis workup. After a long wait, the emergency physician comes to tell them that it appears Amanda has a viral infection. He gives Mrs. Smith detailed discharge instructions, which he patiently explains. Mrs. Smith leaves, carrying a sleepy Amanda and looking very relieved.

THE CHILD IN THE EMERGENCY DEPARTMENT

TODDLERS, PRESCHOOLERS, AND ELEMENTARY SCHOOL-AGE CHILDREN

After infancy, children can be divided into three age groups: toddlers, preschoolers, and elementary school age. Each age group has unique fears, experiences of pain and relationships with their families.

Toddlers (Case Study 2) are probably the most difficult children to examine and treat; they are also the most likely to experience short- or long-term emotional effects from trauma because they remember incidents and their memories are often confused or disoriented.

Preschoolers (Case Study 3) often appear to have a better comprehension of the situation, but may misunderstand common words and frequently distort explanations.

Elementary school-age children (Case Study 4) can comprehend simple situations and requests, and will generally cooperate with examinations or procedures.

The following three minicases are presented to compare and contrast the developmental tasks and psychosocial issues among these three age groups.

CASE STUDIES 2, 3, AND 4 OBJECTIVES

On completion of these case studies, the learner will be able to

- List one developmental task of a child in each of the following age groups: toddlers, preschool, and school-age children
- Compare and contrast the fears and experience of pain for each age group: toddlers, preschool, and school-age children
- Describe nursing interventions that facilitate coping in these age groups
- Recognize and appreciate anxiety experienced by family members with an injured child
- Help family members to cope with their anxiety about the consequences and treatment of their child's injuries

CASE STUDY 2: THE TODDLER IN THE EMERGENCY DEPARTMENT

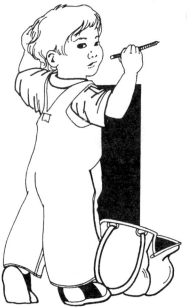

FIGURE 8.2

Colin Put Something Up His Nose

Mrs. Thompson brings her 2-year-old son, Colin, to the emergency department. Colin is active and playful, and does not seem to be in any distress at the moment. He has managed to take a pencil out of his mother's purse and is playing with it. Mrs. Thompson is attentive to him, but seems a bit exasperated. She gently takes away the pencil (see Figure 8.2 Colin and the pencil.), handing him one of his toys, and then tells you, "I think he put something up his nose."

Question

Judging from your brief observation of Colin and his mother, and your knowledge about developmental stages, do you think Mrs. Thompson's assumption is likely to be correct? (Choose one answer.)

____ Yes   ____ No

Answer

Yes. The mother's assumption is likely to be correct. Toddlers are developing autonomy[1] and are learning to explore their world. They experiment with all new objects of interest by banging, tasting, and feeling them, as well as seeing what they will do and where they will go. Toddlers also like to explore their body orifices and may attempt to fit small objects into them. Colin certainly seems to be an active, curious child.

As you attempt to perform your assessment, Colin clings to his mother, cries, and resists your efforts to do a thorough examination.

Question

Is Colin's behavior appropriate for his age? (Choose Yes or No.)

____ Yes   ____ No

Answer

Yes. Colin's behavior is very common at this age. In unfamiliar circumstances, toddlers may be frightened of being separated from familiar people, places, or things. To help them feel secure, they often use "transitional objects" such as a small blanket or toy that they carry with them. Although they are developing a small vocabulary, toddlers are generally able to comprehend only very simple explanations and requests.[2] They are still very egocentric, seeing things only from their unique viewpoint.

A brief examination by the physician reveals unilateral purulent discharge and a glistening mass in Colin's right nostril. On further examination it appears that a foreign body is lodged in the posterior naris, and the decision is made to remove it. Mrs. Thompson is sitting quietly, comforting Colin as they wait. While you prepare equipment, Mrs. Thompson asks whether she will be allowed to stay with Colin during the procedure.

Question

If your emergency department policy allows parents to stay with their children during procedures, should you let Mrs. Thompson stay with Colin? (Choose Yes or No.)

____ Yes   ____ No

Answer

Yes. It would probably work out well for Mrs. Thompson to stay with Colin. It is usually better at this age to avoid separating the child and parent, and it is often helpful for parents to stay in the treatment room during minor procedures (see Table 8.5). Observation of the parent–child interaction may help to decide whether to encourage or discourage a parent from being present. If the parent wishes to stay and is calm and soothing with the child, there is little likelihood of problems. If the parent seems to be in emotional distress, is not able to be reassuring to the child, or asks to leave, the parent should be allowed to do so without censure.

Note: The parent should not be asked to restrain the child or participate in any way other than to comfort the child. Toddlers expect parents to protect them and thus may perceive participation as betrayal. Children may exhibit more distress (crying, fussing, aggressive behaviors) with the parent present, because they feel safe enough to express their emotions. Parental absence would not necessarily reduce children's anxieties and fears. If the parent is threatening or scolding the child, you should explain that the child's behavior is normal and model appropriate comforting measures.

The foreign body will have to be removed from Colin's nose. Pain relief and restraint may be necessary during the removal process.

TABLE 8.5. Helping Children Through Procedures

Method	Appropriate for	Used for
Papoose board	Small children	Short procedures
Topical anesthetic Tetracaine, Adrenaline, Cocaine (TAC), lidocaine	All ages	Small lacerations, foreign body removal from extremities
Analgesia, sedation	All ages	Fracture reduction, crush injuries, burns, large lacerations

The ideal in the emergency department setting is to provide relief from pain (analgesia) and relief from anxiety (sedation) for short periods while examination and treatment occur. Some procedures are very short and may best be performed without sedation or analgesia, but careful assessment should be made of the need for relief before beginning the procedure. You should always consider that any procedure that would cause pain in an adult will cause an equal amount of pain in a child.

The papoose board should be reserved for situations when the child is too large or frantic to be held effectively by emergency department staff. For those children with painful injuries, such as fractures, burns, or crush injuries of a single extremity, adequate medication for pain control with a combination such as morphine sulfate for analgesia and midazolam for sedation is not only humane but may be necessary to gain cooperation for adequate examination and treatment. This medication should be followed by close monitoring of the child's vital signs. Such analgesia is *not* indicated in the child with multiple trauma or a combative child with a head injury. When used, adequate staff and equipment for respiratory support must be available.

Even in children too young to cooperate, all procedures and the use of restraints should be appropriately explained to the parents and the child before beginning. Ask parents if they are willing to participate and make certain that they understand what is expected of them during the procedure. Throughout the procedure, you should continue to monitor the parents' coping skills and assess the parents' reactions. Even with adequate analgesia, children may continue to cry and be combative. It is important that both the child and the parent are told that this is age-appropriate behavior.

As the procedure begins, Colin starts to scream, kick, and bite. Two nurses and the physician try to assist with restraint, but he is frantic.

Question

Which of the following would help Colin and assure successful completion of the procedure? (Circle any that apply.)

1. Stop the procedure briefly and plan a coordinated approach.
2. Encourage Mrs. Thompson to reassure Colin.
3. Ask the physician to order a sedative medication.
4. Ask Colin's mother to help you hold him down.
5. Ask the mother to leave the room.

Answer

The correct answers are (1), (2), and (3). It might be helpful to stop briefly and plan a coordinated approach. Allow time for Colin to calm down and then gently restrain him, using a "mummy" wrap (see Figure 8.3). The most effective person to help Colin cope will be a calm, soothing mother, but you can also help by remaining calm, and restraining him as gently as possible and only as long as necessary. Analge-

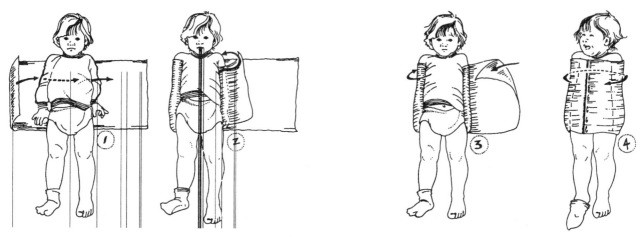

FIGURE 8.3 Using a mummy wrap.

sia, cautiously administered, and a period to gain control, may be necessary. Encourage the mother to offer continuous reassurance. Answers (4) and (5) are incorrect because (a) it is not advisable for parents to assist with restraint because the child may see this as betrayal, and (b) separating the parent from the child will not help him to cope and will only increase his anxiety. Other interventions are listed in Table 8.6.

TABLE 8.6.   Interventions for Helping Children During Painful Procedures

Interventions	Rationale
Let parents remain with child	Relieves fear of separation from parents
Allow child to hold object or keep it in sight	Need security object (transitional object)
Keep explanations simple, use nonthreatening language	Have limited cognitive and comprehension skills
Firm but gentle restraining means	Attempt to escape by kicking, biting
Reassure family and gain their trust; talk calmly, quietly, and confidently	Child becomes upset if parents are upset—emotional contagion theory[3,4]
Examine/treat child in upright position whenever possible	Child feels vulnerable and out of control lying down

Within 10 minutes, the physician has successfully removed the foreign body, a bead. A sweaty, tired Colin is removed from the mummy wrap and handed to his mother. You tell Colin that you know how hard he tried to stay still and give him a sticker to wear on his shirt. Anticipatory guidance for Mrs. Thompson should include explaining to her that toddlers may regress after a visit to the emergency department; his behavior could include clinging to her, whining, wanting the bottle, and so on.[6] You reassure her that if she remains calm and supportive, these behaviors will disappear in a short while.

CASE STUDY 3: THE PRESCHOOLER IN THE EMERGENCY DEPARTMENT

Malia Needs the Best Doctor Available!

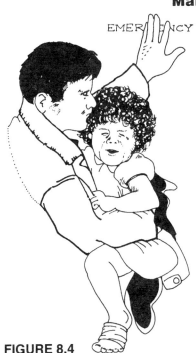

FIGURE 8.4

Four-year-old Malia Alano is carried into the emergency department by her distraught father after she cut her foot on a piece of glass (see Figure 8.4). Her father demands "the best doctor available" to care for his daughter and refuses to let you assess the injury. The father wrapped the laceration at home, and there is no visible active bleeding on the rag wrapped around her foot. Malia is screaming and crying hysterically.

> **Question**
>
> What should you do? (Choose one answer.)
>
> 1. Unwrap the foot carefully, and measure the length of the laceration.
> 2. Ask Mr. Alano to leave Malia with you while he registers her—then you can assess the injury when he's not present.
> 3. Begin by making a "noninvasive" assessment and develop rapport with the father and child.
> 4. Show the father to the waiting area and suggest to him that he return when Malia is calmer.

Answer

It would be best to begin with a "noninvasive" assessment, and develop rapport with the father and child. Beginning with the least-disturbing approach is always a good rule, so making a "noninvasive" assessment and developing rapport with father and child is the most reasonable action to take. Insisting on examining the foot could initiate a vicious cycle of escalating emotions in which the child and parent push each other to higher and higher levels of distress, anger, and anxiety. Asking Mr. Alano to leave Malia to go to the registration area, or remain in the waiting area separates parent and child, which could cause increased anxiety and fear in both the parent and the child. It is usually best to keep parent and child together. Ways to develop a rapport with the father are outlined in Table 8.7.

TABLE 8.7. Developing Rapport with Distraught Parents

Praise the parent for doing a good job of caring for the child and offer reassurance when appropriate.
Empathize with the caretaker. Giving family members an opportunity to talk and explain the problem helps them to feel that the treatment process has started.
Tell parents that you will check back periodically while they are in the waiting room. If this is not possible, tell the parent who to inform if there are changes in the child's condition. This communicates your concern and assures the parent that if something should go wrong, someone is readily available.

Malia is called into the treatment room 1 hour later to be examined by the physician. Mr. Alano is very angry and complains loudly to the physician about the long wait. He says angrily, "My daughter has a bad injury. Other people who came after us were seen first, and they didn't look sick at all."

Question

How should you respond to the father? (Choose one.)

1. Acknowledge his frustration and assure him that his daughter is being treated now.
2. Tell him that if he does not want to wait, he is free to take his daughter elsewhere for treatment.
3. Explain to him that his daughter's injury is not severe and that he had to wait because there were others in the emergency department with serious illnesses.
4. Ask him what it is that he is so angry about and try to determine what is at the root of his anger.

Answer

In a crisis situation, it is usually most helpful to begin by acknowledging the other person's feelings (1); it would help to defuse this father's anger if he felt you were really listening to what he is saying. Answer (2) would not be advisable because it is not in Malia's best interests. Giving your assessment of severity (3) would also not be advisable because the father's perception is that his daughter's injury is very serious; your implication that the injury is not severe will probably not be convincing to him at this point. Answer (4) would not be helpful at this point because he has already explained his concerns; exploring other possible causes for his anger would not be helpful until after his feelings have been acknowledged.

When the physician begins to take the dressing off to examine Malia's foot, she screams, "Don't take it off! My blood will come out!"

Question

Malia is reacting this way because she believes that her skin holds her body together. (Choose True or False.)

____ True   ____ False

Answer

True. Malia is at the stage where she is concerned about body integrity. Preschoolers have an incomplete and distorted understanding of how the body works (see Figures 8.5 and 8.6). They are interested in body surfaces and believe that the skin holds the blood and organs inside the body.[1] Therefore, a cut in the skin might let the blood escape. Often the preschooler will stop crying as soon as the injury is covered so that blood is no longer visible. Remember the "miracle cure" of an adhesive bandage in this age child!

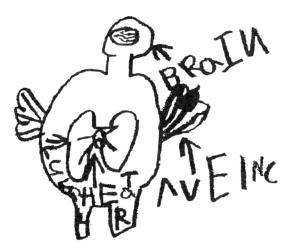

FIGURE 8.5 (above) Five-and-one-half-year-old Chad Thomas's drawing of the inside of his body, showing the brain, heart, heart, lungs, and veins.

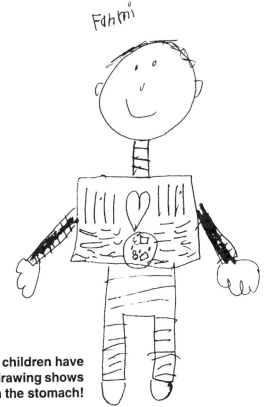

FIGURE 8.6 (at right) By first or second grade, school-aged children have a more sophisticated perception of their bodies. This child's drawing shows the heart, lungs, and chicken, broccoli, rice, and ice cream in the stomach!

The physician examines Malia and explains to Mr. Alano that Malia will need stitches. The father is told that it will be necessary to restrain Malia during the cleaning and suturing of the laceration. Mr. Alano objects to having Malia restrained. "Can't you just put her to sleep so it won't hurt?" he asks.

Question

You respond to Mr. Alano's request by: (Choose one.)

1. Suggesting that the physician order medication to sedate Malia.
2. Explaining the purpose of physical restraint.
3. Requesting that Mr. Alano leave the room.
4. Allowing Malia to sit on her father's lap during the cleaning and suturing.

Answer

It may be helpful to calmly explain to Mr. Alano that restraint is necessary to ensure that Malia does not move and further injure herself during the suturing procedure. Restraint will allow the procedure to be completed rapidly and with the least possible trauma. Reassure the father that he may remain with Malia and help explain to her what is going to happen so that she will not be afraid.

Sitting on her father's lap is appropriate for an examination but not for a procedure that tends to be messy and requires dexterity and skill, so answer (4) would be inappropriate. Malia does not need to be sedated at this time, because the procedure has not started yet and you would like to try other means of helping her first.

Because the laceration is very small, the emergency physician decides to infiltrate with lidocaine, rather than using TAC, a solution used in many emergency settings. (Information on the use of TAC is provided in Table 8.8.)

TABLE 8.8. General Procedure for Using TAC

TAC, a solution containing tetracaine, adrenaline, and cocaine, is used as a topical anesthetic for small lacerations in many emergency settings.
The general procedure is for the solution to be placed on a cotton ball or gauze, which is held tightly on the wound with a gloved hand for 15 min. Parents can assist with TAC application, holding the child to provide a calming effect while preparations are made for suturing. If parents will be assisting, make sure they know what will be expected of them during the procedure.
Caution! TAC must never be used on • _**Fingers, toes, ears, nose, or penis**_ (because of the risk of impaired circulation from vasoconstriction) • _**Mucous membranes**_ (because of rapid absorption)

Question

How do you explain the procedure to Malia?

1. Explain simply, one step at a time as you proceed.
2. Explain the procedure in detail, summarizing the entire process at once.
3. Warn her well in advance that the procedure might hurt.
4. Tell her that if she holds still and doesn't cry, it won't hurt.

Answer

The correct answer is explain simply, one step at a time. It is usually not helpful at this age to describe the entire process at once, nor is it helpful to give any warnings well in advance. Preschoolers are verbal but may be unwilling to talk. They frequently misinterpret common words and distort explanations, and may develop frightening fantasies at this age (see Table 8.9).[2] Answer (4) sets Malia up for failure if she does cry. Unexpected pain may cause increased fear and loss of trust, making further treatment more difficult.

TABLE 8.9. Helpful Communication Techniques to Use With Young Children

Words to use	Words to avoid
Measure or check	Take (as "your blood")
Bacteria, virus	Bugs, germs (implies small insects crawling around)
"The doctor will make you better"	Cut, incision (implies pain, mutilation)
". . . will spray cold feeling medicine on your arm"	Deaden, deadening (instills fear of making something dead)
". . . (cast) will enable you to (run) again"	Fix (implies it's broken and may be thrown away)
Correct anatomic names	Organs (organ music)
Special medicine to help you	Put to sleep (instills fear of dying)
Injection	Shot (being shot with a gun)
Intravenous	IV (ivy or plant)
Reprinted with permission from Irma D'Antonio, RN, PhD.	

Do

- Explain each step of the procedure as it is being done
- Use nonthreatening words
- Talk with Malia beforehand about some of the sensations she will be experiencing

Don't

- Explain procedures more than a few moments beforehand
- Cover a young child's face entirely with sterile drapes during a procedure
- Give Malia the impression that she was "bad" because she cried or struggled.

Malia's father impatiently agrees to the restraint. Malia is restrained on the papoose board, her father sitting next to her. He is obviously upset but he manages to be helpful to Malia, encouraging her. Malia's foot is exposed and cleaned for the procedure.

Question

How can you help Malia cope with the suturing? (Circle any that apply.)

1. Remind her this would not have happened if she had kept her shoes on, and that she should keep her shoes on when she goes outside.
2. Distract her by saying, "Do you have any pets? Tell me about them."
3. Tell her you know she can be very brave and grown-up and not to cry.
4. Talk with her about what she is feeling at each step of the procedure.
5. Tell her that she should try not to fuss because her father is worried about her and will be upset if she cries.

Answer

Both interventions (2) and (4) would help her to focus on something other than her fear and pain. Telling her to be brave may cause her to lose self-esteem if she cries and telling her that her father will be upset may only heighten guilt and anxiety. Injury prevention education is inappropriate at this point.

A variety of techniques for coping with pain can be very effective in calming preschool children during procedures (see Table 8.10).

TABLE 8.10.   Coping Techniques for Preschoolers

Technique	Rationale
Use distraction (story telling, talking, questions about preschool)	A preschooler's attention span and imagination makes him responsive to distracion.
Allow parents to sit near the child to provide comfort	Preschoolers fear separation in a stressful or strange setting; they are more trusting if parents are present
Always tell the child what you are going to do	Builds trust
If something will hurt, tell them in advance	Allows them to relax if they know you will not cause them pain without warning
Give the child something to do during the procedure (blow on party blower, count, tell a story, hold a bandage, pick a word to say repeatedly when they feel upset, practice taking deep breaths)	Builds initiative; provides relaxation; promotes participation and sense of control ("I helped")
Tell the child that you will help him to hold still	Accepting help is a means of coping[3]; helps child gain and maintain control
Reinforce positive coping behaviors	Promotes emotional growth and independence[3]

The procedure is started. During the wound cleaning, you explain everything the physician is doing in simple terms. ("The doctor is going to clean your foot; the soap will feel cool. Now he is going to put the medicine in. You will feel a pinch as he does it.")

Malia is screaming and crying during the cleaning. You are keeping an eye on Malia's father, and he is becoming more and more distressed. He angrily bursts out, "There must be a better way to do this. We're going to a different hospital." He makes a move to release the papoose board.

Question

What is your nursing diagnosis of Mr. Alano's behavior? (Fill in the blank.)

_____

Answer

Mr. Alano appears to be experiencing ineffective individual coping. This nursing diagnosis is defined by an impairment of adaptive behaviors and problem-solving abilities when meeting life's demands and roles.[4] The ineffective coping is related to the situational crisis of Malia's injury and treatment.

Question

What might help Mr. Alano cope in this situation? (Fill in the blanks.)

1. _____

2. _____

Answer

Any of the following would be correct:

1. Reassure Mr. Alano by talking to him and explaining what you are doing and why
2. Explain to him that the procedure will be over shortly and ask for his help in keeping Malia calm
3. Acknowledge his feelings and assure him that he is contributing to making Malia better
4. Avoid separating him from Malia, if at all possible, unless he is making the situation worse

The cause of parents' anger is usually anxiety. Parents may become anxious during procedures because they

- Are concerned that the child may be in pain
- May have had past negative experiences with pain or a similar procedure
- May experience guilt over submitting their child to the procedure—parents are supposed to protect their children, not allow them to be hurt
- May have inadequate knowledge and additional concerns about the procedure
- May have other stressors (other children at home, concerns about health care costs, absence from work, etc.)

To help Mr. Alano with coping, you listen to him and acknowledge his frustration nonjudgmentally. As he calms down and talks with you, you determine that he is very concerned about Malia's pain, and you talk to him about what would be most helpful for Malia right now. You show him that he can have Malia squeeze his hand tightly to help with the pain. Your intervention is effective, and the physician can continue with the suturing. There are now five stitches in Malia's foot, and she is released from the papoose board. She is being held by her father, and is showing some interest and curiosity. The physician asks Malia if she wants to see her stitches. Malia says yes, but Mr. Alano is concerned that she may become upset again if she looks at them.

Question

Whose request should you honor? (Choose one answer.)

1. Malia's
2. Mr. Alano's
3. Both
4. Neither

Answer

You can probably honor both requests. Tell Mr. Alano that you can understand concern but explain to him that once a child is not in pain or afraid that the child is naturally curious. Tell him that if Malia did not want to look at the stitches, she would not have asked to see them. Remind him that preschoolers often imagine things to be worse than what they really are and have great concerns about their body integrity. If Malia did not want to see her stitches, she should not be forced to do so, and her request should be honored.

Malia looks at her new stitches, and proudly shows them to her father. You praise Malia for being so brave and reward her with stickers and a popsicle. Mr. Alano thanks the staff for their patience.

CASE STUDY 4: THE SCHOOL-AGE CHILD IN THE EMERGENCY DEPARTMENT

Ricky is Trying not to Move

Ricky Schafer, a 10-year-old African-American male child, is brought by paramedics to the emergency department with severe pain, fever, and a 3-day history of vomiting. Ricky has a history of sickle cell disease. He was in the care of a teenage baby sitter while his mother was at work. The physician diagnoses Ricky in sickle cell crisis, and she asks you to start an IV line for pain medication and hydration. You have spoken with the mother over the telephone, and she has given her consent for treatment. She will not be able to leave work for a few hours, but she will call the emergency department later to see how Ricky is doing.

You observe Ricky; he is lying very still, making every effort not to move. He closes his eyes when you ask him questions. His vital signs are within normal limits, except for a slightly elevated heart rate.

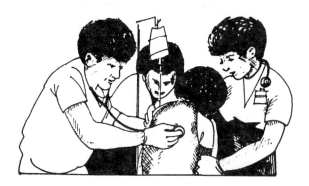

FIGURE 8.7 Ricky and the emergency department staff.

Question

What would be the most appropriate nursing diagnosis at this point? (Fill in the blank.)

_____

Answer

Acute pain related to his sickle cell disease.[1] School-age children are generally reliable in reporting severity and localization of pain. Some children, however, may not tell you they have pain in an attempt to remain in control; they may also fear being given an injection. Observation of movement—guarding against pain, grimacing, and crying or calling out when moved in a certain manner are all indicators of pain. A developmental overview of toddlers', preschool-age, and school-age children's responses to pain is outlined in Table 8.11 (facing page).

Question

Assessment tools to measure pain are not reliable and valid for use with small children. (Choose True or False.)

_____ True   _____ False

TABLE 8.11. Developmental Overview of Children's Responses to Pain[2]

Age	Nonverbal behavior	Verbal behavior	Child's description of pain
Toddler	Withdrawal of extremity; non-specific aggression (hitting, biting, kicking); use of entire body to resist; regression	Crying, screaming	Identifies location: "arm hurts," "leg ouches"; points to abdomen, touches ear
Preschool	Goal-directed aggression; active physical resistance (pushes nurse away, hides); regression	Attempts to postpone; pretends to be another person; uses aggressive statements ("I hate you"; "Go away")	Identifies location and intensity ("My leg ouches a lot!")
School age	Passive resistance (rigid body, clenched teeth or fists); regression	Denial of pain	Identifies location and intensity in more detail; progresses from physical to inclusion of psychological aspects

Answer

False. Pain assessment tools are useful for measuring pain in children as young as 3 to 4 years of age.[3] Some use pictures for children to select; some others use a variety of other techniques to assess pain.[4] To be useful in the emergency setting, the tool must be portable, easy to use, and universally understandable. The Hester Poker Chip Tool has been used for this purpose in the emergency department (see Table 8.12 and Figure 8.8, The Hester Poker Chip Tool). It consists of four red poker chips, which are shown to the child (4 years old or older).

When you explain the Hester Poker Chip Tool to Ricky, he quickly picks all four red poker chips. This further confirms your nursing diagnosis that Ricky is experiencing acute pain, and you reassure Ricky that you will speak with the doctor right away.

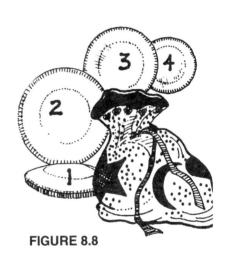

FIGURE 8.8

TABLE 8.12. Hester Poker Chip Tool Procedure

Procedure
Four red poker chips are used to represent "pieces of hurt" (the word "hurt" is used because small children often do not know the word "pain"). The explanations given to the parents and child are as follows:

Tell the parent
"The Poker Chip Tool is a method that uses four red poker chips to measure pain."

Tell the child
"These are pieces of hurt: one is a little bit of hurt, and four are the most hurt you could have. How many pieces of hurt do you have?"

Chart
The number of chips the child chooses is recorded as the amount of hurt.

You discuss your assessment of Ricky's pain with the emergency physician, and she gives you an order for a narcotic analgesic, and you give Ricky his pain medication. Fifteen minutes after the intravenous pain medication is given, you evaluate its effectiveness. Ricky's respirations are 16 and unlabored, his pulse rate is 110 beats/min, and he appears more relaxed, as if he is sleeping.

Question

How can you tell if the pain medication was effective? (Circle all appropriate answers.)

1. Observe for pain behavior.
2. Draw a blood sample to check for therapeutic dosage of pain medication.
3. Ask Ricky if he is in less pain or if he is more comfortable.
4. Readminister the pain scale.

Answer

The correct answers are (1), (3), and (4). Observation, discussion with the child, and readministering a pain tool would all be valid means for assessment. At this age, children can generally tell you if the pain is decreasing and are able to use a rating scale. Observe Ricky for flinching from touch or avoiding movement. Are these behaviors more, less, or about the same as before the pain medication? Do these behaviors get worse or better when Ricky is alone or when he is interacting with others? School-age children are aware of secondary gains with pain; this may be increased in the chronically ill child. In some cases, it may be necessary to separate out the effect of attention or sympathy to assess the pain accurately.

As you reassess Ricky, you notice that he has a slight tachycardia. The tachycardia may be indicative of unresolved pain, but will have to be differentiated from dehydration (3-day history of vomiting), or anemia secondary to a more serious form of sickle cell crisis. His sleeping is not necessarily an indication of the absence of pain but may indicate a tolerable level of discomfort that is not interfering with rest—children may regress into sleep if pain is not alleviated.

Ricky is awake and tells you he is still experiencing pain. It is too soon for another dose of pain medication.

Question

List two techniques to help Ricky cope with pain. (Fill in the blanks.)

1. _____

2. _____

Answer

School-age children have developed several techniques of coping with their pain already. You can help them by encouraging them to use their own techniques and by teaching them additional methods (see Table 8.13).

TABLE 8.13. Interventions for Pain Control for School-Age Children

Technique	Rationale
Prepare by providing sensory and procedure information	Allows child to prepare for procedure
Relaxation exercises (focused breathing, blow out like a kiss, etc.)	Decreases muscle tension
Guided imagery	Distraction
Soft touch/soft talk	Distraction/decreases muscle tension
Progressive relaxation (contract/relax different muscles)	Decreases muscle tension
Hypnosis	Alters perception of pain
Music/videos	Distraction
Storytelling ("Once upon a time . . .")	Distraction
Positive self-talk ("I can make it")	Promotes mastery

Ricky has been in the emergency department for hydration for several hours. The decision is made to admit him to the hospital.

Question

List two major concerns of school-age children regarding admission to the hospital. (Fill in the blanks.)

1. _____

2. _____

Answer

Selected concerns of school-age children are listed in Table 8.14.

TABLE 8.14. Concerns of School-Age Children About Hospitalization

Issue	Intervention	Rationale
Death	Reassurance/comfort	Relieves anxiety
Pain	Explain procedures; always warn if something will hurt	Builds trust, allows child to relax
Fear of unknown setting	Tell what to expect; allow child to use own clothes and toys; introduce child to new nurses	Reduces strangeness of hospital
Separation from parents	Allow parent to stay with child	Reduces fear of unknown and allows someone the child trusts to be present
Loss of control	If possible, encourage child to participate in his care[5]	Conveys a sense of control and decreased dependence[5]

Tips Regarding School-Age Children

1. Following the rules, going to school, and interacting with peers are important; these activities give them a sense of industry.[6] School-age children believe "I am what I learn and do."

2. The concerns of a chronically ill child who has experienced previous emergency department visits and hospitalizations will differ from a child being hospitalized for the first time. For the chronically ill child, visits to the emergency department and hospitalizations are "a way of life," and are normal for them. They cope with intrusive procedures and changes in routines differently from acutely ill children. Chronically ill children anticipate what will happen to them more so than acutely ill children (see Figure 8.9).

   A child's self-esteem is often threatened when he or she has a chronic condition because of the inability to be like his peers and participate in all activities.

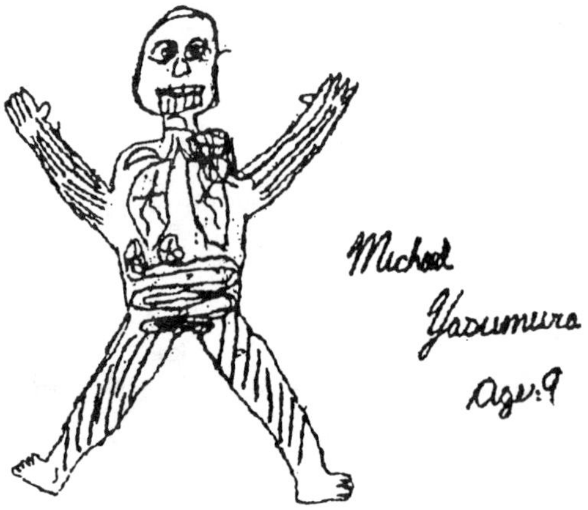

3. Remember, whenever you are interacting with a school-age child

   - Talk directly to the child.

   - When talking to the parents, include the child.

   - Explain all procedures and tell the child what to expect. Refer to benefits of procedure or the positive outcome that follows.[7]

   - Ask the child if he or she has any questions.

   - Make sure the child has understood what you have said (ask him or her to repeat what you said). Use positive phrasing when making comments ("You can" instead of "don't").

   - Treat all questions, fears, and concerns seriously.

FIGURE 8.9   Drawing of a body by nine-year-old Michael shows veins, lungs, and intestines

Ricky is admitted to the hospital. His mother has not yet arrived, but Ricky did speak with her over the telephone. You escort him to his room and introduce him to "his" nurse. You give a report to the receiving nurse about the IV fluids and pain medication Ricky received in the emergency department. You also discuss with him which methods of pain control were effective and encourage Ricky to tell his mother about the fears he had discussed with the emergency department staff.

CASE STUDY 5: THE ADOLESCENT IN THE EMERGENCY DEPARTMENT

PREVIEW

Adolescents are dealing with issues of independence, privacy, and changes in their physical appearance[1] to develop identity.[2] The concerns of this age group are uncertainty about whether or not their bodies, thoughts, and feelings are "normal."[3] They are fearful of death when ill or injured but generally have feelings of being invincible in normal circumstances. Although adolescents understand what is occurring, they are prone either to underplay major injuries or "catastrophize" minor injuries. This is the age of "all or nothing," "black or white," and "here and now" reactions. Teenagers generally do not think in terms of the future or "shades of gray." Patients from this age group are often modest and may resist treatment or examination if modesty issues are violated. They separate easily from parents and may actually provide a more accurate history when parents are not present. There is often active conflict, rebellion, and "breaking away" in the parent–child relationship.

CASE STUDY 5 OBJECTIVES

- List one developmental issue of adolescence
- Explain the concerns that adolescents have with body image
- Describe how adolescents perceive pain
- State one intervention to support the adolescent who requires surgery

CASE STUDY 5

Glen Is in Pain and Wants a *Male* Doctor

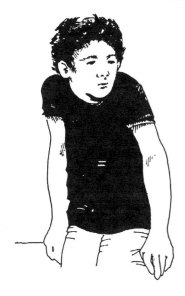

FIGURE 8.10

Glen Miyashiro, a 15-year-old male of Japanese descent, is brought to the emergency department by his father with a complaint of intense scrotal pain (see Figure 8.10). Glen is grimacing and is guarded in his movements when he enters the treatment room. He is irritable and responds to his father's concern and questions with some anger.

You weigh Glen, take his vital signs, and begin taking his history. Glen is reluctant to provide details about the location of his pain. His father speaks up and reports that Glen has been suffering intense scrotal pain for the past 2 hours. You, a female nurse, ask Glen to disrobe to prepare for the examination. Glen seems reluctant to remove his jeans and underwear, and does not want to show you where he has pain. He wants reassurance that no women will come into the room and that only a male doctor will see him.

Question

How should this situation be handled when only female nurses are available? (Choose one.)

1. Assure Glen that he will be able to cover himself with a sheet and that only the physician will examine him.
2. Reassure him that nurses are accustomed to seeing all their patients undressed.
3. Tell him straightforwardly that this is a routine matter and that he will have to remove his clothes if he wants to be examined.
4. Acknowledge his discomfort and tell him that you have a child his age so he doesn't have to feel uncomfortable.

Answer

Allowing Glen as much modesty as possible will lessen his anxiety. You recognize that a triage examination is unnecessary because acute onset of scrotal pain in childhood is an emergent situation requiring rapid evaluation by the physician. You can avoid direct confrontation and needless delay by assuring him a "male-only" examination and a means of maintaining modesty throughout. This action will help develop trust and rapport with Glen. Adolescents have difficulty accepting help from adults because they are developing independence.[1] Insisting or ordering Glen will only increase his resistance and develop mistrust. Mentioning your own children or your own experience may further isolate him, because these statements still do not acknowledge *his* feelings.

Question

Suppose you want to respect Glen's need for modesty, but have only female nurses and a female physician. How would you handle the situation? (Fill in the blank.)

_____

_____

Answer

Acknowledge Glen's modesty. Tell him in a very straightforward manner that you have only female nurses and a female doctor. Be empathetic and understanding. Explain the need for rapid care in his case. Assure him that he can cover himself and that only the physician will examine him. Interventions to promote modesty are listed in Table 8.15.

TABLE 8.15. Interventions To Promote Modesty

Don't make fun of a child's need for modesty by engaging in a power struggle. Teenagers are struggling for autonomy and control, and can resist adamantly.

Maximize privacy by drawing curtains and closing doors so that the adolescent will not feel exposed.

Remain calm, empathetic, and friendly in your interaction while respecting the patient's opinions and feelings. Remember, you will never win a power struggle with a teenager.

You are successful in reassuring Glen. You leave the room, and he disrobes and covers himself. The doctor examines him and makes a tentative diagnosis of testicular torsion. He explains this in a general way to Glen. A surgical consultation is requested. Glen is still in pain and is now quite frightened. You decide that you should stay with him and help him to cope with his discomfort.

Question

Match the appropriate interventions for pain relief with the correct age group.

  1. Infant   _____   Progressive relaxation

  2. Toddler   _____   Rock, cuddle

  3. Preschooler   _____   Rhythmic breathing ("blow out like a whistle")

  4. School age   _____   Counting ("one, two, three, four, five")

  5. Adolescent   _____   Distraction with toy or talking

Answer

The answers are (5), (1), (4), (3), (2), respectively.

For Glen, working with him on progressive relaxation, beginning with his feet and working upward, may help him cope with his pain. You tell him to begin by tightening his toes and feet as much as he can, then relaxing them. As you work upwards, his tension eases somewhat.

The physician is speaking with Glen's father outside the room, explaining the critical nature of the condition and the possible need for surgery. Glen can hear them talking and asks you, "What is wrong with me? It must be very serious if they are talking so much about it. Am I going to die?"

Question

Is this a typical question for an adolescent to ask? (Choose Yes or No.)

_____ Yes _____ No

Answer

The correct answer is Yes. Any type of illness or injury can be of great concern to an adolescent.[1] They are very aware of their bodies, and when cues from the environment suggest a serious situation they may worry about dying. Adolescents frequently think in "all-or-nothing" extremes; some may understand the finality of death but not think it applies to them, whereas others immediately imagine the worst. In this particular case, Glen is clearly very worried. Providing a nonjudgmental atmosphere in which Glen can discuss his concerns with you may help to lessen his isolation and alleviate some of his anxiety. You can also encourage Glen's participation in any discussions with the physician and Mr. Miyashiro regarding Glen's condition. Simple explanations about the anatomy, physiology and treatment of testicular torsion may be helpful (see Figure 8.11). The physician may also want to discuss the situation with Glen in greater depth, and you can help facilitate this.

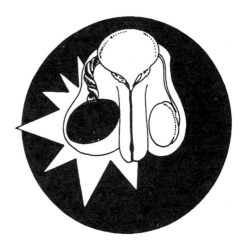

FIGURE 8.11 Testicular Torsion

The surgeon arrives and examines Glen. He recommends surgery to correct the testicular torsion. The surgeon explains to Glen and his father that surgery is necessary. The surgeon explains the condition, the corrective procedure, and the expected outcome. Glen asks appropriate questions and seems accepting of the surgery. To everyone's surprise, Mr. Miyashiro becomes angry, upset, and adamantly refuses to consent to surgical intervention.

Question

How should you respond to Mr. Miyashiro? (Choose one answer.)

1. Explain to Mr. Miyashiro that there is no choice, that this is a life-threatening situation, and that he should sign the consent immediately.
2. Ask Mr. Miyashiro's about his reasons for objecting to the surgery.
3. Tell Mr. Miyashiro that you can initiate proceedings immediately to obtain a court order if he is unwilling to sign.
4. Encourage Glen to convince his father that he needs the surgery.

Answer

It would be most helpful to discuss Mr. Miyashiro's concerns with him. Listen, empathize, and attempt to diffuse negative feelings and resolve conflict peacefully. The parent who has feelings of helplessness, fear, or anxiety may respond with resistance, anger, or by making demands. Rather than opposing Mr. Miyashiro immediately, it may help to address the underlying concerns and emotions. This approach is more likely to result in a better outcome than trying to coerce him into signing the consent form, or encouraging a confrontation between father and son.

Mr. Miyashiro tells you that his wife died from surgical complications just 2 years ago this month. He is holding back tears as he talks about conflict with his son, his guilt for consenting to his wife's surgery, his loneliness, and his feeling of failure as a single parent. He feels that he has been unable to fill the void left in Glen's life by the loss of his mother.

You and the surgeon listen to the father's reasons and empathize with him. The surgeon again explains the consequences of not doing surgery and the relatively low risk involved. You talk with Mr. Miyashiro about the importance of rapid intervention and contrast the difference between his late wife's situation and the current problem with Glen. You discuss the normal parent–child conflict and pattern of "breaking away" in adolescence. Mr. Miyashiro decides he will consent to surgery.

You go into the room to prepare Glen for surgery while his father goes to the admitting office to complete the required forms. Glen reveals a current active sexual relationship with a girl whom his father does not like. He asks, "Could having sex cause this?" He expresses the feeling that maybe the surgery is "like a punishment" that may make him less attractive to girls and unable to perform sexually in the future.

Question

How should you respond to his concerns? (Choose one answer.)

1. Assure him that he is very good looking and tell him that he will not have to worry about being attractive to girls.

2. Tell him that testicular torsion isn't related to sexual activity and that it is not helpful to escalate this into something more serious than it actually is.

3. Acknowledge his fears, encourage him to talk to the surgeon, and give him some written material on testicular torsion.

4. Tell him that although his sexual experimentation is not the cause of his condition, he is young to be having sexual relations, and many problems can result from early sexual experiences.

Answer

Help him to take control by obtaining more information. Glen's concern about scarring reflects normal adolescent anxiety about physical disfigurement and attractiveness. It is common at this age to be concerned about sexual identity and body image. Sexual curiosity and experimentation are normal parts of development and are fraught with guilt and insecurity; adolescents often interpret illness or injury as related to something they have done. Their knowledge of physical function (see Figure 8.12) and illness is frequently incomplete and distorted. Answers (1) and (2) are incorrect because it is not helpful to ignore, judge, or belittle an adolescent's concerns or fears; these attitudes will not promote identity formation. Answer (4) is also incorrect: A judgmental attitude only increases guilt and fear. Providing a

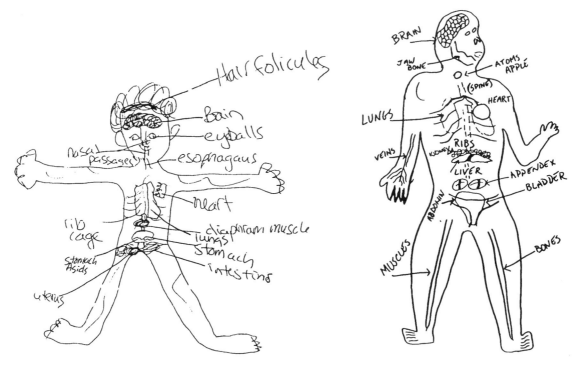

FIGURE 8.12 Human anatomy drawn by Heather, age 14 (*left*), and Cari, age 15 (*right*).

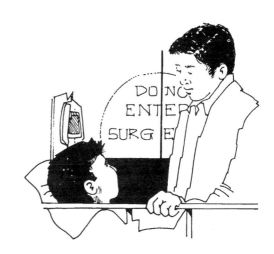

FIGURE 8.13

nonjudgmental atmosphere so that he can ask questions freely may be the best way to assure his obtaining information about his sexuality and sexual practices in the future.

You transport Glen to surgery with his father walking alongside to the operating suite (see Figure 8.13). Glen and his father exchange words of comfort, and you escort the father to the waiting area where he will be able to telephone family members and rest until Glen is out of surgery.

CASE STUDY 6: THE DEATH OF A CHILD IN THE EMERGENCY DEPARTMENT

PREVIEW

The sudden death of a child is a tragedy for the family and extremely stressful for emergency department staff. Today, more pediatric deaths are seen in the emergency department than in previous years. Advanced pediatric life support and advanced trauma life support in the prehospital setting are getting more children to the emergency department in highly compromised states. More premature infants and more "high-tech" children have longer life expectancies and present with life-threatening conditions related to their health status.

Because parents are expected to provide proper care and supervision for children, when a child is seriously ill, injured, or dies, the loss or threat of loss of a child is like the breaking of a special trust. Families will have a range of emotional reactions including anger, grief, withdrawal, denial, and even attempts to bargain. Emergency department staff should have an organized, practical approach to helping families of acutely ill, dying, or deceased children.

The emergency nurse has the opportunity to help the family begin their grieving process. While this case study focuses on the infant with sudden infant death syndrome (SIDS), the support measures can be rendered to parents of any child who dies suddenly and unexpectedly in the emergency department.

CASE STUDY 6 OBJECTIVES

On completion of this case study, the learner will be able to

- Develop strategies to help explain SIDS to bereaved parents
- Apply concepts of grief work through interventions with the bereaved parent
- Identify interventions to assist the family to begin their grieving process following the sudden death of their child

CASE STUDY 6

Little Joshua Is in Full Cardiopulmonary Arrest

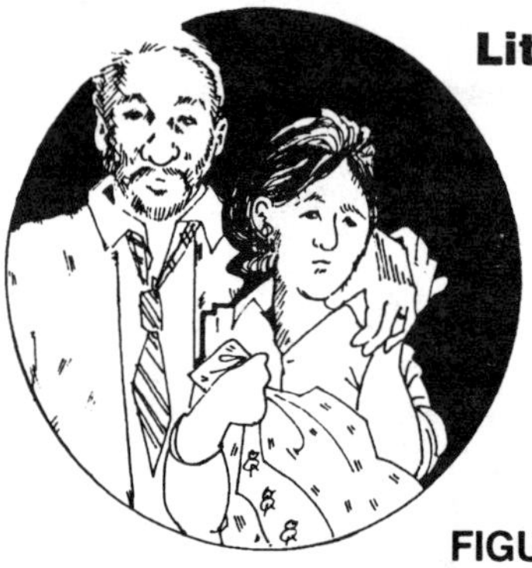

Joshua Stewart, a 3-month-old infant, comes to the emergency department via ambulance in full cardiopulmonary arrest. The distraught parents, Mr. and Mrs. Stewart (see Figure 8.14), have been taken to the doctor's sleeping room (the only private place available in your hospital).

FIGURE 8.14

Question

Parents who have been in similar situations indicate that their most important needs at this point are: (Circle all that apply.)

1. To have contact with another person who has had a similar experience
2. To have privacy
3. To receive emotional support from caring staff members
4. To have as much information as possible
5. To have their physical needs met
6. To speak with the physician
7. To have a staff member identified as their contact person

Answer

The correct answers are (2), (4), (5), and (7). Studies of parents who have lost a family member have indicated that these four: privacy, information, physical comfort, and an identifiable staff person are the essentials for parents at first, usually in that order.[1] When staff members feel that they are not the "right type of person" to provide comfort for these families, it is important to remember that in the early stages of grief, basic comforts such as privacy; access to a telephone and a bathroom; facial tissues; and coffee, tea, or water can be easily provided, and parents consider these of utmost importance.

Once a staff member has been identified as liaison, parents should be asked if they wish a religious counselor to be present (priest, minister, rabbi, etc.) and contact the counselor for them. The family may want a religious ritual (e.g., baptism) performed or a short prayer. If there is no member of the clergy available, a staff member with similar beliefs may be helpful. It should not automatically be assumed that the family will want spiritual counseling—it should simply be offered as a choice.

Table 8.16 shows the steps that are of major importance in assisting families of acutely ill or dying children.

TABLE 8.16.   Assisting Families of Acutely Ill or Dying Children

Provide privacy for the family.

Meet the family's physical needs: comfortable seating, access to telephone and bathroom, facial tissues, coffee, tea or water.

Allow the family in the resuscitation room, if requested.

Provide continuous updated information to parents not present in the resuscitation area as to resuscitation status.

Provide honest answers, and avoid false reassurance.

Provide appropriate support mechanisms with social services, psychology, or chaplaincy.

Allow the family to express grief in whatever way seems helpful to them. Do not attempt to inhibit the grieving process.

Assist with social needs including transportation, religious rites, and family crisis.

Question

If the Stewart family had asked to be in the treatment room during Joshua's resuscitation, should their request have been granted? (Choose Yes or No.)

_____ Yes   _____ No

Answer

The answer is Yes in many cases. It may or may not be appropriate for a family not to witness a resuscitation: the emotional stress and chaos that usually occurs during a pediatric resuscitation may be difficult for a family to manage. Conversely, this may be the child's last moments of life, and emergency department staff should be very careful in making a decision about separating parent and child.

In a study where family members witnessed cardiopulmonary resuscitation, 94% felt they would do it again, and most felt it was helpful both to them and to the patient.[2] If a family requests to be present during a resuscitation, this request should not be denied. If they wish to be present, support person(s), such as clergy, and a social worker or nurse, should remain with the family member(s) at all times to care for them. Being present during at least some part of the resuscitation lessens the isolation of the family. It also offers them an opportunity to say good-bye. There is also some evidence to show that the family's presence in the resuscitation room helps in the grieving process.[2]

In many emergency departments, the family waits in a room near the resuscitation area with a support person (social worker, clergy, or staff member). A physician (or designate) acts as a liaison to keep the family updated with resuscitation proceedings. Medical crisis in a child evokes special feelings and behaviors in parents and hospital staff.

Another staff nurse has been staying with the family most of the time, serving as liaison between the parents and the resuscitation room. Each time she goes to the resuscitation room and returns, the family asks her how Joshua is doing. Although they have been told that Joshua is not breathing on his own and has no heartbeat, their attitude indicates that they expect him to improve. After 45 minutes of unsuccessful resuscitation, Joshua is pronounced dead. The emergency department physician enters the cause of death as possible SIDS. The parents have not been told as yet of Joshua's death.

You and the emergency department physician go into the waiting room to inform Mr. and Mrs. Stewart of Joshua's death. You introduce yourselves and say that you have been taking care of Joshua. Mrs. Stewart asks, "How is Joshua doing?"

Question

Which is the best response? (Choose one answer.)

1. "I'm sorry; Joshua has died."
2. "I'm sorry; we did everything we could, but Joshua is no longer with us."

Answer

The most appropriate response would be answer (1). When informing the parents of their child's death, it is best to be clear and to use the words "dead" or "died." Saying that you were "unable to resuscitate him" or that he "is no longer with us" or "is gone" is unclear and leaves room for misinterpretation. For example, if you tell parents that their child "is gone" the parents may ask where he went if he's not here. Always refer to the infant or child by his or her name, as this reassures parents that you know him or her as a person rather than an illness or problem.

A parent should not be alone when receiving this news. If other family members or friends are not available, a nurse, social worker, or other staff member or volunteer can serve as a support person for the parent when the information is given. Although a health care professional is probably the most appropriate, almost any experienced, kind, understanding, and supportive member of the emergency department staff or trained volunteer can serve in this capacity. The support person must remain with the parent until the extended family or friends arrive.

Question

How the parents are told of their child's death is just as important as what they are told. (Choose True or False.)

_____ True   _____ False

Answer

The correct answer is True. Parents remember *how* they were told about their child's death as well as what was told to them. Therefore, how information is presented to them is just as important as what is said. Parents will not be immediately comforted by your sympathetic words; proceed as gently as possible with what you think needs to be said.[3] The parents need time to respond to what they are being told. Listen to what they say, and answer their questions honestly. The parents also need reassurance that everything possible was done to save their child. They need to know that the emergency department staff worked to their fullest capabilities to save the child.

The emergency physician sits down with Joshua's family and gives them a brief explanation of what was done for Joshua. You remain in the room as the Stewarts respond to the news.

Question

What are two responses the Stewarts might have to the news of Joshua's death? (Fill in the blanks.)

1. _____

2. _____

Answer

The Stewarts' responses might include

1. *Overwhelming shock and sadness.* Some parents may understand the enormity of the event immediately, and respond with extreme grief and anguish.

2. *Anger.* The parents may feel very angry and, lacking any real focus for their anger, direct it toward emergency department personnel. It is best not to respond to the content of what they are saying by attempting to defend staff or procedures at this point, but to respond to the emotional message, acknowledging their anger and pain.

3. *Guilt.* The parents may feel guilty about the child's death, whether or not they were responsible for it. You may wish to acknowledge their feelings and reassure them that there is no basis for this belief. You (or the physician) may say that you know they have questions about whether they may have caused, prevented, or changed the child's death. Reassure the parents when appropriate; ask the parents what they believe caused the death and correct any misconceptions.[3]

4. *Disbelief and denial.* These responses are more likely when parents were not with the child when the illness or injury occurred, or when they have not seen the child during the resuscitation. The pain of a child's death is so great, however, that a parent may continue to deny the child's death for an extended period.

5. *Confusion and questioning.* When a child dies suddenly, parents have not had time to assimilate information about the event. As a means of controlling the situation, they may focus on sorting out the sequence of events and want more information about exactly what happened, and what was done in the emergency department. This may be uncomfortable for emergency department staff, because they, too, may be wondering what more could have been done. The parents' questioning, however, should not be seen as their questioning the abilities of staff members, or the appropriateness of care, but rather as a means of buying time and asserting control. Questions should be answered as honestly as possible.

The emergency physician tells Joshua's family that she suspects that Joshua's death is due to SIDS, but that this will not be known until after some tests have been performed.

Question

The underlying pathology of SIDS is (Choose one answer.)

1. A genetic defect
2. A congenital anomaly
3. A bacterial infection
4. Unknown

Answer

The correct answer is (4). Table 8.17 is a review of the characteristics of SIDS.

TABLE 8.17.   Sudden Infant Death Syndrome[4, 5]

Sudden Infant Death Syndrome
Is the sudden and unexpected death of an apparently healthy infant, for which no medical cause is found
Is a diagnosis determined on autopsy
Is implicated in approximately 1.5–2 deaths per 1,000 live births; this rate varies based on epidemiologic variables such as socioeconomic status, ethnic origin (Native Americans, 10/1,000), maternal drug addiction, young maternal age, discharge from a neonatal intensive care unit, and season of the year (higher in winter)
Occurs at any point during the first year of life (peak incidence is 2–4 months of age)
Occurs in any location at any time of the day or night (highest incidence is between midnight and 8:00 a.m.)

Note: When an infant less than 6 months of age dies, child abuse as well as SIDS must be considered as a possibility, but asking parents about child abuse may produce psychological harm. All parents should receive emotional support, and when the post mortem findings are available, appropriate agencies can become involved if there is abuse.[6] In a case of suspected SIDS, the parents may be told that it appears that their infant has died from SIDS, but that an autopsy is needed to confirm this diagnosis.[4] If there is any reason to suspect abuse or homicide, law enforcement agencies must be involved immediately.

You and the emergency physician ask Mr. and Mrs. Stewart if they want to see Joshua. Mrs. Stewart looks inquiringly at Mr. Stewart, who looks somewhat doubtful. You assure them that they can each make the decision separately (one parent sometimes refuses to protect the other). You tell them that some people prefer to have the memory of the healthy child, others feel they need to hold the child to say good-bye.

> **Question**
>
> It is essential for close family members to see the dead child to progress through the grieving process. (Choose True or False.)
>
> _____ True   _____ False

Answer

False. If the family does not want to see the baby or child, do not force the issue. To help them decide, you may remind them that often what they imagine is worse than what is real. Note, however, that there is no established evidence that forcing a family to see, hold, or touch their dead child aids in the grieving process.[1] The parents should be given as much time as is reasonable to be with their child; other family members, too, may want to visit and to say their good-byes.

Both parents decide to go in to hold Joshua. You ask them to wait just a moment, and you return to the treatment room to determine if anything further needs to be done before they enter.

> **Question**
>
> What are two interventions to prepare Joshua for presentation to his parents? (Fill in the blanks.)
>
> 1. _____
>
> 2. _____

Answer

If the family wants to be with Joshua, he should be prepared for viewing. The following interventions are the most important:

- Remove any bloody or fluid-stained sheets and towels, and clean the child's face and body.
- The baby or small child should be wrapped in a warm blanket; a larger child should be cleaned and covered with a warm blanket. Parents are often concerned, from long habit, about whether the child is kept warm.
- The resuscitation room may be tidied up, but this should not take more than a few minutes. It is more important for the parents to be able to see their child, and parents rarely notice their surroundings in this situation.
- If tubes must be left in place, they should be adequately secured.

> **Question**
>
> What are some strategies for family support during the viewing? (Fill in the blanks.)
>
> 1. _____
>
> 2. _____

Answer

Any of the following strategies would be appropriate:

- Provide a quiet, private room with the lights turned down, if available. This is the best type of situation for the family to be together with their baby or small child.
- If there is deformity from medical procedures or trauma, explain this briefly to the parents before they enter the room to avoid surprises.
- The parents may feel they need your permission to hold, kiss, or hug their child; some may want to comb their child's hair or wash the body. Assure them that they may care for him or her, they only need to be careful not to disturb the endotracheal tube and IV line(s).

As Mr. and Mrs. Stewart come into the room, they move quickly toward Joshua, stopping as they arrive at the bedside. You help them pick him up, explaining that because he is not moving, he may feel heavier to them.

You explain that the endotracheal tube was to help him breathe, and unfortunately it and the IV tubing must stay in place for the time being. To respect the family's need to be alone, you assure them that you are leaving, but you will return in a few minutes, and that if they need you, you will be next door in the emergency department.[7]

The parents stay with Joshua for 2 hours. You check back with them periodically. When they are ready to leave, you ask another nurse to stay with Joshua.

Note: Seeing someone staying with their child may help parents feel that the child is safe; most parents are reluctant to leave the child alone in the room.

Question

Mementos or keepsakes of their child should be offered to parents. (Choose True or False.)

_____ True   _____ False

Answer

True. It may be important to the family to have a memento of some kind. With the young infant, parents may not have many mementos of their baby. If possible, cut a piece of hair from an unobtrusive place on the baby's head; secure it with tape to a piece of paper with the infant's name and date. Place it in an envelope for the parents.[7] With a neonate, no photographs may have ever been taken. The parent may request an instant camera picture of the baby and a copy of the footprints—this should not be seen as an unusual or strange request.[7] Neatly fold any clothing or blankets; return any personal effects (bottles, toys) to the parents. Check with clergy, if present: some religious organizations are willing to send the parents a certificate of baptism or an official acknowledgment of other religious ceremony performed.

You give the Stewarts a lock of Joshua's hair and ask them to return with you to the waiting area.

Question

What other issues will you need to discuss with them? (Fill in the blanks.)

1. _____

2. _____

Answer

Here are some other issues you may need to discuss.

1. ***Organ donation***. Although many physicians and nurses are uncomfortable discussing this, parents may be grateful for the opportunity to have some good come from their child's death. In most urban areas, organ procurement agencies are willing to send a representative to discuss organ donation with the family, if that is needed. One way of opening this discussion could be a statement such as, "I know this is a terrible time for you. Some parents who have gone through this have been comforted to think that some good could come from this tragedy. . . . I wonder if you want to consider tissue donation . . . ." Corneas, skin and bones are commonly retrieved tissues in cases of sudden death. Most unexpected pediatric deaths become coroner's cases, and permission from the medical examiner or coroner is usually required, so special arrangements must be made either to have the autopsy performed rapidly or to allow harvesting of organs before autopsy.

2. *Autopsy.* An autopsy is usually required in unexpected death, most often performed by the coroner or medical examiner. Parents should be informed of the process, for example, "Joshua will stay here with us for a day, and then he will be taken to the coroner's office. After that, the mortuary you choose will be responsible for him."

3. *Mortuary arrangements.* Parents are often in a state of shock and bewilderment after the death of a child, and do not usually have the name of a mortuary readily at hand. It can be very useful to prepare for this in advance by researching and making a list of mortuaries in the vicinity, with prices of funerals, which you can give to the parents. When there is financial need, there is often a mortuary that may offer interment without cost, or at a substantially reduced rate—this information should be available to parents. Their decision does not usually have to be made immediately, but you should include the telephone number of the medical examiner's or coroner's office so they can notify the mortuary. In the rare cases in which an autopsy is not required, you should give them the emergency department or nursing supervisor's number for notification.

4. *Support group information.* Most families in this situation are not able to retain information and do not find it helpful to be told about support groups at this point. If you want to provide this information, the best means is to give parents printed information about support groups or resources in their community. SIDS support groups are available in most areas, and many communities have other resources, such as "HAND" or "Compassionate Friends," which relate to a broader spectrum of need.

5. *Grieving process.* Parents experience intense pain with the death of a child, and although they may feel this pain will continue indefinitely, it usually abates over time. We know this to be true, but it is not helpful to try to inform the family of this fact; rather, it is important to allow them to express their grief and to experience their pain in whatever way they choose at this moment. Medication is not a solution, because it only puts off the pain, and, however much we want to relieve them of their pain, telling them that things will be better does no good whatsoever. Here again, if you want to provide information about the grieving process, a sheet of written information would be the most appropriate means.

6. *Siblings.* The parents may ask you how they should tell the other children about the baby's or child's death. Advise the parents to provide simple, honest answers; the siblings will sense that something is wrong and will be upset when the sibling does not come home. Parents should avoid such terms as "God took Joshua because he was good" or "Joshua is sleeping now." These types of statements may cause a fear of behaving well, religious anxieties, or fears of going to sleep at night. Siblings may believe they "caused" the death by wishing the baby would "go away," being jealous of the baby, and so forth. Reassuring them that they are not to blame will help to alleviate their anxiety. In the event that a sibling did actually participate in the event (shooting, stabbing, drowning, etc.) professional counseling will be needed. Siblings may also want to go to the funeral and may feel left out or hurt if they are not allowed to be present; this may also exacerbate any existing feelings of guilt for the child's death.[3] If there are small children in the family, it is best for a family friend to take care of them at the funeral so that the parents will not have to assume this responsibility.

Table 8.18 (following page) provides a summary of these issues.

Question

Siblings should be excluded from seeing their dead brother or sister. (Choose True or False.)

_____ True   _____ False

TABLE 8.18. Issues to Discuss with the Parents After the Sudden Death of a Child

Issue	Comments
Organ donation	May provide parents with comfort that some good has come out of the tragedy. May require permission from coroner or medical examiner. Requires special arrangements for autopsy.
Autopsy	Parents usually require information regarding the autopsy process. Stress lack of disfiguration. May be mandatory in unexpected death. Most often performed by coroner's or medical examiner's office.
Mortuary arrangements	Because of unexpected death, many parents are not prepared for this. Cost may be an issue. Provide a written list of mortuaries and costs, and include telephone numbers of the coroner's or medical examiner's office, and your emergency department.
Support groups	Most families do not find this useful until later. Provide written information on resources available.
Grieving process	Allow parents to express their grief, however they choose at this moment. Provide nonjudgmental support. Provide a sheet of written information about the grieving process.
Siblings	Siblings will be aware something is wrong, regardless of age. Advise parents to provide simple, honest answers.

Answer

False. Siblings should not be excluded from seeing their dead brother or sister. If siblings are present in the emergency department, it is up to the family to decide whether they should see the deceased. If the children are old enough, they may have a choice themselves. As with the parents, this act should not be forced upon them.[7]

You arrange follow-up for the Stewart family before their departure. Because an autopsy will be performed, the Stewarts will meet with their private physician to discuss the findings. Mr. and Mrs. Stewart leave the emergency department. You have assisted Mr. Stewart in contacting the funeral director, and they have a safe ride home with their extended family.

Note: The family should return to their private physician's office in 4 to 6 weeks (or sooner) to review the autopsy findings.[3] If there is no primary care physician, the emergency physician should accept this responsibility.

Question

After the Stewart family has departed, what can the emergency department staff do to bring some closure to this stressful situation? (Fill in the blanks.)

1. _____

2. _____

Answer

Pediatric deaths are often reviewed from a medical and technical standpoint, but this is not all that is needed. To bring closure to the emotional aspects of the death of a child, staff should be provided with opportunities to

- Take a few minutes to collect themselves following this crisis. Realistically, a busy emergency department cannot stop for nurses and physicians to do this, but some attention should be given to providing at least a momentary pause.

- Talk about their feelings in a nonjudgmental way with other staff members. Each person's grieving process is affected by the staff member's conscious or unconscious identification with the patient, parents, and family.

- Participate in a guided session by an experienced professional. This session may be necessary for staff to share their feelings in particularly traumatic deaths, or in the case of the death of a child of a hospital staff member. Participation is very important to bring closure to the situation and can help prevent staff burnout.

- Take part in a critical incident stress debriefing. When the staff is presented with a very overwhelming incident, a critical incident stress debriefing may be required 24 to 48 hours later.

Emergency department staffs are faced with this kind of tragedy on a regular basis, and must be aware of the long-term effects. The death of an infant or child is invariably painful and difficult for the emergency department staff. Along with the pain, however, emergency department nurses have a unique opportunity to consider the significance of their own lives, the inevitability of death, and the value of compassion.

Joshua's death has been painful for you; you and the rest of the emergency department staff who were involved take some time to discuss your sadness as you clean the resuscitation room.

REFERENCES

Case Study 1

1. Erikson, E. (1950). *Childhood and society*. New York: Norton.
2. Blaesing, S., & Brockhous, J. (1972). The development of body image in the child. *Nursing Clinics of North America*, 7, 587–607.
3. Flavil, J. (1963). *The developmental psychology of Jean Piaget*. New York: Van Nostrad.
4. Mercer, R. (1983). Parent-infant attachment. In L. Sonstegard, K. Kowalski, & B. Jennings (Eds.), *Women's health: Childbearing* (Vol. 2). New York: Grune & Stratton.
5. Aslin, R. (1987). Visual and auditory development in infancy. In J. Osofsky (Ed.), *Handbook of infant development* (2nd ed., pp. 5–97). New York: Wiley.
6. Kulka, A., Fry, C., & Goldstein, F. (1960). Kinesthetic needs in infancy. *American Journal of Orthopsychiatry*, 30, 562–571.
7. Lutz, W. (1986). Helping hospitalized children and their parents cope with painful procedures. *Journal of Pediatric Nursing*, 1, 24–32.

Case Study 2

1. Erikson, E. (1950). *Childhood and society*. New York: Norton.
2. Piaget, J. (1973). *The child and reality*. New York: Grossman.
3. Lutz, W. (1986). Helping hospitalized children and their parents cope with painful procedures. *Journal of Pediatric Nursing*, 1, 24–32.
4. Escalona, S. (1953). Emotional development in the first year of life. In M. J. Senn (Ed.), *Problems of infancy and childhood*. New York: Foundation Press.
5. Visintainer, M. A., & Wolfer, J. A. (1975). Psychological preparation for surgical pediatric patients: The effect on children's and parents' stress responses and adjustment. *Pediatrics*, 64, 646–655.

6. Bernardo, L. (1989). *Caring for your child in the emergency room*. Bethesda, MD: Association for the Care of Children's Health.

Case Study 3

1. Anthony, J. (1968). The child's discovery of his body. *Physical Therapy, 12*, 1103–1114.
2. Freud, A. (1952). The role of bodily illness in the mental life of children. *Psychoanalytic Study of the Child, 7*, 69–82.
3. Ritchie, J., Caty, S., & Ellerton, M. (1988). Coping behaviors of hospitalized preschool children. *Maternal–Child Nursing Journal, 17*, 153–172.
4. Kim, M. J., McFarland, G. K., & McLane, A. M. (1989). *Pocket guide to nursing diagnoses* (3rd ed). St. Louis: Mosby.

Case Study 4

1. Kim, M. A., McFarland, G. K., & McLane, A. M. (1989). *Pocket guide to nursing diagnoses* (3rd ed.). St. Louis: Mosby.
2. Lutz, W. (1986). Helping hospitalized children and their parents cope with painful procedures. *Journal of Pediatric Nursing, 1*, 24–32.
3. McCaffery, M., & Beebe, A. (1989). *Pain: Clinical manual for nursing practice*. St. Louis: Mosby.
4. McGrath, P. A. (1989). Evaluating a child's pain. *Journal of Pain and Symptom Management. 4*, 198–214.
5. Ritchie, J., Caty, S., & Ellerton, M. (1988). Coping behaviors of hospitalized preschool children. *Maternal Child Nursing Journal, 17*, 153–172.
6. Erikson, E. (1950). *Childhood and society*. New York: Norton.
7. Pridham, K., Adelson, F., & Hansen, M. (1987). Helping children deal with procedures in a clinic setting: A developmental approach. *Journal of Pediatric Nursing, 2*, 13–22.

Case Study 5

1. Goldberger, J., Gaynard, L., & Wolfer, J. (1990, March). Helping children cope with health-care procedures. *Contemporary Pediatrics, 7*, 141–162.
2. Erikson, E. (1950). *Childhood and society*. New York: Norton.
3. Pridham, K., Adelson, F., & Hansen, M. (1987). Helping children deal with procedures in a clinic setting: A developmental approach. *Journal of Pediatric Nursing, 2*, 13–22.

Case Study 6

1. Frader, J., & Sargent, J. (1988). Sudden death or catastrophic illness: Family considerations. In S. Ludwig & G. Fleisher (Eds.), *Textbook of pediatric emergency medicine* (2nd ed., pp. 1164–1173). Baltimore: Williams & Wilkins.
2. Doyle, C. J., Pat, H., Burney, R. E., Maino, J., Keefe, M. & Rhee, J. (1987, June). Family participation during resuscitation: An option. *Annals of Emergency Medicine. 16*, 673–675.
3. Frader, J., & Sargent, J. (1988). Sudden death or catastrophic illness: Family considerations. In G. Fleisher & S. Ludwig (Eds.), *Textbook of pediatric emergency medicine* (2nd ed., pp. 1164–1173). Baltimore: Williams & Wilkins.
4. Goodale, L., & Kelley, S. (1988). Sudden infant death syndrome. In S. Kelley (Ed.), *Pediatric emergency nursing* (pp. 52–63). Norwalk, CT: Appleton Lange.
5. Torrey, S. (1988). Apnea. In S. Ludwig & G. Fleisher (Eds.), *Textbook of pediatric emergency medicine* (2nd ed., pp. 78–82). Baltimore: Williams & Wilkins.
6. Ludwig, S. (1988). Child abuse. In S. Ludwig & G. Fleisher (Eds.), *Textbook of pediatric emergency medicine* (2nd ed., pp. 1127–1163). Baltimore: Williams & Wilkins.
7. Jezierski, M. (1989). Infant death: Guidelines for support of parents in the emergency department. *Journal of Emergency Nursing, 15*, 475–476.

APPENDIX

Advance Preparation for an Emergency Department Visit

Before an emergency occurs, some of the following activities help to promote appropriate emergency department use and introduce children to the hospital.

1. Arrange field trips for local day care centers and schools to visit the emergency department during nonpeak hours; (plan an alternative date for them in case the emergency department is too busy on the scheduled day). A "sick doll" clinic and equipment demonstration could be included. Having high school students visit not only teaches them about emergency care but also exposes them to emergency nursing at a time when career choices are important for them.

2. Encourage visits of parents' groups (parent–teacher associations, clubs, etc.) to your emergency department with or without their children. Having very young children visit with their parents is often a reassuring way of introducing them to the hospital setting.

3. Develop a "speakers bureau" of emergency nurses who can visit schools, clubs, and so forth, and talk with children about emergency topics. Topics for discussion can include the emergency department experience, injury prevention, bicycle safety, and so on.

Chapter Nine

Child Maltreatment: Recognition and Management of Pediatric Abuse

Prerequisite Skills

- Ability to perform a basic pediatric assessment and identify variations from normal
- Ability to identify various age-related stages of growth and development in children and recognize behaviors that vary from normal expectations for age
- Baseline knowledge of general priorities of care in the emergency management of injured children
- Baseline knowledge of procedures commonly used in the emergency care of injured children
- Baseline knowledge of, or prior experience with, "family-centered" nursing care
- Baseline knowledge of, or prior experience with multidisciplinary case management

Recognition and Management of Pediatric Abuse

PREVIEW

One of the most difficult emergency situations faced by health care providers is the abuse or neglect of a child. "Child maltreatment" or "abuse" refers to any adult behavior that is destructive to the normal growth, development, and well-being of the child.[1] It includes both action and inaction that results in physical, sexual, emotional, or neglectful abuse of infants, children, and adolescents.[2]

Each year more than 1.5 million U.S. children are the victims of abuse.[3] Child abuse is rarely an isolated event, but is usually recurrent and progressive.[2] Approximately 2,000 children will die annually[1] and a larger number will have permanent physical and emotional aftereffects of child maltreatment,[3] As front-line care providers for children in hospitals and in the home, nurses play a crucial role in the early recognition and management of suspected child abuse. The nurse's role in this process includes

1. Recognizing suspicious findings
2. Contributing to the child's immediate medical and psychosocial care
3. Assisting in ensuring the child's immediate safety.

4. Initiating a continuing investigative process by law enforcement and child protective agencies

5. Being aware of his or her own emotions when confronted with suspected nonaccidental trauma

The following discussion provides information to help you to recognize the subtle signs and symptoms of abuse, to further define your role in child abuse management, and to know the essentials of care for these children and their families.

CASE STUDY 1 OBJECTIVES

Once you have completed this case study, you will be able to

- Correctly triage a victim of suspected physical abuse as emergent, urgent, or nonurgent
- List pertinent historical, behavioral, and physical findings in the assessment of suspected nonaccidental trauma
- Recognize the feelings that health care providers typically experience when confronted with cases of child abuse
- Identify three coping strategies for your own personal reactions to child maltreatment
- Identify demographic and other factors that are associated with an increased risk for child abuse
- Decide, based on a preliminary assessment, whether there is sufficient evidence to warrant reporting suspected abuse
- Identify acceptable nursing documentation for suspected child maltreatment
- Select nursing diagnoses appropriate for the assessment and care of a patient who may have been abused
- Identify three priorities of care in the management of suspected physical abuse
- Choose an appropriate approach for interacting with a family expressing hostility
- State the legal responsibilities of health care providers in cases of suspected child abuse

CASE STUDY 1

Sheralyn Just Isn't Very Playful

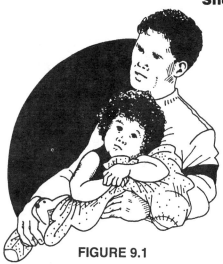

FIGURE 9.1

Sheralyn, a 20-month-old white female, is brought in to the emergency department late Sunday evening by her father, Shawn Dalton, because "she's extremely irritable and not very playful" (see Figure 9.1). Her father tells you Sheralyn has had a slight cold for the past week with occasional coughing and a fever as high as 101.6°F the previous night. He hasn't seen any changes in Sheralyn's appetite or activity level until this evening but seems very upset about her increased irritability. He says, "Her cold must be much worse or else she's really sick. She's crying so much today. Usually she's so playful and into everything."

As you look at Sheralyn, you see her sitting quietly in her father's lap. She has dark curly hair and large, somber dark brown eyes. She is clinging to a worn receiving blanket and appears alert but uninterested in her surroundings. When she is uncovered and moved, she suddenly begins to cry. She continues crying throughout the initial assessment but makes no attempts to resist your efforts. Her respiratory rate seems slightly rapid and irregular, but her respiration does not seem labored. She has slight upper airway congestion and a runny nose. Her skin is pale pink and warm to touch.

TRIAGE DECISION

On the basis of your assessment at this point, you would triage Sheralyn as

Emergent.   A life-threatening situation in need of immediate intervention.

Urgent.   Patient needs care within 1 hour to prevent further deterioration.

Nonurgent.   Patient is able to wait more than 1 hour without further deterioration.

TRIAGE DECISION ANSWER

Sheralyn should be triaged as urgent. While Sheralyn's airway, breathing, and circulation (*ABCs*) appear stable, she has a rapid respiratory rate and a history of fever and upper respiratory infection symptoms. More significantly, her mental status, with the history of increased irritability and decreased playfulness and her passive behavior during your initial examination is not typical for her age and developmental level.

Mr. Dalton, who is well groomed and appears to be in his late 20s, handles Sheralyn carefully. He asks repeatedly why she is crying so much. He focuses his attention on his child and makes little eye contact with staff members. He tries distracting Sheralyn with a small toy and speaking in low, soothing tones. She looks at him but does not appear comforted by his efforts. He attempts to cuddle her close to him, but she pushes away from his chest.

You complete triage vital signs and undress Sheralyn for weighing. Her vital signs are

Pulse	160 beats/min
Respiratory rate	50 breaths/min
Blood pressure	90/52
Temperature (rectal)	38.3°C (101°F)
Weight	10.8 kg (23.8 lbs.)

Under the bright examination lights, you suddenly notice a dark reddish-purple discolored area slightly behind her right ear under her dark curls. Sheralyn's father says she hasn't fallen or had any accidents that could have caused bruising and says he thinks she had a "birthmark" in that area. Then he laughs and says, "If it is a bruise it's probably because Sheralyn is just beginning to walk and doesn't do too well. She probably just ran into a table or something." He seems anxious for you to finish the initial examination and asks, "Do you really think her cold is making her feel this bad?" He answers your direct questions in a monotone, volunteers little additional information, and avoids any eye contact with you.

Question

Because you are uncertain about Sheralyn's possible "bruise" and her father seems unconcerned about it, it is not necessary to mention it to the physician or document it in your assessment notes. (Choose True or False.)

_____ True   _____ False

Answer:

False: The bruise should be documented. Though the area of possible bruising is subtle, it still warrants further investigation. The bruise may be due to other causes, but it is important to remember that injuries resulting from child maltreatment can range from very subtle physical findings to very obvious injuries. The presentation of child maltreatment may be direct (i.e., parent or child openly disclosing the abuse) or indirect (i.e., total denial of knowledge of the cause of obvious injuries).

Physical abuse and neglect cases most commonly present indirectly with complaints of unrelated or vague symptoms (e.g., "not acting right" or "unresponsiveness") and no adequate explanation for traumatic injuries.[4] Direct disclosure may be more common in sexual abuse cases, where a family member will often voice concerns about the possibility of abuse on presentation to the emergency room or shortly thereafter.[5,6]

Question

The most important findings in Sheralyn's assessment have been obtained

1. Through taking her history
2. From her triage vital signs
3. From your limited physical exam
4. By the behavior of Sheralyn and her father

(Choose one answer.)

(a) 1, 2, 3, and 4   (c) 1 and 4

(b) 1 and 2   (d) 2 and 3

Answer

History, vital signs, physical examination, and behavior (a) are all important sources of information in this situation. Early recognition and management of suspected child maltreatment involves putting together subtle clues from a group or "pattern of indicators that arouse suspicion" and warrant prompt further investigation (see Table 9.1 and Figure 9.2).[1,7,8]

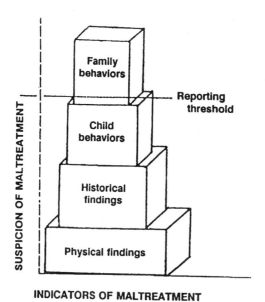

INDICATORS OF MALTREATMENT

FIGURE 9.2   The "pattern of indicators" for suspected child maltreatment.

Note: Many factors must be considered in cases of suspected maltreatment. A wide variety of illnesses, as well as health care treatments (e.g., coin rubbing, moxibustion) of diverse cultures may appear deceptively similar to child abuse.

TABLE 9.1. Common Indicators of Child Maltreatment[1,7,4,8,9]

Family behaviors
Inappropriate parent/child interaction Extremes of reactions to hospital staff (e.g., hostile or unconcerned) Unrealistic expectations of child
Child behaviors
Extremes of behavior (e.g., withdrawn or acting out) No opposition to painful procedures Developmental delays Inappropriate sexual behavior Somatic complaints (e.g., chronic headaches, sleep disorders, enuresis) Suicidal behavior and threats Drug or alcohol abuse
Historical findings
Story inconsistent with physical findings or developmental level Delays in seeking medical treatment Direct disclosure Repeat visits to emergency department
Physical findings
Multiple injuries in various stages of healing Injury type or location inconsistent with child's developmental level Characteristic pattern reflective of object used to cause injury (e.g., belt marks) Signs of poor overall care Genital bleeding or discharge in prepubescent children

---

Question

Think about the history, physical findings, and parent–child behaviors, and list any three items from Sheralyn's assessment thus far which may have raised your suspicions about the possibility of child abuse. (Fill in the blanks.)

1. _____

2. _____

3. _____

Answer

Any of the following answers would be appropriate:

- Suspicious area of possible bruising to the head.

- Lack of credible history for possible bruising to the head. If the child truly had a birthmark the father would probably be aware of its location. A toddler learning to walk would probably bruise the forehead on a table, not the area behind the ear.

- Sheralyn's behavior for her age or developmental level. The history of extreme irritability and lack of playfulness, the lack of curiosity about the emergency department setting, the passiveness during vital sign measurement, and the resistance to being comforted by her parent are all atypical toddler behaviors.

- Change in father's behavior once the possible bruised area was noticed (i.e., his increased anxiety and decreased willingness to volunteer information).

When you take Sheralyn and her father to the waiting room and provide Sheralyn with some toys, Mr. Dalton appears slightly less anxious. Soon you are able to escort them to the treatment area. While walking through the halls with the pretty little girl and her quiet, controlled father, you momentarily attempt to collect your thoughts. Questioning your initial suspicions, you wonder if it really could be a birthmark that you noticed on Sheralyn's head. Suddenly you remember a case of suspected abuse earlier this week and wonder how that turned out. You're still not sure whether you've overreacted, but you feel very angry at parents who can injure their own children.

Question

Feelings of confusion, denial, embarrassment, empathy for the child, and anger are common among health care providers who are confronted with situations like Sheralyn's. (Choose True or False.)

_____ True   _____ False

Answer

All of these feelings are common among professionals confronted with child abuse[1,4,5] and may be related to the ethical dilemmas common to suspected abuse cases.[10] Among these dilemmas are the need to protect the child, the desire to treat the entire family justly, the uncertainty of the diagnosis, the possibility of violating patient/client privacy and confidentiality, and the risk of separating a child from their family.[10–12] The ability of professionals to cope effectively with these issues is critical to working successfully with suspected child abuse victims and their families.

Question

What are some of the coping strategies that may be used by professionals confronted with a child who may have been abused? (Fill in the blanks.)

1. _____

2. _____

3. _____

Answer

Any of the strategies listed in Table 9.2 may be helpful for coping.

TABLE 9.2. Professional Coping Strategies: Managing Reactions to Child Maltreatment

- Acknowledge personal feelings, and recognize their potential effect on care of abuse victims and families.[1,7,13]

- View the family as the patient and the child as the victim, emphasizing assessment and treatment rather than punishment.[7,8,12]

- Avoid placing blame. Your responsibility is not to *prove* that abuse occurred or identify the perpetrator but to file a report of *suspicion.*[8,11]

- Share responsibility for recognition and management of suspected abuse with other multidisciplinary team members (e.g., physicians, nurses, social workers, child protection, and law enforcement personnel).[7,8,11,14]

- Develop and use a written protocol for child abuse management to focus attention on safe care of the child and family.[1,8,15]

- Learn more about child abuse and become involved in local prevention efforts to help combat feelings of powerlessness and frustration.[1,3,7,16]

Once Sheralyn and her father are settled in the treatment area, you notify the physician of the child's presence and begin Sheralyn's emergency department record. Talking with her father more in detail, you learn that they live in one of the "better neighborhoods" in town. You also note how articulate and well educated he seems.

Question

When considering the possibility of child maltreatment, you know that the greatest likelihood of child abuse is in (Choose one answer.)

1. An African American, Hispanic, or Asian family
2. A family from a lower socioeconomic group
3. A family from an urban setting
4. None of the above

Answer

The answer is (4); the incidence of child abuse does not vary by any of the above factors including race, socioeconomic level, sex, or urban versus rural settings.[3,8] The problem is widespread in all segments of the population, but poor and minority abuse cases tend to be reported more frequently.[3,4,11,16] (See Appendix A for facts on child abuse in the U.S.)

When Dr. Martin arrives and is introduced to Sheralyn and her father, Mr. Dalton readily volunteers that "Sheralyn has a cold that seems to be getting much worse because she is acting really fussy." Dr. Martin assures him that he will look her over carefully, and the unit clerk takes Mr. Dalton to the registration area to finish the emergency department paperwork. You quickly summarize Sheralyn's vital signs and history for Dr. Martin. You mention your concerns about the discolored area posterior to her ear and Mr. Dalton's conflicting explanations for this. You then prepare to assist with the physical examination.

Question

In view of her age and Sheralyn's presenting complaints, it will be in Sheralyn's best interest for Dr. Martin to perform an abbreviated physical exam, focusing primarily on her respiratory and neurologic status, to complete the exam as quickly as possible. (Choose True or False.)

_____ True   _____ False

Answer

False. Dr. Martin should perform a full physical examination. Because child maltreatment can affect any body system and may present with a wide range of physical findings, it is of extreme importance that a very detailed and thorough head-to-toe physical assessment be completed on all children presenting with any potential signs of child abuse.[1,7–9,11] Multiple indications of injuries, such as bruises in various stages of healing may be found in the course of a thorough physical examination (see Table 9.3).[1,4,8,12]

TABLE 9.3.   Physical Assessment FindingsSuggestive of Child Maltreatment

Any positive physical finding that is inconsistent with the history provided or the child's developmental level
Bruises, lacerations, contusions, burns, or scars in multiple sites and of differing ages
Swelling, tenderness, or limited mobility of extremities, especially in infants who are not walking
Signs and symptoms of hypovolemic shock with inadequate history
Signs of blunt trauma to the abdomen (e.g., pain, distention, rigidity) with inadequate history
Unexplained alterations in mental status, unresponsiveness, coma, or death
Signs of malnutrition, poor hygiene, or untreated illnesses
Genitourinary injuries or sexually transmitted diseases in prepubescent children

DOCUMENTING INJURY IN CHILD MALTREATMENT

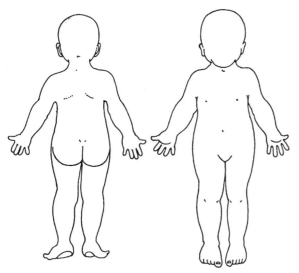

FIGURE 9.3   For documentation, it is helpful to use a line drawing to show location of injuries.

On examination, Sheralyn appears well-developed, well-nourished, and alert but irritable. Her pupils are equal and reactive to light. The bruiselike area behind her right ear is reddish-purple and measures 2 × 3 cm. It appears slightly swollen and tender. There is slight rhinorrhea from the nares. The tympanic membranes are dull and intact bilaterally without drainage.

Sheralyn's respiratory rate is still rapid despite the fact that she is no longer crying and has passively allowed herself to be examined. Respirations are somewhat irregular, but no retractions are noted. Two parallel, slightly curved greenish-yellow areas, 1/2 cm x 2 1/2 cm are noted on the left posterior lateral aspect of the chest. The abdomen is soft and nondistended.

There are no obvious injuries or areas of swelling of the bones or joints, and no apparent limitations in range of motion. The left forearm appears slightly curved in comparison with the right forearm.   The left lateral thigh reveals a small 1 cm × 3/4 cm healed oval lesion suggestive of either an infected insect bite or an old burn. The external genitalia and rectum appear normal for a 20-month-old female. The diaper is wet with urine, but there is no sign of discharge or bleeding.

Question

Based on your knowledge of what is normal for a toddler, identify any two findings from Sheralyn's assessment which may warrant further examination. (Fill in blanks.)

1. _____

2. _____

Answer

Any of the following would be correct:

- Passive behavior during examination
- Persistent rapid/shallow respirations
- Possible bruise behind the right ear
- Greenish-yellow marks on posterior rib area
- Healed lesion on left lateral thigh
- Slightly curved left forearm

Question

Indicate any of the following which you would need to document in Sheralyn's emergency department record. (Mark each correct answer.)

_____ 1. Objective, specific descriptions or sketches of the physical findings.

_____ 2. Descriptions of Sheralyn's behavior in the emergency department.

_____ 3. Your suspicion that the father may have injured Sheralyn.

_____ 4. Mr. Dalton's actual explanation for the suspected bruise in quotation marks.

_____ 5. Detailed, objective descriptions of Mr. Dalton's behavior with Sheralyn and the emergency department staff.

Answer

The emergency department documentation should include all of the preceding entries except the third one.

It would be a mistake to document any suspicions you may have about Mr. Dalton. The medical record is one of the most important pieces of evidence in the legal proceedings associated with suspected child abuse.[7,17,18] It is essential for health care providers not to take on the role of criminal investigators in attempting to determine guilt, but to document observations accurately, in detail, and objectively (see Table 9.4, following page and Figure 9.3, previous page).[1,7,9] A useful rule is to document *only* what you can actually

- **See**
- **Hear**
- **Smell**
- **Taste**
- **Touch**

TABLE 9.4.   Documentation Guidelines for Suspected Child Maltreatment[1,4,7–9,18]

• Include only objective information, not personal opinion, gossip or conjecture

• Record a history of the injury
  1. Date, time, and place of occurrence
  2. Entire sequence of events with associated times
  3. Time lapses between occurrence and arrival for medical care
  4. Both the child's and the caretaker's accounts in their exact words in quotation marks

• Describe actual behaviors of the child and family
  1. In response to the injury
  2. In response to each other
  3. In response to the hospital setting and staff
  4. Which demonstrate the child's current developmental level

• Describe positive physical findings in qualitative and quantitative detail
  1. Number and location
  2. Measured size
  3. Shape and symmetry
  4. Color
  5. Distinguishing characteristics (especially clues to injury cause)
  6. Evidence of previous injuries

• Use sketches, body diagrams, or photographs as necessary to clarify narrative descriptions

Once Dr. Martin has completed his examination, he explains to Sheralyn's father that she does have a respiratory infection but he can't tell how serious it is until he gets some X-ray films. Dr. Martin also asks if Sheralyn has had any other illnesses or injuries that could account for her not "feeling well." Mr. Dalton glances quickly at you and says "none that I know about, but she climbs and is into everything right now. You know how kids are at her age, always falling off beds or chairs or something."

Following Dr. Martin's initial orders you begin to make preparations for a chest X-ray film. He follows you into the hall and also orders a skeletal survey including full views of skull, ribs, and extremities.

Question

Dr. Martin has probably requested the skeletal survey for the primary purpose of (Choose one answer.)

1. Determining whether Sheralyn's physical growth is appropriate for her age
2. Ruling out an intracranial hemorrhage because of the bruise to the head
3. Determining if there are multiple fractures in various stages of healing.
4. Evaluating childhood lymphoma as an underlying cause for Sheralyn's persistent cold.

Answer

Dr. Martin probably has requested the skeletal survey to determine whether there are multiple fractures. When there is a suspicion of child abuse, it is very important to consider alternative causes of injury to minimize risk of misdiagnosis. Multiple fractures in various stages of healing are common indicators of chronic injury from recurrent abusive episodes. Together with the other positive historical, physical, and behavioral findings, these X-ray film results support the suspicion of physical abuse (see Table 9.5).[1, 4]

TABLE 9.5.   Diagnostic Tests: Suspected Child Maltreatment[1, 2, 11]

Potential diagnostic tests:
Complete blood count, coagulation studies
Urinalysis
Toxicology screens
Skeletal survey/bone scan
CT scans/ultrasounds
Cultures for sexually transmitted diseases
Specific diagnostic tests ordered dependent on:
Child's presenting symptoms and vital signs
Nature of the suspected abuse
Local legal requirements
*Refer to Appendix B for a complete list of diagnostic tests and findings associated with child abuse.

By now Sheralyn and her father have been at the hospital for approximately 3 hours. During this time, Mr. Dalton has become increasingly anxious and has phoned Sheralyn's mother, Erica. She arrives at the emergency department with her own mother about the time that the X-ray films are completed. The two women appear quite upset but are able to ask questions, listen to answers, and provide additional information about Sheralyn's care. There is noticeable lack of interaction among the three adults. Although they take turns staying with Sheralyn without conflict, they do not look directly at one another.

The tension in the room is palpable, but no angry words are spoken. Occasionally one of them goes outside. You find yourself wondering about the family system, and whether the "family tension" might be related to Sheralyn's injuries.

Question

The Daltons' behavior shows that family dysfunction is most likely the cause of Sheralyn's possible abuse. (Choose True or False.)

_____ True   _____ False

Answer

False. Family dysfunction may or may not be related to abuse. Child maltreatment has been associated with a complex group of factors that include societal, cultural, familial, and situational influences, as well as characteristics of both the child and the parents.[1, 7, 11,19,20,21] A ***combination*** of these risk factors appears to be more important than any one factor in actually triggering abusive episodes (see Figure 9.4, following page).[3,7,11] (See Appendix C for a summary of the risk factors associated with child abuse.)

When the films are completed, Dr. Martin calls you over to the X-ray film view box. The chest film shows clear lung fields but fractures of the left lateral ribs 4 through 7 that are less than a month old. The skeletal survey also reveals a right parieto-occipital skull fracture and an old fracture of the left humerus which appears healed at a slight angulation.

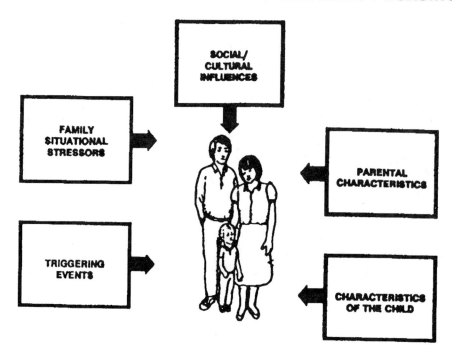

FIGURE 9.4 Family unit and contributing factors.[1]

Note. From S. Ludwig, Child abuse. In G. Fleisher & S. Ludwig (Eds.), *Textbook of Pediatric Emergency Medicine* (2nd ed., pp. 1127–1163). © 1988, Baltimore: Williams & Wilkins. Reprinted by permission.

With the results of the examination and X-ray films, you meet with Dr. Martin briefly to plan for Sheralyn's immediate and long-term care.

Question

Which are the most *immediate* nursing diagnoses for ongoing assessment and care of Sheralyn and her family? (Indicate with an **X** the most immediate.)

_____ Posttrauma response related to abuse

_____ Potential for impaired gas exchange

_____ Potential for further injury because of environment.

_____ Altered family process

Answer

The correct answers are potential for impaired gas exchange and potential for further injury due to environment.

Although Sheralyn has shown only mild tachypnea and irregular respirations on presentation, possibly related to her head injury or apparent upper respiratory infection, the respiratory status in young children must always be of primary concern. In addition, Sheralyn's fractured ribs have the potential for contributing to impaired gas exchange because of pain and splinting.

Interventions should include use of oxygen by cannula, mask, or hand-held blow-by, depending on tolerance. The amount of pain she is experiencing should also be assessed, and comfort measures such as repositioning should be considered.

There is cause for serious concern for Sheralyn's safety because physical abuse tends to be recurrent and progressive in nature.[1–4,11] Sheralyn should be in a location where she and her family can be observed until law enforcement or child protective services can assume the responsibility. (See Appendix D for morbidity and mortality in child maltreatment.)

Considering Sheralyn's irritability and the positive finding of the skull fracture, the risk of significant intracranial injury is also of concern. She will require careful continuing observation of her neurologic status for any possible deterioration, as CNS injuries are the leading cause of significant morbidity and mortality in young children who are physically abused.[1,2,4,8] Also of great significance is the combination of all of the presenting injuries, in terms of both their number and extent, in such a young child (see Table 9.6).[3,4,8]

TABLE 9.6.   Child Maltreatment Management Priorities[1,2,4,5,12]

1. Assess and stabilize *ABC*s
2. Manage potential respiratory distress and shock
3. Protect child from further immediate injury
4. Assess, prioritize, and treat presenting injuries and illnesses*
5. Prepare the child and the family for medical procedures
6. Initiate multidisciplinary discharge and follow-up care plans
a. Ensure immediate safe disposition
b. Arrange for child and family community referrals
i. Health care needs
ii. Psychosocial needs
iii. Child protection agency and law enforcement
c. Discharge and follow-up teaching for continuity of care
7. Document all assessments and care rendered
8. Complete local child abuse legal requirements
*See Appendix E for potential nursing diagnoses.

Dr. Martin phones the local child protection agency and the police. Once they arrive, you ask the staff at the nurses' station to watch Sheralyn temporarily, and you accompany Dr. Martin to the examining room to talk with the family.

Dr. Martin introduces himself to the newly arrived family members, and starts by explaining that he does not think that Sheralyn's "cold" is causing her irritability but that she has been physically injured. The reasons to suspect abuse are outlined for the family.

1. Skull fracture, rib fractures, and arm fractures of different ages

2. Skin lesions (bruises and scarring of at least two different ages) suggesting chronic injury

3. No clear history for any of the injuries

Dr. Martin tells the family that he is concerned about Sheralyn's injuries and the risk of further injury, and that he has made a report to the county's child protection agency. He introduces the child protection worker. He emphasizes his concern for Sheralyn's safety and the emergency department staff's legal obligation to report all suspicious findings for further investigation. Because of Sheralyn's need for continued observation due to her skull fracture, he suggests that she be admitted to the hospital.

Question

Even if Sheralyn had not needed further medical care, as a suspected child abuse victim, it would still be necessary to admit her to the hospital to ensure her immediate safety. (Choose one answer.)

_____ True   _____ False

Answer

False. A victim of child abuse may not necessarily require admission. Depending on the circumstances, hospital admission is only one of the options for safe disposition of suspected child abuse cases from the emergency department. Other options might include

- Transfer to another medical facility (if required diagnostic or therapeutic services are not available locally)
- Discharge to another responsible guardian other than the parent
- Discharge home (provided that adequate supervision and support are immediately available to the family)[1,4,8]

Generally, hospital admission is indicated *only* when there are injuries or illnesses that require more intensive medical care, when additional information is needed from a more thorough evaluation, when there are no safe alternatives for discharge, or when there is reason to believe that the child cannot be adequately protected if discharged (see Table 9.7).[1,2,11] If hospitalization is necessary and the family is resistant, involvement of the police, local child protection agency, or courts may be needed to prevent the family from discharging the child against medical advice.[1,4,8,12] Check your local child protection legislation for specifics regarding protective holds for suspected child abuse victims.

TABLE 9.7.   Factors for Consideration: Emergency Department Disposition of Suspected Child Maltreatment[1,2,4,8,22]

How vulnerable is the child for further injury (age, nature of trauma, family characteristics/interaction)?

Is an alternative safe environment available for discharge?

Does the suspected perpetrator have access to the child in the home?

Is this the first episode of minor injury without indication of family instability or responsibility?

Is a concerned relative or friend available for family support?

Has the triggering event for the abusive episode been resolved?

Will the local child protection agency (or police) respond to the suspected abuse report within 24 hours of notification for home investigation?

Note: If any doubt exists, the child's safety must be of paramount concern. When safety cannot be ensured otherwise, short-term hospitalization can provide time for a more thorough evaluation and planning.

Question

Your role as a nurse in ensuring Sheralyn's safe disposition from the emergency department includes all of the following *except:* (Choose the exception.)

1. Active participation in ongoing assessments of the child and her family
2. Ensuring that pertinent information is shared among all members of the multidisciplinary team (including the physician, child protection agency workers, police, social workers, and the court as necessary)
3. Expressing your sympathy and concern to other family members about the father's possible maltreatment of Sheralyn
4. Providing explanations as necessary to assist team members in understanding the significance of the specific medical and psychosocial information gathered thus far

---

Answer

The exception is (3). This assumes guilt on the part of the father. Assessment, communication, and coordination activities are all extremely important nursing responsibilities in ensuring safe disposition of suspected child abuse cases.[8,14,15] Any concern expressed should be nonjudgmental and should include the entire family. Health care providers should avoid drawing conclusions about the case and taking sides with some family members against others because responsibility has not as yet been determined. It is now the task of law enforcement and mental health professionals to assure the child's safety, determine accountability, and provide necessary long-term counseling.

When the family is confronted with the abuse suspicions and informed of the need to hospitalize Sheralyn, her mother begins to cry softly. Mr. Dalton's posture becomes very stiff, and he glares at all of you. The baby's grandmother begins asking questions in a hostile manner including, "Who is to pay for all the tests and this hospital stay?" and "Why are *we* being accused of hurting the baby?" Dr. Martin quietly answers any questions that he can. You try to be empathetic and supportive, but you are beginning to feel overwhelmed by this family.

Question

The best response to the grandmother's hostile remarks would be to:
(Choose the best response.)

1. Focus your attention on Sheralyn and allow the grandmother to regain control of her emotions.
2. Have hospital security stand by until she has regained control of her emotions.
3. Acknowledge the grandmother's feelings, answer her questions, and point out your common concerns for Sheralyn's immediate needs.
4. Ask Sheralyn's mother to calm the child's grandmother down or send her home.

Answer

It would be best to acknowledge the grandmother's feelings, answering questions simply and honestly, and focusing on your common concerns for the child's immediate needs (see Table 9.8). These are the best approaches for working with families who are demonstrating behaviors reflective of intense emotions.[1,4,7,8] Focusing on Sheralyn tends to depersonalize the grandmother, and calling for security may escalate the situation. Asking other family members to help may cause divisiveness.

TABLE 9.8.   **Caring for Families Experiencing Child Maltreatment**[1,7,12,22,23]

Recognize that families may be seeking help for themselves as well as for the child.
Anticipate a wide range of emotional responses from families confronted with suspected child maltreatment.
Demonstrate a nonjudgmental attitude.
Avoid extremes of reactions in your responses (e.g., direct confrontation or simply ignoring the family).
Keep all discussions childfocused and nonaccusing.
Deescalate intense emotional reactions by focusing on your mutual concern for the child.
Give the parent simple, concrete instructions for things to do to help the child.
Avoid competition with the family for the child's attention or affection.
Emphasize the differences in responsibility between the hospital and the child protection agency.

The parents reluctantly agree to Sheralyn's admission. You are relieved that you did not need to get the police involved to prevent the parents from leaving against medical advise with the child. In your state, posthospitalization placement of the child is the responsibility of the physician and child protective services, and you know that you may help to assure appropriate decisions by accurately communicating your assessment findings. You quickly wonder if you have completed all of the necessary legal responsibilities for this case.

Question

The legal responsibilities associated with Sheralyn's care that are common to all U.S. jurisdictions include all of the following *except:* (Choose the exception.)

1. Supplying mandated reporting of suspicions of abuse to appropriate local agency
2. Maintaining detailed, objective documentation of the reasons for suspected abuse
3. Providing possible legal testimony if the case goes to court
4. Obtaining child abuse photographs

Answer

Obtaining child abuse photographs is not a responsibility in all jurisdictions. Although many local jurisdictions use photographs in suspected abuse cases, they are not legally admissible in all states and may not be allowable without parental consent.

All jurisdictions have a mandated child abuse reporting law that identifies nurses and other health care providers as "mandated reporters." These laws require mandated reporters to document and report the reasons for their suspicions, and to be available for potential legal testimony. In cases of unsubstantiated abuse, immunity from civil prosecution is generally given to any mandated reporter who files a suspected abuse report in good faith.[1,4,8,22,24]

Each local jurisdiction has unique legislation regarding child protection and the specific mechanisms for how to file the suspected child abuse report.[1,7,8,24,25] It is particularly important for the emergency nurse to become familiar with their own local laws and institutional policies (see Table 9.9, facing page).

For additional information regarding who to contact about your state's child protection legislation, call the **National Child Abuse Hotline, 1-800-422-5543**.

You wait with the Dalton family for the admitting nurse who will take Sheralyn upstairs. The child protection worker has brought crayons and paper to entertain Sheralyn until the nurse arrives. As you look at this family, you know what a long, difficult road lies ahead for them and how often this situation can tear a family apart. You hope that Sheralyn will find a way to cope with the many psychological and physical problems resulting from abuse, and that she and her family will be able to obtain the caring, empathetic, professional help so necessary to recover from this frightening situation.

TABLE 9.9. Legal Responsibilities: Suspected Child Maltreatment[1,4,7,8,22,24,26]

General requirements (common to all jurisdictions)	Specific requirements (per local jurisdictions)
Mandated reporting of suspected child maltreatment	Specific definition of "abuse" Specific agency to report to Specific information required in report Who should file the report and how
Mechanism for provision of immediate safe environment for child if parents refuse hospitalization	Specific agency to contact Specific provisions that can be made
Detailed objective documentation of reasons to suspect abuse	Specific forms for documentation Who may have access to medical records and written reports on suspected child abuse
Forensic evidence collection	How to collect and handle evidence What to collect (i.e., rape kits, photographs, tapes, etc.) Maintaining "Chain of Evidence" What is considered "legally admissible"?
Consents for treatment of minors No consent required for reporting child abuse suspicions	When are they required? Special provisions if consents are unavailable Who obtains the consents? Which form should be used?
Legal testimony by persons who filed the report of suspected abuse or witnessed the evidence of abuse suspicions	Who will be required to testify When and how testimony is given Who provides legal counsel to assist with preparation of court proceedings

CASE STUDY 2 OBJECTIVES

On completion of this second case study, you will be able to

- Choose interviewing techniques that promote child and family privacy, confidentiality of information, and family-centered care in cases of suspected sexual abuse
- List pertinent assessment findings in the recognition of suspected child sexual abuse
- List procedures and tests that are appropriate for verifying a diagnosis of sexual abuse
- Identify approaches for preparation of the child and the family for the sexual abuse examination
- Identify the functions and limitations of the nurse's role during the discharge interview process.
- Identify the legal requirements for reporting cases of sexual abuse

- Describe the psychosocial implications of disclosing sexual abuse
- Describe necessary discharge referrals for the child and the family with suspected child sexual abuse

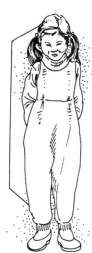

FIGURE 9.5

CASE STUDY 2

Gwyn Says Her Bottom's Itching

Seven-year-old Gwyn is brought to the emergency department on your evening shift after her mother returns home from work (see Figure 9.5). Gwyn's mother, Sharon Altman, seems reluctant to discuss her concerns with you in the public area of the desk. She indicates that she is worried about a discharge staining her daughter's panties, then stops talking and looks away from you. Gwyn is standing distanced from her mother and has not said anything at all. Her facial expression is strained and somewhat tense.

Question

At this point it would be most important to: (Choose one answer.)

1. Encourage Mrs. Altman to give you more specific information about Gwyn's problem
2. Note the information and wait to discuss the mother's concerns further in a more private setting
3. Ask Gwyn to give you a more detailed description of the discharge in her panties
4. None of the above

Answer

Because of the sensitive nature of the situation, it would be most appropriate to note the available information, but delay any potentially embarrassing questions until you are in a more private setting.[1–3] The child and family should be treated discreetly when in the triage area, and taken to a private location as soon as possible.

Once they are in an examination room, Gwyn's mother becomes more talkative. Gwyn has complained of vaginal itching for several days and now she has a discharge. The mother has applied vaseline to Gwyn's vaginal area but that hasn't helped much. Her mother asks you "What could have possibly caused such a nasty discharge in a child Gwyn's age? Is it true that bubble baths irritate little girl's bottoms?"

Question:

Possible causes for Gwyn's symptoms could include all of the following *except:* (Choose the exception.)

1. Pinworms
2. Systemic illnesses (i.e., chickenpox, measles)
3. Chemical irritants (i.e., powders, lotions, soaps)
4. Syphilis or gonorrhea transmitted from bedsheets, bathtubs, or public toilets

Answer

Although syphilis and gonorrhea can cause vulvovaginitis in children, there is no evidence that such infections are transmitted differently in children than they are in adults. Indirect contact with inanimate objects does *not* appear to be a mode of transmission for these sexually transmitted diseases.[4–6]

In addition to specific and nonspecific genital and pelvic infections, other possible etiologies for vulvovaginitis in the prepubertal child include pinworms, foreign bodies, polyps, tumors, systemic illnesses, vulvar skin diseases, atopic or allergic dermatitis, and traumatic injuries.[6]

The physician, Dr. Alan Phillips, has been reviewing Gwyn's old records and discovers a report of suspected abuse from 2 years prior. When you share the initial triage information, he decides that Gwyn should be carefully evaluated for signs of sexual abuse as a possible cause of her vulvovaginitis.

Question

A thorough physical examination is the most important means for determining whether Gwyn has been sexually abused. (Choose True or False.)

_____ True   _____ False

Answer

False. A thorough physical examination is not the most important means for determining sexual abuse (see Table 9.10). As with other types of suspected child maltreatment, physical examination findings must be interpreted in the context of the history and the presenting behaviors of the child and family.[1,2,3,5,7,8]

The only physical findings that can be considered as "proof" of sexual abuse in a prepubescent child are acquired syphilis, acquired gonorrhea, or sperm on a microscopic examination.[1,3,4,9,10] It is extremely important to note that *normal* physical examination findings are *common* in suspected sexual abuse and can only be used to rule out injury, not to invalidate historical or behavioral signs of abuse.[1,3,4,11]

TABLE 9.10. Indicators of Suspected Child Sexual Abuse[1,2,4,5,7,8,11]

Physical findings
Injuries to genitorectal area, breasts, thighs, buttocks, or lower abdomen
Genitorectal swelling, scars, or hyperpigmentation
Symptoms of sexually transmitted diseases
Pregnancy in young adolescents
Genital discharges or unusual odors
Torn, stained underclothing
Nonphysical findings
Direct or indirect disclosure of the possibility of abuse
Nonspecific physical complaints (e.g., pain, frequency of urination, difficulty sitting)
Inappropriate sexual behavior (e.g., excessive sexual curiosity or knowledge)
Abrupt behavioral changes
Somatic complaints (e.g., sleep disorders, enuresis)
Suicidal behavior or threats

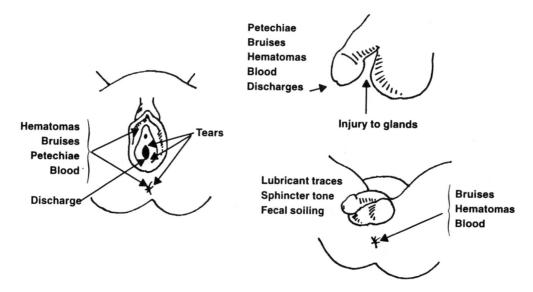

FIGURE 9.6 Physical findings suggestive of sexual abuse. Adapted with permission from Jones, Yamaouchi, & Lawson. (1987). , p. 9; Paul, D. M. (1975). The medical examination in sexual offenses. *Medicine, Science, and the Law, 15,* 154–162.

Question

To obtain the necessary cultures, determine the cause of Gwyn's vulvovaginitis, and evaluate Gwyn for signs of sexual abuse, it will be necessary for Dr. Phillips to perform a full pelvic examination including internal visualization with a speculum and a bimanual examination. (Choose True or False.)

_____ True   _____ False

Answer

False. A full pelvic examination is not necessary. In prepubescent girls, the sexual abuse examination is generally a thorough physical examination including a detailed visual inspection (with minimal manipulation) of the external genitalia.[1,4,12,13] Cultures are indicated when there is evidence of vulvovaginitis or to rule out sexually transmitted diseases.[1,3,4,13] "Rape" or "Sexual Assault" Kits may be necessary for forensic evidence collection if sexual contact has occurred within the past 72 hours and the child has not bathed (check your local abuse legislation.)[1,3,12,13] These procedures can usually be completed via external visualization and minimal manipulation of the genitalia.[3,4]

In prepubescent females, a full internal pelvic examination is unnecessary when

1. The external genitalia is without evidence of trauma or vaginal bleeding.
2. The hymen is intact.
3. A reliable account of the abuse rules out genital sexual contact.

In addition, pelvic instrumentation (e.g., use of speculums or otoscopes) should be avoided in prepubescent females. The vagina and cervix are visually inspected to the extent possible through the hymenal orifice for evidence of trauma. If the internal pelvic examination appears necessary because of bleeding or suspicion of traumatic injuries, it is preferable to postpone the examination and arrange for evaluation under general anesthesia.[1,3,4,12,13]

The thought of obtaining the necessary cultures and the genitorectal portion of the physical examination on Gwyn makes you uncomfortable. You realize that you're not exactly sure how to prepare Gwyn for the physical examination. What if Gwyn has been abused? How will she react to the procedures?

Question

Providing age-appropriate explanations will help Gwyn discriminate between a genital examination and the abusive act and will minimize her risk of additional emotional trauma. (Choose True or False.)

_____ True   _____ False

Answer

True. Giving age-appropriate explanations is often very helpful. In children who have been sexually abused, the genitorectal portion of the physical examination may be incorrectly perceived as similar to the abuse and equally as traumatic.[1,13,14] Careful preparation of the child (see Table 9.11) and the family is an important means of minimizing fears. Adequate preparation can prevent the need for sedation, cancellation of the examination, or the use of restraints. All of these options increase the risk of contributing to the child's sense of powerlessness.[13]

Children use information to solve problems and deal with their fears just as adults do. Therefore, children who are being evaluated for suspected sexual abuse need information about what will happen during the procedure, what sensations they are likely to experience during the procedure, and concrete suggestions for things they can do to feel "more comfortable" during the procedure.[13,15]

TABLE 9.11.   Preparation of the Child for the Sexual Abuse Examination[1,3,13,15,16]

Give explanations with the parent present while the child is still dressed
Use "matter-of-fact" approach and include all "head-to-toe" aspects of a physical examination
Use actual terms that the child uses to describe body parts
Introduce familiar procedures first (e.g., listening to the heart rate) and proceed to less familiar
Explain what sensations are likely (e.g., "this shouldn't hurt," "like someone pushing on you")
Teach the child deep breathing and controlled relaxation as means of coping with "unpleasant sensations"
Allow the child to "rehearse" the examination, handle equipment, and practice relaxation
Consider whether the young child will cope better if the parent is present for the examination

After you talk with Gwyn and her mother about the examination, you ensure that all the equipment and supplies that might be needed are in the room and easily accessible. Gwyn has already handled most of the equipment and is in a gown, covered with a sheet sitting up on the examination table when Dr. Phillips enters the room and introduces himself.

Question

Because Dr. Phillips has all the needed supplies and you have already completed your teaching with Gwyn and her family, the most appropriate use of your time now will be to: (Choose one answer.)

1. Go to the nurses' station to begin your documentation.
2. Begin your assessment on a new patient in another room.
3. Escort Mrs. Altman out of the room to ensure Gwyn's privacy.
4. Stay with Gwyn throughout the examination and help as necessary.

Answer

It is important for you to stay with Gwyn during the entire examination. During a suspected sexual abuse examination, it is necessary for the nurse to remain present in the room during the entire examination to avoid possible misinterpretation of the examination procedures by either the child or the parent.[1,3,13,14] The presence of a familiar caregiver may also help the child and the family cope with the examination procedures, decrease the discomfort of the examination, and ensure the success of the sexual abuse examination.[13,15] (Specific roles for the nurse in assisting with the sexual abuse examination are discussed further in Appendix F.)

Dr. Phillips performs the general physical examination. During the genitorectal portion of the examination, there are no external signs of trauma, but it is clear that some sort of irritant is present. The examination is apparently uncomfortable and Gwyn begins to squirm and to whine that she is "tired of this."

Question

Because Gwyn is losing control and is apparently unable to successfully complete the examination, your best approach at this time would be to (Choose one answer.)

1. Ask Dr. Phillips for an order to sedate her.
2. Call for help to temporarily restrain Gwyn then finish the examination as quickly as possible.
3. Schedule Gwyn for an immediate examination in the operating room under general anesthesia.
4. Stop momentarily until Gwyn rests and is able to use the relaxation techniques and participate again.

Answer

A pause may be helpful at this point. It is normal for any child to lose composure and temporarily regress in behavior under stress. A temporary delay will give Gwyn time to regain her composure while you reinforce your instructions on how to relax. Because the examination is causing discomfort, it is also important to prioritize the remaining parts and complete them as efficiently and quickly as possible.

The use of sedation or gentle restraint should be "last resorts" as they can contribute to an increased sense of powerlessness in an abused child, [13] and could also potentially alter the muscle tone and size of the vaginal orifice. With the absence of genital injuries, Gwyn's situation does not warrant the invasiveness of a full speculum examination under anesthesia. (For information about equipment that would be needed for a full sexual assault examination, see Appendix G.)

Once the examination is completed, Dr. Phillips confides in you that he suspects Gwyn has gonorrhea. He asks you to phone the on-call social worker to be present when he speaks with the mother. After she arrives, Dr. Phillips introduces her to Gwyn's mother and takes them to his office. He explains that Gwyn has a vaginal infection but that the exact type won't be known until the culture results are available in a couple of days. He also states that Gwyn can be started on antibiotics and sent home, but first he needs a little more information about the history of Gwyn's discharge and its likely cause.

Question

A primary purpose for this discussion with Gwyn's mother should be to gather enough information to determine whether Gwyn can be safely discharged home. (Choose True or False.)

_____ True   _____ False

Answer

True. More information would be helpful in determining whether Gwyn will be safe. As with other forms of child abuse, in suspected sexual abuse it is preferable to discharge the child home if the child's safety is ensured and there are no medical problems which warrant hospitalization. Before discharge, some effort must be made to determine the likelihood that the child will be safe from immediate harm at home.[1,4,13] (Review Table 9.7 for factors to consider in the safe disposition of suspected child abuse cases.)

While Dr. Phillips is talking with Gwyn's mother, you help Gwyn finish dressing and wait with her in the examining room for her mother. She appears to be more comfortable than she was earlier and begins to ask you questions about the equipment in the room.

Question

Because she is less anxious and you are in a private setting without her parent, should you use this time to directly question Gwyn for details about her suspected sexual abuse? (Choose Yes or No.)

_____ Yes   _____ No

Answer

No. It would not be appropriate for you to question Gwyn. The interview of a child for suspected sexual abuse has serious psychological and legal implications and is therefore best handled by specially trained professionals. Ideally the child should also not be asked to repeat the account of the abuse more than once. Therefore, unless the child's immediate safety is being jeopardized, the detailed interview of the child should generally be delayed until the professional with most experience in sexual abuse interviewing and counseling is available.[2,3,4,8]

Question

While you are alone with Gwyn, she suddenly makes the statement, "I know that my itchy bottom is because of the 'yucky' things that my brother Paul makes me do." (Indicate with an **X** any of the following which would be appropriate responses.)

_____ Listen attentively and document Gwyn's exact words.

_____ Allow Gwyn to tell the story in her own way, and do not press her for details.

_____ Ask Gwyn if the "yucky" things Paul did hurt her bottom.

_____ Tell Gwyn you are proud of her for telling you.

_____ Remind Gwyn that she really shouldn't talk like that.

Answer

The correct responses are to listen attentively and document Gwyn's exact words; allow Gwyn to tell the story in her own way and do not press her for details; and tell Gwyn you are proud of her for telling you.

Occasionally a child will spontaneously begin to disclose the details of an abusive episode. In such situations, the best approach is to listen attentively and allow the child to say things in his or her own way. Avoid any responses or questions that could provide "leading" information about how the child might feel or information about adult sexuality that the child doesn't already know. Also to be avoided are any responses that make the child feel guilty about the disclosure or at blame for what has happened.[1,2,3,13,14]

Gwyn's mother returns to the examining room and says that Dr. Phillips told her they could go home after all the paperwork is completed. You excuse yourself momentarily and join Dr. Phillips and the hospital social worker in the emergency department conference room and share the information Gwyn has just disclosed. You ask about the plan of care for Gwyn and whether or not the child protection agency needs to be called. Dr. Phillips says that filing the report needs to be delayed until the culture results confirm that Gwyn has gonorrhea.

Question

Your best response to Dr. Phillips's suggestion that the suspected abuse report be filed at a later time would be to: (Choose one answer.)

1. Recognize that he is ultimately responsible for all of Gwyn's care and not press the issue any further

2. Suggest that he talk to Gwyn and her mother again, and ask if she would like the report filed now or later

3. Remind Dr. Phillips that abuse suspicions need not be confirmed before a report is filed

4. Talk to the nursing supervisor at the end of the shift and let her file the report then if it is necessary

---

Answer

Dr. Phillips needs to be reminded that the *suspicion* of possible abuse is reason enough to file the report and that the report's purpose is to initiate a more thorough investigation to determine whether abuse has actually occurred.[3,4,7,14,17–19] In situations with disclosure, it is especially important to begin the investigation as soon as possible to determine if the perpetrator poses further risk to the child.

In the event that team members disagree, the nurse is still legally obligated as a mandated reporter to file a report if there is a reasonable suspicion of abuse.[7,17,19,20] Contact with the appropriate child protection agency as soon as possible also facilitates involvement of all of the appropriate multidisciplinary team members in the family's discharge and follow-up care.[1,9,13,21] If in doubt, it is never wrong to call the local child protection agency for help in deciding how to handle a particular situation.

Based on your concerns, the social worker makes a call to the child protective agency. In addition, she offers to talk with Gwyn's mother to determine if Gwyn is at risk of further contact with her brother if she is discharged home.

Question

Should Gwyn's mother be told about mandated sexual abuse reporting and the possibility that they will be contacted by a child protection worker for further information? (Choose Yes or No.)

_____ Yes   _____ No

Answer

Yes. Gwyn's mother should be informed. If there are reasons to suspect abuse, these should be concisely summarized for the family (e.g., "because of Gwyn's age, the possibility that she has a sexually transmitted disease . . .," and "Gwyn's comments about her brother . . ."). Then the family may be told that it is required by law that suspicious findings be reported for further investigation.[1,3,7]

After an emotional discussion with Gwyn's mother, it is determined that the brother in question is in the navy and is no longer in the home. Because Gwyn's mother appears to believe the child and be supportive, the decision is made that Gwyn can be safely discharged home.

While completing Gwyn's discharge paperwork, Dr. Phillips discusses the following home care instructions with Gwyn and her mother:

- The family will be contacted with the results of Gwyn's tests and any further instructions for her care in 2 to 3 days.

- Gwyn should be seen again within 1 week by Dr. Phillips to reevaluate the infection and her continuing health care needs and to arrange for psychosocial counseling as necessary.

- Mrs. Altman should make certain that Gwyn takes all of the medication as prescribed, keep the child's perineal area clean and dry, and maintain Gwyn's normal routines and activities.

- Either the hospital social worker or a local child protection agency will be in contact with the family, probably within the next 24 hours.

- The social worker will be available to assist with arrangements for professional psychosocial counseling for the family if necessary.

Question

Emergency department management priorities for suspected child sexual abuse should focus on prompt diagnosis, humane treatment of presenting illnesses or injuries, and ensuring that appropriate referrals are made for continuing care. (Choose True or False.)

_____ True   _____ False

Answer

This statement is True. The primary goals of sexual abuse management in the emergency department are to identify and report the abuse, to avoid any additional secondary trauma associated with the examination or disclosure, to manage presenting physical and psychological problems, to ensure the child's immediate safety, and to provide the abuse victim and the family with referrals for long-term care (see Table 9.12, following page).[1,10,12,13,22]

You review the discharge instructions and give Gwyn's mother a clinic appointment card along with the emergency department phone number. You walk the Altmans to the door, say good-bye, and remind the mother to call if she needs anything. As you return to the desk, you take one last look at the child and her mother. If Gwyn really is a victim of sexual abuse, you can't help wondering how things will turn out for this family.

TABLE 9.12.   Emergency Management of Suspected Child Sexual Abuse[1,4,10,12,13,16]

1. Assess, prioritize, and treat presenting injuries and illnesses

2. Assess child's safety and ensure protection

3. Adequately prepare the child and the family for all procedures

4. Initiate treatment as indicated for

    a. Sexually transmitted disease prophylaxis and treatment

    b. Pregnancy prevention

    c. Acute psychosocial problems

5. Provide support and reassurance to the child and the family

6. Initiate multidisciplinary discharge and follow-up care plans

    a. Ensure safe disposition

    b. Complete legal responsibilities and documentation

    c. Arrange child and family community referrals

    d. Discharge and follow-up teaching for continuity of care

    e. Follow-up appointments for medical and psychosocial care needs within 1–2 weeks

---

Question

The reaction of Gwyn's mother to the disclosure of sexual abuse will be almost as significant as the abusive incident in the child's subsequent long-term psychological outcome. (Choose True or False.)

_____ True   _____ False

Answer

The correct answer is True. All abuse victims face the risk of long-term psychological sequelae as a result of their experiences. However, the best psychological outcome for sexually abused children is most likely when parents can work through their initial reactions and show concern for the child in ways that demonstrate acceptance and approval of the child's behavior and disclosure. In addition, parents should acknowledge that the child is without blame for what has happened, be willing to protect the child from further abuse, and try to resume as normal a lifestyle as possible.[1,7,13] (For more information on working with parents of child sexual abuse victims, refer to Appendix H.)

ACKNOWLEDGMENTS

The authors would like to acknowledge the editorial contributions of members of the Central Arkansas ENA Chapter, David Holman, BSN, CEN, and Carolyn Adcock of the Arkansas EMS for Children Project; and Mary Lou Smith, PhD, of the ACH Nursing Education Department. In addition, we truly appreciate the support, guidance, encouragement, and endless patience of Debra H. Fiser, MD, UAMS, Department of Pediatrics, Division of Critical Care Medicine; Rhonda M. Dick, MD, Division of Emergency Medicine; Jerry Jones, MD, Children at Risk Program; and Ella Christopher, BSN, ACH Division of Nursing.

REFERENCES

Case Study 1

1. Ludwig, S. (1988). Psychosocial emergencies: Child abuse. In G. Fleisher & S. Ludwig (Eds.), *Textbook of pediatric emergency medicine* (2nd ed., pp. 1127–1163). Baltimore: Williams & Wilkins.
2. Scherb, B. J. (1988). Suspected abuse and neglect of children. *Journal of Emergency Nursing, 14,* 44–47.
3. National Committee for Injury Prevention and Control (B. Guyer chairperson). (1989). Child abuse. In *Injury prevention: Meeting the challenge.* New York: Oxford, pp 213–222.
4. Kerns, D. L. (1985). Child abuse. In T. A. Mayer (Ed.), *Emergency management of pediatric trauma* (pp. 421–434). Philadelphia: Saunders.
5. Kelley, S. J. (1985). Interviewing the sexually abused child: Principles and techniques. *Journal of Emergency Nursing, 11,* 234–241.
6. Ricci, L. R. (1986). Child sexual abuse: The emergency department response. *Annals of Emergency Medicine, 15,* 711–716.
7. Whaley, L. F., & Wong, D. L. (1987). Health problems of early childhood. In *Nursing care of infants and children* (2nd ed., pp. 681–700). St. Louis: Mosby.
8. Kelley, S. J. (1988). Child abuse and neglect. In S. J. Kelley (Ed.), *Pediatric emergency nursing* (pp. 1–26). Norwalk, CT: Appleton & Lange.
9. Mittleman, R. E., Mittleman, H. S., & Wetli, C. V. (1987). What child abuse really looks like. *American Journal of Nursing, 87,* 1185A–6B, 1199D, 1199F.
10. Levinson, R. M., Graves, W. L., & Holcombe, J. (1984). Cross-cultural variations in the definition of child abuse: Nurses in the United States and the United Kingdom. *International Journal of Nurising Studies, 21,* 35–44.
11. Bittner, S., & Newberger, E. (1981). Understanding child abuse and neglect. *Pediatrics in Review, 2,* 197–207.
12. Bourg, P., Sherer, C., & Rosen, P. (1986). Child abuse: Nonaccidental trauma. In *Standardized nursing care plans for emergency departments* (pp. 197–202). St. Louis: Mosby.
13. Dennis, L. I. (1988). Adolescent rape: The role of nursing. *Issues in Comprehensive Pediatric Nursing, 11,* 59–70.
14. Mundie, G. E. (1984). Team management of the maltreated child in the emergency room. *Pediatric Annals, 13,* 771–776.
15. Muchlinski, E., Boonstra, C., & Johnson, J. (1989). Planning and implementing a pediatric sexual assault evidentiary examination program. *Journal of Emergency Nursing, 15,* 249–255.
16. Krowchuk, H. V. (1989). Child abuser stereotypes: Consensus among clinicians. *Applied Nursing Research, 2,* 35–39.
17. George, J. E., & Quattrone, M. S. (1988). Reporting child abuse: Duties and dangers. *Journal of Emergency Nursing, 14,* 34–35.
18. Tammelleo, A. D. (1988). If you suspect child abuse. *RN, 51,* 57–59.
19. Anderson, C. L. (1987). Assessing parenting potential for child abuse risk. *Pediatric Nursing, 13,* 323–327.
20. Finkelhor, D. (1984). *Child sexual abuse* (pp. 54–61). New York: Free Press.
21. DeJong, A. R. (1988). Maternal responses to the sexual abuse of their children. *Pediatrics, 81,* 14–20.
22. Stanley, S. R. (1989). Child sexual abuse: Recognition and nursing intervention. *Orthopedic Nursing, 8,* 33–40.
23. Leatherland, J. (1986). Do you know child abuse when you see it? *RN, 49,* 28–30.
24. DeJong, A. R., Emans, S. J., & Goldfarb, A. (1989). Sexual abuse: What you must know. *Patient Care, 23,* 145–148, 151, 155-158.
25. Rhodes, A. M. (1987). The nurse's legal obligations for reporting child abuse. *MCN, 12,* 313.
26. Rhodes, A. M. (1987). Identifying and reporting child abuse. *MCN, 12,* 399.

Case Study 2

1. Ludwig, S. (1988). Psychosocial emergencies: Child abuse. In G. Fleisher & S. Ludwig (Eds.), *Textbook of pediatric emergency medicine* (2nd ed., pp. 1127–1163). Baltimore: Williams & Wilkins.
2. Kelley, S. J. (1985). Interviewing the sexually abused child: Principles and techniques. *Journal of Emergency Nursing, 11,* 234–241.

3. DeJong, A. R., Emans, S. J., & Goldfarb, A. (1989). Sexual abuse: What you must know. *Patient Care, 23*, 145–148, 151, 155–158.

4. Ricci, L. R. (1986). Child sexual abuse: The emergency department response. *Annals of Emergency Medicine, 15*, 711–716.

5. Whaley, L. F., & Wong, D. L. (1987). Health Problems of Early Childhood. In *Nursing care of infants and children* (2nd ed., pp. 681–700). St. Louis: Mosby.

6. Emans, S. J. (1986). Vulvovaginitis in the child and adolescent. *Pediatrics in Review, 8*, 12–19

7. Stanley, S. R. (1989). Child sexual abuse: Recognition and nursing intervention. *Orthopedic Nursing, 8*, 33–40.

8. Sgori, S. M., Porter, F. S., & Blick, L. C. (1982). Validation of child sexual abuse. In S. M. Sgori, F. S. Porter, & L. C. Blick (Eds.), *Handbook of clinical intervention in child sexual abuse* (pp. 39–79). Lexington, MA: Lexington Books.

9. Bittner, S., & Newberger, E. (1981). Understanding child abuse and neglect. *Pediatrics in Review, 2*, 197–207.

10. Jones, J. G. (1982). Sexual abuse of children: Current concepts. *American Journal of Diseases of Children, 136*, 142–146.

11. Emans, S. J., et al. (1987). Genital findings in sexually abused, symptomatic, and asymptomatic girls. *Pediatrics, 79*, 778–785.

12. Muchlinski, E., Boonstra, C., & Johnson, J. (1989). Planning and implementing a pediatric sexual assault evidentiary examination program. *Journal of Emergency Nursing, 15*, 249–255.

13. Jones, J. G., Yamaouchi, T., & Lawson, L. (1987). *Physician's guide to the evaluation and management of sexually abused children.* Little Rock: Arkansas Children's Hospital.

14. Kelley, S. (1988). Professionals' attitudes toward child sexual abuse. *Nursing Times, 84*, 56.

15. Lawson, L. (1987). Preparation of sexually abused children for genitorectal examination. *Clinical Research, 35*, 62A.

16. Kelley, S. J. (1988). Sexual abuse of children. In S. J. Kelley (Ed.), *Pediatric Emergency Nursing* (pp. 27–51). Norwalk, CT: Appleton & Lange.

17. Bourg, P., Sherer, C., & Rosen, P. (1986). Child abuse: Nonaccidental trauma. In *Standardized nursing care plans for emergency departments* (pp. 197–202). St. Louis: Mosby.

18. George, J. E., & Quattrone, M. S. (1988). Reporting child abuse: Duties and dangers. *Journal of Emergency Nursing, 14*, 34–35.

19. Tammelleo, A. D. (1988). If you suspect child abuse. *RN, 51*, 57–59.

20. Rhodes, A. M. (1987). The nurse's legal obligations for reporting child abuse. *MCN, 12*, 313.

21. Mundie, G. E. (1984). Team management of the maltreated child in the emergency room. *Pediatric Annals, 13*, 771–776.

22. Mittleman, R. E., et al. (1987). What child abuse really looks like. *American Journal of Nursing, 87*, 1185A–1186B, 1199D, 1199F.

SUGGESTED READINGS

Recognition and Management of Pediatric Abuse

1. Anderson, C. L. (1987). Assessing parenting potential for child abuse risk. *Pediatric Nursing, 13*, 323–327.

2. Barkin, R. M., & Rosen, P. (Eds.). (1984). *Emergency pediatrics.* St. Louis: Mosby.

3. Bittner, S., & Newberger, E. (1981). Understanding child abuse and neglect. *Pediatrics in Review, 2*, 197–207.

4. Bourg, P., Sherer, C., & Rosen, P. (1986). Child abuse: Nonaccidental trauma. In *Standardized nursing care plans for emergency departments* (pp. 197–202). St. Louis: Mosby.

5. Bryan, J. (1988). *Detecting and reporting suspected child abuse.* Little Rock, AR: Arkansas Child Sexual Abuse Education Commission.

6. Cohen, S. A. (1982). *Pediatric emergency management: Guidelines for rapid diagnosis and therapy.* Maryland: Brady.

7. Crittenden, P. M., & Morrison, A. K. (1988). An early parental indicator of potential maltreatment. *Pediatric Nursing, 14*, 415–417.

8. DeJong, A. R. (1988). Maternal responses to the sexual abuse of their children. *Pediatrics, 81*, 14–20.

9. DeJong, A. R., Emans, S. J., & Goldfarb, A. (1989). Sexual abuse: What you must know. *Patient Care, 23,* 145–148, 151, 155–158.

10. Dennis, L. I. (1988). Adolescent rape: The role of nursing. *Issues in Comprehensive Pediatric Nursing, 11,* 59–70.

11. Emans, S. J. (1986). Vulvovaginitis in the child and adolescent. *Pediatrics in Review, 8,* 12–19.

12. Emans, S. J., et al. (1987). Genital findings in sexually abused, symptomatic, and asymptomatic girls. *Pediatrics, 79,* 778–785.

13. Eisenberg, N., Owens, R. G., & Dewey, M. E. (1987). Attitudes of health professionals to child sexual abuse and incest. *Child Abuse and Neglect, 11,* 109–116.

14. Fillmore, A. (1987). Sexual molestation of children: Becoming aware. *Health Visit, 60,* 325–327.

15. Finkelhor, D. (1984). *Child Sexual Abuse* (pp. 54–61). New York: Free Press.

16. Fleisher, G., & Ludwig, S. (Eds.). (1988). *Textbook of pediatric emergency medicine* (2nd ed.). Baltimore: Williams & Wilkins.

17. Flynn, E. M. (1987). Preventing and diagnosing sexual abuse in children. *Nurse Practitioner, 12,* 47, 51–52, 54.

18. George, J. E., & Quattrone, M. S. (1988). Reporting child abuse: Duties and dangers. *Journal of Emergency Nursing, 14,* 34–35.

19. Helfer, R. E., & Kempe, C. H. (1980). *The Battered Child* (3rd ed.). Chicago: University of Chicago Press.

20. Herman-Giddens, M. E., & Frothingham, T. E. (1987). Prepubertal female genitalia: Examination for evidence of sexual abuse. *Pediatrics, 80,* 203–208.

21. Hodge, D. III, & Ludwig, S. (1985). Child homicide: Emergency department recognition. *Pediatric Emergency Care, 1,* 3–6.

22. Hosch, I. A. (1987). Munchausen syndrome by proxy . . . parent fabricates an illness to make their child appear unhealthy. *MCN, 12,* 48–52.

23. Johnson, C. F., et al. (1986). Child abuse diagnosis and the emergency department chart. *Pediatric Emergency Care, 2,* 6–9.

24. Jones, J. G. (1982). Sexual abuse of children: Current concepts. *American Journal of Disease in Children, 136,* 142–146.

25. Jones, J. G., Yamaouchi, T., & Lawson, L. (1987). *Physician's guide to the evaluation and management of sexually abused children.* Little Rock: Arkansas Children's Hospital.

26. Kelley, S. (1988). Professionals' attitudes toward child sexual abuse. *Nursing Times, 84,* 56.

27. Kelley, S. J. (1985). Interviewing the sexually abused child: Principles and techniques. *Journal of Emergency Nursing, 11,* 234–241.

28. Kelley, S. J. (1988). Child abuse and neglect. In S. J. Kelley (Ed.), *Pediatric Emergency Nursing* (pp. 1–26). Norwalk, CT: Appleton & Lange.

29. Kelley, S. J. (1988). Physical abuse of children: Recognition and reporting. *Journal of Emergency Nursing, 14,* 82–90.

30. Kelley, S. J. (1988). Sexual abuse of children. In S. J. Kelley, *Pediatric Emergency Nursing* (pp. 27–51). Norwalk, CT: Appleton & Lange.

31. Kelley, S. J. (1988). *Pediatric Emergency Nursing.* Norwalk, CT: Appleton & Lange.

32. Kerns, D. L. (1985). Child Abuse. In T. A. Mayer (Ed.), *Emergency management of pediatric trauma* (pp. 421–434). Philadelphia: Saunders.

33. Kottmeier, P. K. (1987). The battered child. *Pediatric Annals, 16,* 343–351.

34. Krowchuk, H. V. (1989). Child abuser stereotypes: Consensus among clinicians. *Applied Nursing Research, 2,* 35–39.

35. Lawson, L. (1987). Preparation of sexually abused children for genitorectal examination. *Clinical Research, 35,* 62A.

36. Leatherland, J. (1986). Do you know child abuse when you see it? *RN, 49,* 28–30.

37. Levin, A. V. (1987). Child abuse: Challenges and controversies. *Pediatric Emergency Care, 3,* 211–217.

38. Levinson, R. M., Graves, W. L., & Holcombe, J. (1984). Cross-cultural variations in the definition of child abuse: Nurses in the United States and the United Kingdom. *International Journal of Nursing Studies, 21,* 35–44.

39. Ludwig, S. (Ed). (1988). Psychosocial Emergencies: Child Abuse. In G. Fleisher & S. Ludwig (Eds.). *Textbook of pediatric emergency medicine* (2nd ed., pp. 1127–1163). Baltimore: Williams & Wilkins.

40. Mittleman, R. E., et al. (1987). What child abuse really looks like. *American Journal of Nursing, 87*, 1185A–1186B, 1199D, 1199F.

41. Mott, S. R., Fazekas, N. F., & James, S. R. (Eds.). (1985). *Nursing care of children and families: A holistic approach*. Menlo Park, CA: Addison-Wesley.

42. Muchlinski, E., Boonstra, C., & Johnson, J. (1989). Planning and implementing a pediatric sexual assault evidentiary examination program. *Journal of Emergency Nursing, 15*, 249–255.

43. Mundie, G. E. (1984). Team management of the maltreated child in the emergency room. *Pediatric Annals, 13*, 771–776.

44. National Committee for Injury Prevention and Control (B. Guyer, Chairperson). (1989). Child Abuse. In *Injury prevention: Meeting the challenge* (pp. 213–222). New York: Oxford Press.

45. Owens, R. (1988). Pediatric Trauma: The basics. In *Children are different: A supplemental course text to pediatric advanced life support* (pp. 40–41). Little Rock: University of Arkansas Medical School.

46. Rhodes, A. M. (1987). Identifying and reporting child abuse. *MCN, 12*, 399.

47. Rhodes, A. M. (1987). The nurse's legal obligations for reporting child abuse. *MCN, 12*, 313.

48. Ricci, L. R. (1986). Child sexual abuse: The emergency department response. *Annals of Emergency Medicine, 15*, 711–716.

49. Rivara, F. P., Kametsuka, K. M., & Quan, L. (1988). Injuries to children younger than 1 year of age. *Pediatrics, 81*, 93–97.

50. Rodriquez-Trias, H. (1983, January). Abused or neglected children in the emergency department. *Topics in Emergency Medicine, 4*, 51–56.

51. Scherb, B. J. (1988). Suspected abuse and neglect of children. *Journal of Emergency Nursing, 14*, 44–47.

52. Sgori, S. M., Porter, F. S., & Blick, L. C. (1982). Validation of child sexual abuse. In S. M. Sgori, F. S. Porter, & L. C. Blick (Eds.), *Handbook of clinical intervention in child sexual abuse* (pp. 39–79). Lexington, MA: Lexington Books.

53. Stanley, S. R. (1989). Child sexual abuse: Recognition and nursing intervention. *Orthopedic Nursing, 8*, 33–40.

54. Sykes, M. K., Hodges, M. C., Brooms, M., & Thereatt, B. J. (1987). Nurse's knowledge of child abuse and nurses' attitude toward parental participation in the abused child's care. *Journal of Pediatric Nursing, 2*, 412–417.

55. Tammelleo, A. D. (1988). If you suspect child abuse. *RN, 51*, 57–59.

56. U.S. Department of Health, Education and Welfare. (1978). *Federal standards for child abuse and neglect: Prevention and treatment programs and projects* (Publication No. 105-76-1190). Washington, DC: Office of Human Development Services.

57. U.S. Department of Health and Human Services. (1984). *National study on child abuse and neglect*. Denver: American Humane Association.

58. Whaley, L. F., & Wong, D. L. (1987). Health problems of early childhood. In *Nursing care of infants and children* (2nd ed., pp. 681–700). St. Louis: Mosby.

59. Whitehead, P., et al. (1987). NAPNAP policy statement on child abuse and neglect. *Journal of Pediatric Health Care, 1*, 42.

60. Wong, D. L. (1987). False allegations of child abuse: The other side of the tragedy. *Pediatric Nursing, 13*, 329–333.

APPENDIX A

Child Maltreatment Incidence and Demographics[4]

- Available statistics are from suspected child abuse reports
- All child maltreatment statistics are questionable due to
  - Variations in reporting requirements
  - Massive underreporting
  - Unsubstantiated reports
- Best estimate of actual annual U.S. incidence
  - 1.5 million (25.2/1000) children are victims of abuse
    - Neglect = 63%
    - Physical, emotional, or sexual abuse = 47%
- Most commonly *reported* type of abuse
  - Physical abuse
- Fastest growing type of abuse:
  - Sexual abuse (estimated 200,000 cases annually)
- Most commonly occurring types of abuse
  - Emotional abuse
  - Neglect
- An estimated 10% of patients < 5 years old who present to emergency departments for injuries are child abuse victims.
- Substantiated child abuse incidence rates show no significant differences for
  - Males vs. females
  - African Americans vs. whites
  - Urban vs. rural populations
- Abuse reporting is biased with overreporting of ethnic or racial minorities and economically disadvantaged.

APPENDIX B
Diagnostic Tests Associated with Suspected Child Maltreatment[1,5,7,8,11,21,29]

Laboratory studies	Comments—Rationale
CBC	
Hct, Hbg	Rules out shock; anemia
	Rules out organic cause for bruising or bleeding
Coagulation Studies	
PT, PTT, platelets	Elevated levels may be the first indicator of abdominal injury
	Elevated levels are indicative of extensive soft tissue and muscle injury
Serum	
Amylase	Rules out STD, all ages, suspected sexual abuse
CPK	
Syphilis serology	Rules out pregnancy, all postmenarche girls with history suggesting sexual abuse
HCG	Rules out forced or voluntary ingestions and chemical abuse
Toxicology screen	Rules out renal trauma, dehydration, ingestions, sexual abuse
Urine	
RBCs, specific gravity, toxicology screen, culture, pregnancy test, Sperm	Culture for gonorrhea, chlamydia, and other STDs is especially important with suspected sexual abuse
	Microscopic examination for sperm; may be omitted if > 72 hr since abuse incident or child has bathed
Cultures	
Wounds, Throat, Vaginal, Rectal	
Vaginal secretions	Trichomonas, yeast, or gardnerella infections
Vaginal wet prep	
(saline and KOH) with whiff test	
Radiology studies	
Skeletal x-rays; skull, ribs, extremities	Rules out fractures, common findings are multiple fractures of varying ages
Bone scans	Detects remote injury and extremely recent injuries
Ultrasound, CT scans, MRI	Important in determining subtle intracranial and internal abdominal injuries

APPENDIX C
Risk Factors Associated with Child Maltreatment[1,3,4,11,19–21]

- Sociocultural influences
  - Perception of family sanctity
  - Values and norms about discipline, punishment
- Family conditions
  - Poverty, unemployment
  - Crowded living conditions
  - Absent extended families
  - Single biologic parent
  - Chronic stress situations
  - Poor family relationships
  - Violence common in family interaction
- Parent traits
  - Lack of parenting knowledge
  - Unrealistic expectations of children
  - History of abuse as a child
  - Difficulty controlling impulses (anger, etc.)
  - Low self-esteem
  - Alcohol, drug abuse
  - Character or psychiatric disorders
- Child characteristics
  - Real or imagined "difficult" temperament
  - Handicapping conditions
  - Chronic health problems
  - Developmental delays
  - Nonbiologic offspring
  - Behavioral idiosyncracies
  - Physical idiosyncracies
  - Vulnerability (i.e., size, age, temperament)
  - Poor bonding with parent
- Triggering events
  - Difficulties in normal child rearing (e.g., potty-training)
  - Sudden changes in family lifestyle (job loss)
  - Arguments, family conflict
  - Acute alcohol or drug abuse

APPENDIX D
Child Maltreatment Mortality & Morbidity Facts[1,3,4]

- Population at greatest risk
  - Birth to 5 years (75% of fatalities are < 1 year old)
  - Children with history of previous abuse
- Mortality causes
  - Neglect accounts for approximately 50% of all reported deaths from child maltreatment.
  - Physical abuse accounts for 47% of reported child maltreatment deaths.
  - Child homicide: One of the five leading causes of death in childhood; accounts for 1 of 20 deaths in children < 18 years.
- Most common fatal injuries
  - CNS injuries: leading cause of death from physical abuse.
  - Abdominal injuries: second leading cause of death from physical abuse.
- Types of associated morbidity
  - Growth and developmental delays
  - Physical and mental disability
  - Motor and sensory impairments
  - Serious psychological disability
  - Suicide
  - Drug, alcohol abuse
  - Socially disruptive behavior
- Societal consequences
  - Eighty percent of juvenile offenders report being victims of abuse.
  - Intergenerational tendency of abuse: Abuse victims are 6 times more likely to abuse their own children.
  - Estimated costs: $500 million annually in therapeutic costs.
  - Estimated costs: $600 million annually for foster care or juvenile detention.
  - Estimated annual loss of 93,000 years of potential life and productivity because of child homicides, translating to annual income loss of $1.2 billion.
  - Inestimable cost in human suffering.

APPENDIX E
Nursing Diagnoses: Child Maltreatment[2,3,12]

- Emergent (Lifethreatening)
  - Potential for, or actual alteration in airway patency related to trauma, altered mental status
  - Potential for, or actual alteration in ventilation related to neuromuscular, or skeletal impairment
  - Potential for, or actual alteration in ventilation related to pain, anxiety, decreased energy or fatigue
  - Potential for, or actual decrease in cardiovascular output related to hypovolemic state (hemorrhage, dehydration)
  - Potential for, or actual fluid volume deficit related to active loss (hemorrhage, diarrhea, vomiting), inadequate intake (malnutrition)
  - Potential for, or actual alteration in safety of child's environment related to suspected child abuse
- Urgent
  - Potential for, or actual alterations in comfort (pain) related to injury
  - Potential for, or actual ineffective coping with anxiety related to crisis situation
- Follow-up (Long-term care, discharge planning)
  - Potential for, or actual alterations in child, family psychosocial health related to ineffective coping mechanisms, inadequate support systems, ineffective interaction patterns and role behaviors, or disturbances in self-concept
  - Potential for, or actual parental knowledge deficit regarding child development and care
  - Potential for, or actual alterations in normal growth and development related to abuse

APPENDIX F
Assisting with the Genitorectal Examination: Suspected Child Sexual Abuse[29]

Essential steps	Comments—rationale
Assemble supplies and equipment as necessary.	High-quality examination light, Wood's lamp, nonsterile examination gloves, disposable paper, measuring strips, nonbacteriostatic normal saline, Rape Kit (or laboratory supplies for culture and specimen collection).
Complete patient and family teaching to insure adequate preparation for the procedure.	To decrease risks of additional psychological trauma or altering of the physical findings (constriction or relaxation of vaginal orifice musculature), it is preferable to complete the examination with minimal use of sedation or restraints.
Ensure patient and family privacy.	Maintain two familiar staff members in the room; a parent may be allowed to stay if it is helpful to the child.
Assist as necessary with the normal pediatric physical examination of the head, neck, chest, abdomen and extremities.	To rule out injuries to other body systems and avoid attention being focused on the genitorectal aspect of the examination, a thorough head-to-toe physical examination is always indicated in suspected sexual abuse.
Assist the child into a position of comfort during the genitorectal portion of the examination that will maximize visualization of the external genitalia.	Stirrups are generally unnecessary for prepubertal girls. The "frog-leg" position, knees bent and turned outward and heels together may be assumed by the school-aged child lying supine on the examination table with the head raised slightly to maximize comfort. In infants, toddlers, or preschoolers, the position can be maintained with minimal restraint while the child is sitting in the mother's lap.
Ensure adequate lighting for direct visualization of the external genitalia.	An optical visor with a magnification of 2× and focal length of 10 inches is ideal for this purpose.
Assist as necessary to maintain the child's position while the examiner observes for perineal injuries.	Most genital injuries in females involve the labia majora, posterior fourchette, perihymenal area, or hymen.
Before obtaining cultures or proceeding to a more invasive examination, assist with the measurement of the hymenal orifice in prepubertal females.	Once the labia are gently spread, there should be a pause to allow the hymenal orifice to dilate maximally as the child relaxes. While slight lateral traction is maintained, the nurse positions a small disposable paper measuring strip with 1mm increment markings laterally over the hymen. The examiner gives directions for movement of the strip until it is centered correctly and notes the diameter of the hymenal orifice. (To avoid unintentional "paper cuts" to the genital area, the edges of the disposable measuring strip should be moistened slightly with nonbacteriostatic saline before use.
In postmenarcheal girls where clinically indicated, assist as necessary with the internal pelvic examination.	In prepubertal girls, with hymen intact, vaginal bleeding absent, and external vulva without evidence of major trauma, the internal pelvic examination is unnecessary. If the internal pelvic examination appears necessary due to bleeding or suspicion of internal pelvic injuries, it is preferable to postpone the examination and arrange for exploration and surgical repair under general anesthesia. In all prepubertal girls, pelvic instrumentation, including the use of speculums or otoscopes, should be avoided. Inspect the vagina and cervix visually to the extent possible through the hymenal orifice for evidence of vaginal wall trauma (bruising) or evidence of penetration into the rectum or abdomen.

APPENDIX F (Continued)

Essential steps	Comments—rationale
For both male and female patients, assist child into a position of comfort to maximize visualization of the rectal, anal area.	The "frog-leg" position previously described or lying on the side with knees bent and tucked up against the child's chest. Observations are made for loss of normal reflex tightening of anal sphincter or anal gaping and for the presence of tears, hematomas, fissures, or skin tags. When there is reason to suspect recent sexual contact (< 1 day), in the presence of anal gaping or suspected rectal or anal injuries, a digital rectal examination for sphincter tone may be performed. If external perianal trauma or bleeding is present, or if instrumentation and more invasive procedures (e.g., anoscopy or colonoscopy) are indicated, they are generally postponed until the child is taken to the operating room or under controlled circumstances under anesthesia.
As specified by local policy and child's clinical situation, assist with obtaining photographs of any external genitorectal injuries.	The use of photographs requires a signed parental consent form. For photographs to be of any value, photographic equipment of at least 35mm is generally required. Photographic processing should be completed in such a way as to maintain confidentiality of patient information.
As specified by local policy and child's clinical situation, assist with obtaining specimens for laboratory studies to confirm sexual activity, check for infection, and help support the child's identification of the abuser.	The least invasive procedures should be done first. More invasive and painful procedures should be done last with the child appropriately informed and supported. "Sexual Assault Kit" may be omitted if: it has been > 3 days since the abuse occurred; a highly reliable history of the type of sexual activity precludes the presence of evidence; or the child has bathed or douched. Cultures commonly done for gonorrhea and chlamydia; local institutional and public health infectious disease guidelines should be used to determine local requirements; culture sites; vaginal orifice (urethra in boys), rectum, oropharynx; moisten swabs with sterile nonbacteriostatic normal saline to decrease discomfort. Chlamydia culture may cause discomfort, so it should be done last. Use sterile wire or plastic (not wood) swab with a dacron (not cotton) tip, introduce into cervical canal (or vaginal orifice) and rotate with slight pressure to obtain cellular material. Avoid culturing discharge as the organism is likely to be found only in cellular material abraded onto the swab.
Assist the child to straighten legs, sit up and complete the remainder of the examination.	
Praise the child for participating so well. Tell the child as soon as possible that the examination is complete.	Avoid criticisms of the child's behavior during the examination.
Assist the child to dress and be comfortable.	
Label any specimens and assure appropriate handling and delivery to laboratory or designated area for forensic evidence.	
Maintain local infectious disease guidelines for disposal of supplies and disinfection of equipment.	
Complete documentation per local requirements.	

APPENDIX G
Sexual Assault Kit Equipment and Supplies[29]

Purpose	Equipment	Consumable supplies
Physical examination	Optical Visor (2 × magnification) Wood's Lamp Fiberoptic light source	Nonsterile examination gloves Disposable 1-cm measuring strips marked in 1 mm

Cultures and smears		**Chlamydia**
		   Chlamydia transport medium
		   Rayon culturette with *non-wooden* shaft
		 Gonorrhea
		   Charcoal transport medium
		   Minitip culturette for vaginal and penile cultures
		 Gram stain
		   Glass slides
		 Herpes
		   Viral transport medium
		   Needle for incising vesicle
		 Wet prep
		   Glass slides
		   Cover slips
		   Potassium hydroxide
		   Nonbacteriostatic normal saline without preservatives

Blood tests		Check local laboratory index

APPENDIX H
Working with Parents of Child Sexual Abuse Victims[29]

- Crisis (initial disclosure) phase
  - Use reflective listening, "echoing," and open-ended statements to encourage expression of feelings.
  - Acknowledge that a wide range of feelings (e.g., anger, fear, sadness, guilt, shame, desire for revenge, feelings of being overwhelmed, and overly protective) are common and normal responses to child sexual abuse.
  - Focus intense emotions toward meeting the immediate needs of the child.
  - Give simple, concrete instructions for things to do to help the child including such things as seeing that the child is fed, bathed, and readied for bed.
  - Stress the need to believe the child's story and reiterate that the child is not responsible for what has happened.
  - Discuss the physical findings and planned medical follow-up and provide as much reassurance as possible that the child will recover.
  - Explore the need for sources of anticipated financial, social and legal support, and identify them for the family.
- Recovery (follow-up) phase
  - Caution the parent that the child may have some behavioral changes after the abuse disclosure (fears, clinging, sleep disorders, bedwetting, somatic complaints, or school problems). As the family routine returns to normal, so should the child's behavior. Persistent or extreme behavioral problems may warrant assistance from a professional.
  - Parents should maintain as many "family routines" as possible, especially regarding discipline. Affection to the child can be moderately increased.
  - Caution the parent against interrogating the child about the abuse and the need to protect the child from the questions of others. Allow the child to voluntarily share the experiences at their own pace.
  - Advise parents not to overreact to what a child discloses, but to reassure the child that the disclosures are believed and they are not at fault in what happened.
  - Make parents aware of the available psychological evaluation and counseling for themselves, the child, and their family. If available, a group of parents with similar experiences may be of help.

Index

Continuing Education Information

Accreditation: ENA is accredited as a provider of continuing education in nursing by the American Nurses Credentialing Center's Commission on Accreditation. Accreditation refers to recognition of educational activities only and does not imply Commission on Accreditation approval or endorsement of any product.

ENA's programs meet the requirements for continuing education credit in all of the following states with mandatory continuing education regulations: Alabama (#ABNP0026), California (CEP2322) and Florida (#27F0390).

Continuing Education Contact Hours (CECH) Information: To receive 10.8 CECH in the Category of Clinical for this independent study, you must complete and return the scannable Independent Study CECH/Evaluation form and complete the test with a 70% pass rate. This form is the last page of this book. PLEASE READ ALL THE DIRECTIONS VERY CAREFULLY.

To receive CECH for this study, follow these directions.

1. In order to ensure correct reading of the form: use No. 2 pencil only, darken circles completely, erase cleanly any marks you wish to change, and do not make any stray marks on the form.

2. Print your name and street address in the appropriate boxes on side one and fill in the appropriate circles.

3. Fill in the month, day, and year of completion of the study.

4. Fill in the class code. **The class code for the Pediatric Emergency Nursing Manual is 10600.**

5. Fill out the evaluation of this study by using the number code to rate each area. The key can be found on side 1 of the Independent Study CECH/Evaluation form. For the Objectives evaluation, please evaluate whether each objective is met. If all are met, evaluate how well they were met on the scan form. For those objectives that were not met, make a comment accordingly in the Comments section on side 2 of the form. The Audio-Visual evaluation is not applicable to this study, therefore fill in the 0 (zero) circle. The Presentation evaluation is not applicable to this study, therefore fill in the 0 (zero) circle.

6. On side 2, fill in your city, state, zip code, and telephone number.

7. Identify the time it took to complete this study by filling in the appropriate boxes and circles.

8. Use the answer sheet portion of the scan form to mark the appropriate answers to the enclosed quiz. The test must be passed by 70% to obtain CECH.

9. Comments are welcome in the identified area on the back side.

CECH Certificates: After completion, mail the scannable form along with $10.00 to:

> Emergency Nurses Association
> Department: Educational Services
> 216 Higgins Road
> Park Ridge, IL 60068

A certificate will be sent after scoring of the form to verify passing of a minimum of 70%. No certificate will be provided without completion of all information on the scannable form.

If you have any questions regarding the form or for information on obtaining scannable forms for CECH at the additional cost of $10.00 per form, please call the Department: Education Services at 1–800–2–GET–ENA.

ENA uses forms that are electronically scanned to process CECH information. These forms cannot be duplicated. For further information, please call Department: Educational Services at ENA.

ASSESSMENT AND TRIAGE OF THE PEDIATRIC PATIENT

1. Which of the following components of the initial assessment can best help the emergency nurse determine whether a sleeping child is acutely ill?
   (a) Respiratory rate, respiratory effort, and skin color
   (b) Skin temperature, respiratory effort, and fontanel firmness
   (c) Response to the environment, capillary refill, and peripheral pulses
   (d) Skin color, heart rate, and skin temperature

2. Which of the following factors in addition to fever can affect the respiratory rate of a child whose illness is considered nonemergent?
   (a) Hypoxia and irritability
   (b) Agitation and anxiety
   (c) Irritability and lethargy
   (d) Acidosis and hypothermia

3. A six-month-old infant should be considered developmentally normal for her age if she:
   (a) has a flat fontanel, can roll over, has taken her bottle well.
   (b) has begun to hold her bottle, can crawl and sit from prone position.
   (c) has normal vital signs, a normal size according to the growth chart, and has begun drooling.
   (d) can roll over, grasp the stethoscope, and squeal with delight.

4. Which of the following methods is likely to be the most effective for administering medication to a child younger than 2 years old?
   (a) Tell the child the medication will make him/her feel better
   (b) Use a medication syringe to slowly inject the medication in the posterior portion of the cheek
   (c) Tell the child the medication is candy
   (d) Hold the child's nose so the child will open his/her mouth

5. Initial assessment of a febrile 6-month-old infant reveals that although the infant's mother is providing comforting measures, the infant continues to cry uncontrollably. When placed on an exam table, the infant stops crying and immediately falls asleep. Of the following, the emergency nurse's first impression would be that the infant may be:
   (a) exhibiting signs of child abuse.
   (b) exhibiting paradoxic irritability.
   (c) tired and hungry.
   (d) having difficulty breathing due to nasal congestion.

6. A 3½-year-old child is "acting funny" after he ate a "green pill" he found on the playground. The child is alert but quite agitated and does not seem to recognize his parents. The patient should be triaged as:
   (a) emergent.
   (b) urgent.
   (c) nonurgent.
   (d) clinic.

7. A 12-month-old infant who has a temperature of 104°F (40°C) would be expected to have a pulse and respiratory rate that are:

   (a)   both above normal.

   (b)   both below normal.

   (c)   normal pulse and below-normal respirations.

   (d)   Above-normal pulse and below-normal respirations.

8. An 8-week-old infant has had a low-grade fever, fussiness, and poor appetite for the past 2 days. The infant is awake, sucking on a pacifier, and has pink skin. She has a rectal temperature of 101.6°F (38.7°C). Which of the following statements about the patient is true?

   (a)   The patient is not ill and should be triaged as nonurgent.

   (b)   Because this is the patient's first illness, the parents panicked and should receive additional discharge teaching.

   (c)   The patient may have a serious illness and may require a septic workup.

   (d)   Acetaminophen should be administered and the patient reevaluated before treatment proceeds.

9. Information about which of the following would be considered the most important for making triage decisions?

   (a)   Presence of underlying illness, mother's past medical history, length of illness

   (b)   Presence of underlying illness, child's significant past medical history, and history of present illness

   (c)   Child's significant past medical history, length of hospitalization at birth, and mother's past medical history

   (d)   Family history of past illnesses, presence of underlying illness, and length of illness

10. Which of the following statements most accurately describes most febrile children?

   (a)   They are often cranky, irritable, sleepy, and tachypneic.

   (b)   They often have very serious illnesses that require intervention.

   (c)   They require acetaminophen and immediate evaluation by a physician.

   (d)   Those with temperatures over 104°F (40°C) require emergent management.

11. A 6-month-old infant should have already received which of the following immunizations?

   (a)   DTP, OPV

   (b)   DTP, OPV, Hib

   (c)   DTP, OPV, MMR

   (d)   DTP, OPV, Hib, MMR

12. A 2-year-old girl arrives in the emergency department in her mother's arms crying inconsolably. As the emergency nurse attempts to obtain vital signs, the child grasps her mother's neck and refuses to let go. Which of the following techniques would be most useful in helping obtain the child's cooperation?

   (a)   Allowing the mother to remain with the child, obtaining the vital signs as quickly as possible and offering to give the child a toy if she will quit crying

   (b)   Distracting the child with a toy or stethoscope, allowing the mother to remain with the child

   (c)   Asking the child to be a "big girl" and hold still for just a few minutes, distracting the child with a toy or stethoscope

   (d)   Obtaining the vital signs as quickly as possible, offering to give the child a toy if she will stop crying

RESPIRATORY ASSESSMENT AND INTERVENTION

13. In the absence of a significant history, which is the most likely cause of upper airway obstruction in an injured child?

    (a) Bronchospasm   (c) Tissue swelling and edema

    (b) The patient's tongue   (d) Aspirated mucous or vomitus

14. Croup is most commonly characterized by:

    (a) rapid onset, no fever, patient age between 2 and 6 years.

    (b) harsh, barking cough, 1 to 2 days of upper respiratory symptoms prior to illness, drooling.

    (c) harsh, barking cough, rapid onset, patient age under 2 years.

    (d) harsh barking cough, 1 to 2 days of upper respiratory symptoms prior to illness, no fever.

15. A 4-year-old child who swallowed a piece of hard candy has a complete airway obstruction. To clear the airway, the emergency nurse should administer:

    (a) three back blows, followed by six to ten abdominal thrusts.

    (b) four back blows, followed by four chest thrusts.

    (c) five back blows, followed by five chest thrusts.

    (d) six to ten abdominal thrusts (Heimlich maneuver).

16. A pulse oximetry reading will provide information about:

    (a) how well the patient is ventilating and oxygenating.

    (b) arterial carbon dioxide and pH levels.

    (c) the degree of oxygen saturation of the hemoglobin.

    (d) readings equivalent to all of the parameters of arterial or capillary blood gases.

17. Which of the following signs or symptoms are considered common side effects of nebulizer treatment with an adrenergic drug?

    (a) Tachycardia, nausea, vomiting   (c) Blurred vision, nausea, weakness

    (b) Drowsiness, thirst, tachypnea   (d) Bradycardia, dizziness, nausea

18. In a child, stridor is a classic sign of:

    (a) upper airway obstruction.   (c) bronchial obstruction.

    (b) lower airway obstruction.   (d) transmitted airway sounds.

19. In a child, which of the following is considered a late sign of respiratory distress?

    (a) Wheezing   (c) Anxiety

    (b) Cyanosis   (d) Retractions

20. The best method to keep a child in respiratory distress calm is to:

    (a) ensure the child and parent stay together.   (c) administer oxygen.

    (b) help the child to lie down.   (d) administer a sedative.

21. Atropine is used during controlled intubation to:

    (a) paralyze muscles.   (c) prevent bradycardia.

    (b) produce sedation.   (d) prevent increased intracranial pressure.

22. Which of the following interventions is recommended for children who receive aerosolized racemic epinephrine?

    (a) Obtaining vital signs every 15 minutes

    (b) Administering IV fluids and cardiac monitoring

    (c) Observing the patient for 3 to 4 hours or admitting the patient

    (d) Performing intubation if the patient's condition does not improve

CARDIOVASCULAR ASSESSMENT AND INTERVENTION

23. Besides fluid volume deficit, which of the following factors can affect capillary refill time?

    (a) Body temperature and medications

    (b) Ethnicity and medication

    (c) Body temperature and age

    (d) Ethnicity and age

24. The first clinical signs of compensated shock in a child are most commonly:

    (a) low blood pressure and delayed capillary refill.

    (b) increased heart rate and skin mottling.

    (c) increased respiratory rate and delayed capillary refill.

    (d) delayed capillary refill and cool extremities.

25. Can bone marrow obtained during insertion of an intraosseous infusion catheter be used for laboratory analyses?

    (a) No analyses can be performed on bone marrow.

    (b) Only hemoglobin and blood gas analyses can be performed on bone marrow.

    (c) Most laboratory studies can be performed on bone marrow.

    (d) Only electrolytes and blood chemistries can be performed on bone marrow.

26. Which of the following should be used to establish an IV line in a 3-year-old child?

    (a) 16-gauge over the needle catheter

    (b) 20-gauge over the needle catheter

    (c) 24-gauge over the needle catheter

    (d) 25-gauge butterfly

27. For a child who weighs 10 kg, the appropriate dosage for cardioversion would be how many Joules?

    (a) 2.5 to 5   (c) 50 to 60

    (b) 5 to 10   (d) 100 to 150

28. What is the appropriate rate and depth of cardiac compressions for a 3-year-old child?

    (a) A rate of 80 to 100/min and a depth of 1 to 1-1/2 inches.

    (b) A rate of 80 to 100/min and a depth of 3/4 to 1-1/2 inches.

    (c) A rate of 110 to 130/min and a depth of 1-1/2 to 2 inches.

    (d) A rate of 120 to 140/min and a depth of 1 to 1-1/2 inches.

29. The physician orders dextrose to be given to a child via an intraosseous line. The emergency nurse should give 50% dextrose:

   (a) rapidly through the intraosseous line.

   (b) through an intravenous line rather than through the intraosseus line.

   (c) diluted with normal saline solution through the intraosseous line.

   (d) via slow infusion (over 10 minutes).

30. A 3-month-old infant arrives at the emergency department in supraventricular tachycardia (SVT) with a heart rate of 280 beats/min. The patient is lethargic, tachypneic, has mottled skin and delayed capillary refill. Initial intervention includes administration of oxygen by mask at 10 L/min and establishing IV access. The next step in intervention is to prepare for:

   (a) Valsalva maneuvers.   (c) administration of fluid bolus.

   (b) cardioversion.   (d) administration of verapamil.

31. A 3-month-old infant is lethargic, cool to touch, and extremely pale. He is also crying softly. He has a heart rate of 280 beats/min and rapid respirations. The parent states that the infant has had difficult feedings for the last 2 days. Cardiac monitor reveals a rapid rhythm with a narrow QRS. The patient's conditions is most likely caused by:

   (a) inadequate cardiac output.   (c) hypoxemia.

   (b) excessive stroke volume.   (d) ventricular irritability.

32. A 3-year-old child is in full cardiopulmonary arrest after being submerged in a swimming pool for approximately 10 minutes. As a member of the resuscitation team, the emergency nurse is responsible for venous access. Two attempts to initiate peripheral lines in the patient's arms have been unsuccessful. The nurse should attempt:

   (a) scalp vein cannulation.   (c) intraosseous catheterization.

   (b) subclavian catheterization.   (d) lower extremity catheterization.

33. A 6-month-old infant has had diarrhea and vomiting for the past 24 hours. The last stool contained blood and mucous. The parents state, "Our baby just isn't right. He's usually such a good boy, but he has been so irritable." Assessment reveals that the infant is pale, has dry lips, and is whimpering softly. He has rapid respirations and has not opened his eyes during the triage assessment. His rectal temperature is 100.4°F (38°C). The patient's conditions should be triaged as:

   (a) emergent.   (c) nonurgent.

   (b) urgent.   (d) clinic referral.

34. A 4-year-old child who weighs 38 lbs needs a fluid bolus as treatment for hypovolemic shock. How many mL of fluid should be given?

   (a) 200   (c) 380

   (b) 340   (d) 720

35. A 6-month-old child in full arrest is brought to the emergency department with an intraosseous line in place. The skin surrounding the insertion site is cool and the area is swollen. The emergency nurse should:

   (a) do nothing as this is a normal finding.

   (b) prepare to remove the intraosseous line.

   (c) flush the intraosseous line with heparinized saline solution.

   (d) apply antibiotic ointment and an occlusive dressing to the site.

ASSESSMENT AND MANAGEMENT OF NEUROLOGIC EMERGENCIES

36. The priority assessment of a patient who has ingested a toxic substance should be to:

   (a) assess neurologic status.

   (b) assess oxygenation and ventilation.

   (c) determine how much was ingested.

   (d) attempt to prevent or minimize absorption of the toxic substance.

37. Which of the following solutions is appropriate for use in gastric lavage of a 6-year-old child?

   (a) Tap water   (c) 0.45% normal saline solution

   (b) Sterile water   (d) 0.9% normal saline solution

38. A child undergoing gastric lavage should be placed in what position?

   (a) Head-down prone position to avoid aspiration

   (b) Left lateral decubitus Trendelenburg's position to aid in gastric emptying and protect against aspiration

   (c) A position of comfort to encourage patient cooperation

   (d) Supine, with the head of the bed slightly elevated

39. Which of the following substances could be appropriately used to disguise the taste of charcoal powder?

   (a) Jam or jelly   (c) Cherry syrup or sorbitol

   (b) Ice cream or sherbet   (d) Cocoa powder or milk

40. Which of the following are general characteristics of a febrile seizure?

   (a) Fever of less than 12 hours duration, patient age under 6 years, generalized seizure activity

   (b) Fever of more than 12 hours duration, patient age under 1 year, generalized seizure activity

   (c) Patient age under 6 years, focal findings, postictal state

   (d) Low-grade fever, generalized seizure activity, postictal state

41. A comatose 5-year-old child is brought to the emergency department. Results of which of the following assessments would be most useful as part of the primary neurologic assessment?

   (a) Deep tendon reflexes   (c) Cranial nerve assessment

   (b) Glasgow Coma Scale   (d) Radiologic evaluation for skull fractures

42. A child who sustains a forceful blow to the temporal region of the head is most likely to have what type of skull fracture?

   (a) Depressed   (c) Diastatic

   (b) Compound   (d) Linear

43. The most important reason to hyperventilate a child who has a serious head injury is to:

   (a) correct severe hypoxia.   (c) increase respiratory drive.

   (b) reduce possible hypercarbia.   (d) induce respiratory acidosis.

44. Which of the following arteries is most commonly injured as a result of a linear fracture in the parietal-temporal area?

   (a) External carotid artery   (c) Middle meningeal artery

   (b) Middle cerebral artery   (d) Anterior communicating artery

45. Mannitol may be indicated for patients with severe head injuries and associated increased intracranial pressure in order to:

    (a) expand intravascular volume.

    (b) increase renal output.

    (c) temporarily decrease intracranial pressure.

    (d) increase circulation to the brain.

46. What is the most significant complication following administration of activated charcoal to a child?

    (a) Gastric distention   (c) Aspiration

    (b) Charcoal toxicity   (d) Tarry stools

47. A nonintubated patient undergoing a head CT scan should be monitored primarily for changes in:

    (a) cardiac rhythm.   (c) pupillary response.

    (b) respiratory status.   (d) neuromuscular activity.

48. A patient has a grand mal seizure while undergoing a CT scan. The emergency nurse should first:

    (a) ensure the CT scan is completed.   (c) administer an anticonvulsant.

    (b) ensure the patient has an adequate airway. (d) monitor the patient's neurologic status.

49. Which of the following would be considered a desired verbal response in a 2-year-old who has sustained a head injury?

    (a) Crying and restlessness

    (b) Appropriate words and lusty cry

    (c) Moaning and grunting

    (d) High-pitched cry, but unresponsive to a parent's voice

50. The emergency nurse must ensure a patent IV line in a child whose neurologic status is rapidly deteriorating. The initial solution of choice is:

    (a) D_5W.   (c) 0.9% normal saline.

    (b) $D_{10}W$.   (d) lactated Ringer's solution.

MEDICAL EMERGENCIES

51. What early clinical signs might be expected in a 6-month-old infant with cerebral edema secondary to meningitis?

    (a) Change in heart rate   (c) Change in blood pressure

    (b) Bulging fontanel   (d) Cushing's triad

52. Precipitating factors of sickle cell crisis include which of the following:

    (a) dehydration, illness, stress.

    (b) high altitude, hyperthermia, hypoxia.

    (c) exposure to cold, allergy, major burns.

    (d) emotional upset, low altitude, hypercapnia.

53. Which of the following diagnostic tests are most likely to be ordered to confirm a diagnosis of vaso-occlusive crisis?

    (a) Blood culture and CSF analysis

    (b) Reticulocyte count and CBC

    (c) BUN and creatinine

    (d) Urinalysis and urine culture

54.. A patient with sickle cell disease has chest pain and obvious difficulty breathing. The patient's signs and symptoms are most likely caused by:

    (a) costochondritis.

    (b) pulmonary embolism.

    (c) myocardial infarction.

    (d) pulmonary vaso-occlusive crisis.

55. A 2-year-old child is brought to the emergency department after a submersion incident in bath water. The emergency nurse's primary concern is the possibility of:

    (a) bacterial infection.

    (b) electrolyte disturbances.

    (c) hypoxemia.

    (d) hypervolemia.

56. Which of the following factors positively affects emergency treatment of a serious submersion injury?

    (a) Cold water submersion, age under 3 years

    (b) Salt water submersion, time under water

    (c) Fresh water submersion, age under 10 years

    (d) Warm water submersion, cleanliness of water

57. Which of the following febrile children should be most closely monitored upon arrival at the emergency department?

    (a) A 3-year-old boy who cries when he cannot see his mother

    (b) A 6-year-old girl who complains of an earache for the past two days

    (c) A child whose maternal grandmother is a diabetic

    (d) A child who is taking antirejection medication following a renal transplant

58. Infection in small infants most commonly presents as:

    (a) a high fever.

    (b) irritability.

    (c) petechial rash.

    (d) low blood pressure.

59. The best way to prepare to start an IV line in a child in vaso-occlusive crisis would be to:

    (a) gather different sizes of IV catheters.

    (b) reassure the child that it will not hurt.

    (c) swaddle the child so that he or she cannot move during the procedure.

    (d) ask the most experienced emergency nurse to perform the procedure.

60. Emergency department staff are notified that a child who was submerged in a lake is en route to the hospital. The emergency nurse should locate and have ready to use:

    (a) a hypothermia thermometer.

    (b) a cooling blanket.

    (c) bilirubin lights.

    (d) a scale that weighs in pounds (lb).

61. A small child is brought to the emergency department after being submerged in a swimming pool for 20 minutes. The best site for drawing blood for arterial blood gas analysis would be the:

    (a) carotid artery.

    (b) brachial artery.

    (c) radial artery.

    (d) femoral artery.

ASSESSMENT AND INTERVENTION OF NONTRAUMATIC
SURGICAL EMERGENCIES

62. A patient who has abdominal pain is believed to have appendicitis. Which of the following patient complaints would increase the nurse's suspicion?

   (a) Fever and lethargy

   (b) Vomiting and diarrhea

   (c) Pain with movement and constant periumbilical pain

   (d) Intermittent pain in the right lower quadrant and loss of appetite

63. A child who has abdominal pain is believed to have appendicitis. The best way to assess the degree and type of the pain would be to ask the patient to:

   (a) describe how much pain he or she is having.

   (b) describe where the pain is located as the nurse palpates the abdomen.

   (c) bend over and touch his or her toes.

   (d) jump down from the examining table.

64. Which of the following signs is most indicative of a possible surgical emergency in a patient who has abdominal pain?

   (a) Fever   (c) Paradoxical irritability

   (b) Bilious vomiting   (d) Intermittent abdominal pain

65. Which of the following IV fluids is commonly recommended for a child who has signs and symptoms of dehydration?

   (a) 0.45% normal saline solution

   (b) 0.9% normal saline solution

   (c) 5% dextrose in 0.9% normal saline solution

   (d) 5% dextrose in 0.45% normal saline solution

66. Which of the following statements about intussusception is true?

   (a) A barium enema is generally used to confirm a diagnosis of intussusception.

   (b) Most children with intussusception require bowel resection.

   (c) Intussusception is unlikely if the patient has no signs of bilious vomiting and bloody diarrhea.

   (d) Intussusception involves a twisting of the small bowel.

67. Which of the following questions to the parents of a child believed to have pyloric stenosis would be most helpful in confirming the diagnosis?

   (a) "Has there been blood in your child's stool?"

   (b) "Was the child born prematurely?"

   (c) "Have any other family members had this type of problem?"

   (d) "What type of formula is the child being given?"

68. Assessment of peritoneal irritation in a toddler is most likely to reveal:

   (a) guarding.

   (b) rebound tenderness.

   (c) pain exacerbated by movement.

   (d) diminished bowel sounds.

69. A 10-week-old infant is lethargic, has pale, cool skin, and has poor perfusion as a result of vomiting. Initial intervention includes administration of 20 mL/kg of lactated Ringer's solution. The patient now has a palpable blood pressure of 40/min, heart rate of 180 beats/min, and respirations of 68/min. The emergency nurse should next:

    (a)   administer 2 to 4 mL/kg of $D_{25}W$.

    (b)   administer another bolus of 10 to 20 mL/kg of lactated Ringer's solution.

    (c)   obtain additional information about the patient's medical history.

    (d)   prepare for diagnostic procedures.

70. A 4-week-old infant has been vomiting and increasingly irritable for the past 2 days. Assessment reveals that the infant cries frequently, but no tears are produced. The parent states that the patient has had a dry diaper for the past 12 hours. The most appropriate nursing diagnosis would be:

    (a)   Fluid volume deficit.

    (b)   Pain.

    (c)   Altered nutrition: Less than body requirements.

    (d)   Ineffective airway clearance.

71. A 5-year-old child has abdominal pain and has been vomiting. Assessment reveals a blood pressure of 96/40 mmHg, a heart rate of 140 beats/min, and respirations of 28/min. The child has pale, cool skin and a temperature of 99.7°F (37.6°C). The emergency nurse should prepare to:

    (a)   establish IV access.

    (b)   administer 20 mL/kg of D_5W.

    (c)   administer pain medication.

    (d)   administer broad spectrum antibiotics.

TRAUMA ASSESSMENT AND INTERVENTION

72. Which of the following parameters should be used to assess the effectiveness of fluid resuscitation in a 2-year-old child?

    (a)   Capillary refill, heart rate, temperature of extremities

    (b)   Heart rate, pupillary reaction, blood pressure

    (c)   Glasgow Coma Scale, capillary refill, blood pressure

    (d)   Heart rate, Glasgow Coma Scale, pupillary reaction

73. Which of the following signs associated with a basilar skull fracture are most likely to appear in a patient with a head injury?

    (a)   Battle's sign

    (b)   Low systolic blood pressure

    (c)   Rapid respirations

    (d)   Fixed, dilated pupils

74. The most common chest injury in a child who has been injured in a motor vehicle crash is:

    (a)   a flail chest.

    (b)   rib fractures.

    (c)   a pneumothorax.

    (d)   a pulmonary contusion.

75. Which of the following fractures carries special risk for children?

    (a)   Skull

    (b)   Femur

    (c)   Humerus

    (d)   Epiphyseal plate

76. A urine output of how many mL/kg/hr would indicate that fluid replacement is adequate in a pediatric burn patient?
    - (a) At least 0.5 mL/kg/hr
    - (b) At least 1 mL/kg/hr
    - (c) At least 5 mL/kg/hr
    - (d) At least 30 mL/kg/hr

77. Which of the following medications might be ordered before a burn patient is transported to a pediatric burn center?
    - (a) Topical lidocaine
    - (b) Silver sulfadiazine
    - (c) Intravenous antibiotics
    - (d) Tetanus toxoid

78. Of the following statements, which should the emergency nurse consider when assessing the younger child?
    - (a) Small children need closer evaluation for airway obstruction
    - (b) Small children are less likely to have ingested drugs
    - (c) Small children are at higher risk for hypothermia from exposure
    - (d) Circulatory status is more difficult to assess in young children

79. The best way to immobilize a child's cervical spine is to use:
    - (a) manual traction.
    - (b) sandbags and tape.
    - (c) an appropriately sized stiff-neck collar and rolled towels or IV bags.
    - (d) rolled towels or IV bags placed on either side of the head and tape across the forehead.

80. Unequal breath sounds after intubation of a child trauma patient could indicate which of the following emergent conditions?
    - (a) Pneumothorax or hemothorax
    - (b) Obstruction of a bronchus by blood
    - (c) Intubation of the esophagus
    - (d) Intubation of the right main bronchus

81. What is the most common type of burn in a toddler?
    - (a) Sunburn
    - (b) Scald burn
    - (c) Electrical burn
    - (d) Thermal burn

GROWTH AND DEVELOPMENT: PSYCHOSOCIAL ASPECTS OF PEDIATRIC EMERGENCY NURSING

82. The best way to explain a painful procedure, such as suturing a laceration, to a 3-year-old child would be to:
    - (a) use simple language, giving one step at a time.
    - (b) explain the procedure in detail, summarizing the entire process at once.
    - (c) warn the child well in advance that the procedure might hurt.
    - (d) tell the child that if he or she holds still and does not cry, it won't hurt.

83. An adolescent boy who is to undergo examination of his genitals states that he is embarrassed about undressing in front of a female nurse. If only female nurses are available, the emergency nurse should assure the patient that:

    (a) he may remain covered with a sheet until he is examined.

    (b) nurses are accustomed to seeing patients undressed.

    (c) this is a routine procedure and that he will have to remove his clothes if he wants to be examined.

    (d) other children his age have learned not to be embarrassed, and he should not feel uncomfortable.

84. The underlying pathology of SIDS is due to:

    (a) genetic defect.   (c) bacterial infection.

    (b) cardiac anomaly.   (d) unknown causes.

85. Which of the following interventions would be most helpful for a toddler about to undergo a painful procedure?

    (a) Establishing a position of authority

    (b) Asking the parents to help restrain the child

    (c) Allowing the child to hold an object or keep it in sight

    (d) Encouraging the parents to leave the treatment room during the procedure

86. A 16-month-old infant sustains a minor laceration on the right hand that requires suturing. The patient kicks, screams, and cries violently at any attempt to take her from her mother. The patient's behavior is most likely a result of:

    (a) possible child abuse.

    (b) Fear of mutilation and/or disfigurement.

    (c) normal developmental reaction.

    (d) a distorted understanding of how the body works.

87. A 2-year-old boy comes to the emergency department after falling off his brother's upper bunk bed. The patient is crying about his "hurt" and holding his left arm. He resists examination of his injured arm by kicking and hitting. He will not sit on the stretcher and sucks his thumb when he is not fighting. The child's behavior is most likely due to:

    (a) a normal response to pain.   (c) abnormal developmental task.

    (b) separation anxiety.   (d) maladjusted relationship with parents.

88. A 4-year-old child must undergo surgical removal of a needle in her foot. The emergency nurse must explain the procedure to the patient. Which of the following statements would be most appropriate?

    (a) "The doctor will make a cut on your foot and pull out the needle."

    (b) "The doctor will deaden your foot first so you won't feel anything."

    (c) "You will need to keep your foot very clean so no bugs will get inside the cut."

    (d) "The doctor will make your foot better."

89. A 14-year-old girl is being prepared for an emergency appendectomy. The emergency nurse finds her sobbing after her parents leave the examination room. She takes hold of the nurse's hand and asks, "Please tell me the truth, I have to know the truth. I am going to die, aren't I?" The patient asks this question as a result of:

    (a) normal adolescent fear.   (c) separation anxiety.

    (b) awareness of secondary gains.   (d) appropriate adolescent coping for pain.

Questions 90 and 91 refer to the following information:

A 2-year-old child is in full cardiopulmonary arrest as the result of a gunshot wound to the head. The patient's parents are in the "quiet room" awaiting word on their child's condition.

90. The highest priority nursing intervention for the parents at this time is:
    (a) arranging for the parents to speak with the physician.
    (b) arranging for the parents to speak with the police officers.
    (c) providing as much information as possible.
    (d) providing brochures from support groups for parents with similar experiences.

91. The child is pronounced dead by the physician and her parents are told. The father appears confused and asks the nurse to explain what happened, including every procedure and every intervention attempted during resuscitation. He also wants to know what more could have been done. The nurse answers his questions as honestly as possible. As a result of the nurse's intervention, the child's father can be expected to:
    (a) leave the emergency department and state that his lawyer will be contacting the nurse soon.
    (b) begin to cry and ask to see the child.
    (c) pick up a nearby lamp and throw it into the wall.
    (d) turn to his wife and say, "This is all your fault. You killed her."

CHILD MALTREATMENT:
RECOGNITION AND MANAGEMENT OF PEDIATRIC ABUSE

92. The greatest likelihood of child abuse is likely to occur in which of the following groups?
    (a) Black, Hispanic, or Asian families
    (b) Families from lower socioeconomic groups
    (c) Families from an urban setting
    (d) Families from any socioeconomic group

93. The principal reason a skeletal survey is often ordered in cases of possible child abuse is to:
    (a) determine whether a child's physical growth is age appropriate.
    (b) detect the presence of intracranial hemorrhage due to violent shaking.
    (c) detect multiple fractures in various stages of healing.
    (d) rule out various growth abnormalities.

94. The legal responsibilities associated with the care of a child common in all U.S. jurisdictions include all of the following actions *except:*
    (a) mandated reporting of suspicions of abuse to appropriate local agency.
    (b) maintaining detailed, objective documentation of the reasons for suspected abuse.
    (c) possible legal testimony if the case goes to court.
    (d) obtaining child abuse photographs.

95. A child believed to have been sexually abused loses control during examination by the physician. The nurse's best approach at this time would be to:
    (a) ask the physician for an order to sedate the child.
    (b) call for help to temporarily restrain the child, then finish the examination as efficiently and quickly as possible.
    (c) schedule the child for an immediate examination in the operating room under general anesthesia.
    (d) stop momentarily and wait until the child regains control.

96. A 2-year-old girl is brought to the emergency department by her mother's boyfriend. He reports that the child sat on a light bulb 30 minutes ago. Assessment reveals a 4×5 cm partial-thickness burn with redness and purulent drainage to the right buttock. The patient is quiet, alert, and her vital signs are within normal limits. The emergency nurse should first:
    (a) perform a thorough physical examination.
    (b) perform burn care and apply a dressing.
    (c) document abuse on the patient's chart.
    (d) teach the boyfriend home-wound care.

Questions 97 and 98 refer to the following information:

A 6-month-old infant is brought to the emergency department by his father. The father reports that the infant "sleeps a lot" and has been vomiting. Assessment reveals that the patient appears healthy, has vital signs within normal limits, and arouses with moderate stimuli. The mother arrives at the emergency department and says to the father, "What have you done to my baby now?" The mother states that the infant had a skull fracture a week ago, but does not know how it happened. A CT scan reveals a new skull fracture and a small subdural hematoma.

97. The most appropriate course of action would be to:
    (a) anticipate the need for additional diagnostic tests.
    (b) prepare to admit the infant.
    (c) discharge the infant to the mother only.
    (d) discharge the infant to a relative.

98. The most appropriate nursing diagnosis would be?
    (a) Pain.   (c) Potential for injury.
    (c) Altered parenting.   (d) Altered cerebral tissue perfusion.

99. A 6-month-old infant is brought to the emergency department by his mother. The child is appropriately dressed. Physical examination and initial diagnostic work-up are within normal limits, with the exception that the infant's immunization record is not up to date. Results of a toxicology screen are positive for benzodiazepine. The emergency nurse suspects abuse because:
    (a) the mother appears upset.
    (b) the infant has on a clean, worn sleeper.
    (c) developmental ingestion is unlikely.
    (d) the infant's immunization schedule is behind.

100. A 12-year-old boy is brought to the emergency department with an injury to the right forearm. He is quiet when questioned about the mechanism of injury, but his mother quickly states he fell into the door frame. The emergency nurse should:
    (a) send the patient and his mother to registration.
    (b) escort the patient to an examining room alone.
    (c) ask the patient how he fell into the door frame.
    (d) ask the physician to speak to the patient's mother.